Agnès Rocamora is Reader in Social and Cultural Studies at the London College of Fashion, University of the Arts London. She is the author of *Fashioning the City: Paris, Fashion and the Media* (I.B.Tauris 2009) and a co-editor of *The Handbook of Fashion Studies* (2013) and of *Fashion Media: Past and Present* (2013). She also co-edits the *International Journal of Fashion Studies*.

Anneke Smelik is Professor of Visual Culture on the Katrien van Munster chair at the Radboud University Nijmegen, Netherlands. Her books include *Delft Blue to Denim Blue: Dutch Fashion* (I.B.Tauris, 2016) and *Performing Memory in Art and Popular Culture* (2013). She is project leader of the research programme 'Crafting Wearables: Fashionable Technology'.

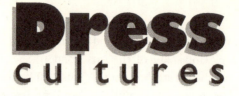

Dress cultures

Across a digital world in which the same T-shirt can be designed in New York, manufactured in Hong Kong, boycotted in London and consumed by a global network of wearers, how do we locate individuality and cultural distinctiveness among the capitalist interplay of logo and subculture? As consumer citizens in a retail society, how does what we buy correlate with our age, gender, ethnicity and class, and how is uniqueness expressed among the proliferation of seemingly infinite choice?

Dress Cultures aims to foster innovative theoretical and methodological frameworks to understand how and why we dress, exploring the connections between clothing, commerce and creativity in global contexts.

Published and forthcoming in the Dress Culture series:

Queries, ideas and submissions to:

Reina Lewis: reina.lewis@fashion.arts.ac.uk
Elizabeth Wilson: mail@elizabethwilson.net
At the publisher, Philippa Brewster: philippabrewster@gmail.com

Thinking through Fashion

A Guide to Key Theorists

Agnès Rocamora and Anneke Smelik (editors)

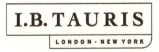

I.B. TAURIS

LONDON · NEW YORK

Published in 2016 by
I.B.Tauris & Co. Ltd
London • New York
Reprinted 2016
www.ibtauris.com

HB ISBN: 978 1 78076 733 8
PB ISBN: 978 1 78076 734 5
eISBN: 978 0 85773 986 5
ePDF: 978 0 85772 662 9

A full CIP record for this book is available from the British Library
A full CIP record is available from the Library of Congress
Library of Congress Catalog Card Number: available

Typeset by Out of House

Printed and bound by CPI Group (UK) Ltd, Croydon, CR0 4YY

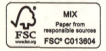

CONTENTS

FIGURES

ACKNOWLEDGEMENTS

The editors and publishers wish to thank the copyright holders for permission to reproduce the images in this book. Every effort has been made to trace rights holders, but if any have been inadvertently overlooked the publishers would be pleased to make the necessary arrangements at the first opportunity. As editors we are very grateful to series editors Reina Lewis and Elizabeth Wilson for their enthusiastic response to the idea for this book. Their continuous support and critical reviews of the draft have been invaluable. We would also like to thank Philippa Brewster at I.B. Tauris for her encouragement and for having so efficiently and smoothly helped us through the process of bringing the book to its conclusion. Our gratitude also goes to the authors, who have patiently, constructively and swiftly responded to our feedback and that of the reviewers. Finally, many thanks to Roos Leeflang for her dedicated preparation of the manuscript.

1

THINKING THROUGH FASHION
An Introduction

Agnès Rocamora and Anneke Smelik

'To think is to voyage.'
(Deleuze & Guattari, 1987: 482)

PART I: THEORIZING FASHION

The role of the veil in the definition of contemporary Muslim identities; the representation of women in fashion magazines; the cultural history of men's underwear; the rise of fashion blogs; the origins of catwalk shows and their participation in the definition of modernity; the creative economy and globalized circulation of African fashion: these are a few only of the topics the growing academic literature on fashion has covered (see, for instance, respectively, Lewis, 2013; Jobling, 1999; Cole, 2009; Rocamora, 2012; Evans, 2013; Rabine, 2002). Common to all the texts is the desire to make sense of fashion, to unpack, comprehend and analyse the social and cultural dynamics of fashion, dress and appearance. Indeed, the field of fashion has now become a major topic of enquiry in social and cultural theory, with many analyses devoted to an understanding of this complex arena. Numerous enlightening interrogations of its many layers have shown that fashion offers a rich platform from which to reflect on key social and cultural issues, from practices of consumption and production through to identity politics.

Thinking through fashion, like thinking through any cultural processes and experiences, is an exciting and challenging exercise. It is dependent on one's ability to critically engage with a vast array of theories and concepts, often from thinkers who, unlike in some other fields of cultural criticism, have not themselves written about fashion. The aim of the present book is to accompany readers through the process of thinking through fashion. It seeks to help them grasp both the relevance of social and cultural theory to the fields of fashion, dress and material culture, and, conversely, the relevance of those fields to social and cultural theory. It does so by guiding them through the work of selected major thinkers, introducing key concepts and ideas, discussing, when relevant, how they have been appropriated by other authors to engage with the topic of fashion, and looking at other ways they can be appropriated to reflect on this topic.

Thinking through Fashion uses the word fashion in the broad sense of the term, that is, as also referring to dress, appearance and style. We understand fashion as both material culture and as symbolic system (Kawamura, 2005). It is a commercial industry producing and selling material commodities; a socio-cultural force bound up with the dynamics of modernity and post-modernity; and an intangible system of signification. It is thus made of things and signs, as well as individual and collective agents, which all coalesce through practices of production, consumption, distribution and representation. The study of fashion necessarily covers a wide terrain, ranging from production to consumption and systems of meaning and signification, and scholars need an equally wide array of methodologies and theories from many disciplines. Thus whilst the study of dress, appearance and style was dominated by costume historians, art historians and museum curators until the early 1980s, it was also receiving the attention of anthropology, linguistics and cultural studies (Burman and Turbin, 2003; Mora et al., 2014). Cultural studies, in particular, was instrumental in the broadening of the field of fashion studies to wider social, cultural and economic concerns (Breward, 2003). Cultural studies is inherently interdisciplinary and influenced by most of the theorists discussed in the present volume.

Gradually the term 'fashion studies' has come to refer to the study of fashion in its broad meaning, covering many areas of research across many disciplines, from history (including costume history), philosophy, sociology, anthropology through to cultural studies, women's studies and media studies (Mora et al., 2014). It has brought together a range of approaches, from an object-based approach focused on the materiality of fashion, to a concern with fashion's more intangible dynamics and underpinnings such as globalization, post-colonialism or its key role as a creative industry (see, for instance, on globalization, Maynard, 2004; Rabine, 2002, on post-colonialism, Hendrickson, 1996; Root, 2013 on fashion and the creative industries, Rantisi, 2004; Santagata, 2004).

Fashion studies, then, is by definition an interdisciplinary field. Even if scholars work in a particular discipline, say art history or material anthropology, they will always need to know or at least be aware of adjacent disciplines. This book helps to orient students and scholars to possible different backgrounds to 'thinking through fashion'. When researchers choose to focus on a particular dimension of fashion, for example production rather than consumption, or representation in the media rather than the wear and tear of material clothes, they will need to choose the appropriate methodologies and theories to carry out the research effectively and analyse the results. By providing evaluative introductions to key theorists in the context of fashion, the book provides readers with an accessible overview of relevant theories and concepts in order to help them 'think through fashion' more deeply and critically.

The underlying premise of *Thinking through Fashion* is that theorists provide invaluable tools to 'think through fashion', and that engaging with theory is essential in order to understand and analyse fashion. In the *Collins Dictionary of Sociology*, David Jary and Julia Jary define theory as: 'any set of hypotheses or propositions, linked by logical or mathematical arguments, which is advanced to explain an area of empirical reality or type of phenomenon' (1995: 686). To theorize fashion means to develop propositions and arguments that advance the understanding of its logic and manifestations. Theory aims to explain the many practices (Williams, 1983) involved in the making of fashion: practices of representation, of production and of consumption.

The conceptual dimension of theory has left it open to the accusation of being abstract, removed from the real world. However, 'The true difficulty of theory', as Eagleton notes, 'springs not from this sophistication, but from exactly the opposite – from its demand that we return to childhood by rejecting what seems natural and refusing to be fobbed off with shifty answers from well-meaning elders' (1990: 34–35). In other words, the student or scholar of fashion needs to look at the field of fashion with fresh eyes, clearing her or his mind of preconceived ideas and prejudices. This is why theory can help us better understand the dynamics of fashion. It allows us not to take for granted its many manifestations, but to instead question its obviousness or naturalness and give us the means to achieve the critical distance necessary to a full understanding of its layered complexity. In her chapter on Bruno Latour, Joanne Entwistle, for instance, shows how his notion of 'actant' can help us reconsider the role of non-humans in the making of fashion. In Francesca Granata's discussion of Mikhail Bakhtin, the idea of the grotesque helps us understand the transgressive work of designers. Agnès Rocamora shows how Pierre Bourdieu's notion of field reminds us that creativity is a collective process; that a fashion collection does not simply originate in the mind of an isolated individual removed from the social world but is the product of various social, economic and cultural forces. And Peter McNeil explains how Georg Simmel's theorizing of everyday life as informed by dualism helps us understand the logic of fashion, at once fuelled by the desire to be like someone else, but also different from someone else or, to put it differently, fashion is as much about sameness as it is about difference.

Theory also involves the careful attention to and command of concepts in one's analysis and interpretation of a topic. As Stuart Mills observes, '"Theory" has to do, above all, with paying close attention to the words one is using, especially their degree of generality and their logical relations' (2000 [1959]: 120). Indeed, 'specialized terminologies' (Hills, 2005: 40) are involved in one's practice of theory. These are the terminologies of the disciplines that a theoretical framework belongs to and engages with. This book focuses on social and cultural theory, the type of theory that informs the work of thinkers from the social sciences and humanities, which include disciplines such as history, philosophy, sociology, anthropology, cultural studies and media studies.

The boundaries between disciplines are not always clear cut, and the work of many thinkers straddles one or two disciplines. Michel Foucault, for example, is often referred to as a historian, but also as a philosopher. Pierre Bourdieu's early career is informed by ethnography, but he later established himself in the field of sociology, and both disciplines underpin his thinking. The practice of theory then often involves engagement with a variety of 'sister' disciplines and attendant concepts. The work of all of the thinkers discussed in *Thinking through Fashion* can be related to, brought into dialogue with, other theories and ideas, concepts and arguments, which they appropriate to support their point and further the understanding of a particular phenomenon. Theorizing does not happen in a vacuum. It does not consist in one's formulation of arguments out of the blue, but in critical dialogue with existing works and theories; and 'with the objective of offering new tools by which to think about our world' (Barker, 2011: 37–38). As Michel de Certeau puts it: 'in spite of a persistent fiction, we never write on a blank page, but always on one that that has already been written on' (1988: 43).

This is also why, as Hills observes, theory 'always refers the reader to a set of texts beyond what is currently being read, gesturing towards a vast intertextual web of material' (2005: 39). This web spreads across space – as in the many journals and books where theories can be found – but also across time. The work of Karl Marx for instance, although developed in the nineteenth century, informs the work of later authors, such as Pierre Bourdieu and Jean Baudrillard, who in his early work also cited that of Michel Foucault but later moved away from it (Best and Kellner, 1991); the work of Mikhail Bakhtin has influenced that of Gilles Deleuze; Judith Butler's thought is indebted to psychoanalysis and Foucault's theory of discourse and truth. The theories and concepts of past authors continue to live in the work of their contemporaries.

Because *Thinking through Fashion* is organized around the idea of individual thinkers as historical subjects, we have followed a simple chronological order of date of birth. Although the idea of a linear unfolding of time can allow one to grasp the past and the context and origins of some theories and concepts, it fails to capture the idea that the past and the present always intersect in the practice of theory. Our contributors, therefore, whilst introducing individual theories as historical subjects in their moment in time, also emphasize the cross-fertilization of ideas. The book thus highlights the intellectual proximity of authors distanced by history, an approach that also informs our discussion of strands and developments in theory in the next section.

Authors alive at the same time might follow a different timeline to fame and recognition. One has to keep in mind that some authors became known or acknowledged earlier than older authors. Also, there can be a discrepancy between the moment when a piece of work was written by its author and the moment it receives attention by other scholars, and in other languages. For example, the work of Mikhail Bakhtin was written in Russia in the 1930s and 1940s, but only received wider attention in Western Europe in the 1960s. Another example is the work of many French post-structuralist authors – such as Foucault and Derrida – who rose to prominence through the translations of American scholars. This phenomenon has been called the 'transatlantic connection' or rather 'disconnection' (Stanton, 1980) and has also been addressed as 'travelling theories' (Said, 1982). Theoretical work can be produced and received at different times in different countries, depending on trends in thinking, the availability of translations or social and cultural influences. These are the sorts of a-synchronicities that run alongside the linear organization by date of birth. As our thematic discussion in the next section demonstrates, although authors may be separate in time, their theories and ideas and the uses that are made of them can bring them close to each other.

Historical time, as Caroline Evans (2000: 104) notes, drawing on Walter Benjamin, is not 'something that flows smoothly from past to present but [is ...] a more complex relay of turns and returns, in which the past is activated by injecting the present into it'. This is equally true of theory; there, as in historical time, 'the old and new interpenetrate' (Benjamin, cited in Evans, 2000: 102). Thus, the reader may well decide to read the book from beginning to end but could equally enter it through any chapter, or leap from one chapter to another – from Marx to Baudrillard, or from Freud to Butler – to then move on to yet another one. The 'turns and returns' will become apparent as the reader progresses through the whole collection, which presents theory as a constellation of ideas and concepts that flow across time and space and sediment in various guises in the work of various authors.

The didactic organization into chapters devoted to single authors aims to capture the significance of their thought to an understanding of the field of fashion, dress and material culture, as it does the importance of this field for a critical engagement with these authors' ideas. As editors we are highly aware that any collection involves a process of selection, which means acts of both inclusion and exclusion. This collection is intended to be selective rather than comprehensive. We decided to focus mainly on authors whose concepts and ideas have been both central to modern Western social and cultural theory and have been invaluable in thinking through fashion. This book introduces theories that we think are at this point in time essential to conduct the stimulating and demanding work of 'thinking through fashion'.

All the thinkers included in this book are the product of the Western tradition of thought and sciences, associated with western modernity. From the seventeenth and eighteenth centuries, but especially with the consolidation of the Industrial Revolution in the nineteenth century, new social, cultural and economic developments brought about new theories of the world. Thinkers such as Marx and Simmel attempted to make sense of the changes affecting society and developed theories that could help us comprehend shifting ways of being. Fashion was one of the topics some thinkers engaged with – Simmel (1971 [1904]) for instance devoted a whole paper to it – for in the west fashion was itself seen as a paradigm of modernity. The French poet Baudelaire famously described modernity as 'the transitory, the fugitive, the contingent' (1999: 518). This definition is equally applicable to fashion, and indeed he did see in fashion the perfect expression of modernity (Evans, 2003; Lehmann, 2000; Rocamora, 2009; Vinken, 2000).

Although fashion has been seen as paradigmatic of Western modernity, it does not mean that it is the preserve of the Western world (Mora et al., 2014; Niessen et al., 2003; Rabine, 2002). There are indeed multiple co-existing modernities (Eisenstadt, 2000), and the presumed temporal sequence and geographical inscription of pre- or non-modernity, modernity, post-modernity has been problematized by various scholars (Chakrabarty, 2000; Gaonkar, 2001; Gilroy, 1993) to point to the co-existence of different modes of modernization not only across the globe but also within the imperial and metropolitan centre. Elizabeth Wilson (2003), for example, has demonstrated the uneven take-up of fashion in Europe.

By virtue of focusing on western thinkers whose thought has been central to thinking about Western modernity and the fashion that grew out of it, much of the book is devoted to Western fashion. Similarly the knowledge and expertise of most of the fashion scholars brought together in this book lie in their study of fashion as consumed and produced in the west. Most are based in Anglo-American or Western institutions and have English as their first language, which will have further slanted the book towards a Western focus. The fact that it is aimed at an English-reading audience, written in that language and with no provisions for the translation of chapters that may have been submitted in other languages also undoubtedly limits its geographic extent.[1] We welcome follow-up books that would shed light on systems of thoughts and fashion not framed by those of Western modernity.

Strands and Developments in Theory

To think – to develop, test and evaluate theories – is an act that occurs within a certain context; as we wrote above, theorizing does not happen in a vacuum. The following section situates the key theorists in the broader context in which their thought emerged and circulated. In social and cultural theory it is common to speak of strands, movements or schools of thought that unite different thinkers across historical periods and academic disciplines, for example Marxism, feminism or structuralism. As cultural studies can be seen as the defining framework for the emerging field of fashion studies (Breward, 1995, 2003), we trace the development of theory from this particular vantage point. Incorporating a wide range of disciplines, cultural studies was formed by critical and cultural theory and mostly by theories of language (Cavallaro, 2001; Barker, 2011).

The Linguistic Turn

The starting point for our mapping exercise is Roland Barthes. He was the first theorist to bring structural linguistics to the study of popular culture, that is to say he further developed the structuralist ideas of Ferdinand De

Saussure (1996 [1916]) on semiotics, the science of signs (from the Greek *semeion*; sign). A sign is the smallest element that carries a meaning, consisting of a signifier (in French, *signifiant*), the material carrier of meaning, and a signified (in French, *signifié*), the content to which the reference is made. Saussurian semiotics upholds a binary opposition between signifier and signified, but also emphasizes the arbitrary relation between them: there is no intrinsic relation of the sounds and letters of a word and the object they signify (for a fuller explanation see the chapters on Barthes and Baudrillard). This focus on arbitrariness has been useful for an understanding of a text – or image, music or piece of clothing – as a convention, a construction that is made by humans without a natural or essential meaning tied to it.

This development is intimately bound up with the so-called 'linguistic turn'; a term that was invented by the American philosopher Richard Rorty (1967). Rorty claims that the linguistic turn marks a paradigm shift in the Western system of thought in which linguistics, semiotics, rhetoric and other models of textuality came to form the most important framework for critical reflections on contemporary art and culture. Saussure's writings on semiotics helped develop a structuralist analysis of the 'grammar' of any system, and Barthes was the first to apply it to fashion in *The Fashion System* in the early 1950s (published in English in 1967), and, more successfully, to all kinds of expressions of popular culture in *Mythologies* (1973 [1957]). The linguistic turn heralds the beginning of the success of a semiotic reading of any kind of sign system, be it food, a commercial, dress, film or a literary novel, for example in the work of anthropologist Lévi-Strauss on myth, the early Barthes on fashion, or Metz on cinema (Sim, 1998).

The idea that language is paradigmatic for meaning is then central to structuralism and post-structuralism as it was mostly developed by French thinkers in the 1960s and 1970s, of whom Roland Barthes, Jean Baudrillard, Jacques Derrida and Michel Foucault are discussed in *Thinking through Fashion*. Mikhail Bakhtin is sometimes hailed as one of the predecessors, while Judith Butler's work can also be situated in that tradition; while on the contrary, a post-structuralist French thinker such as Gilles Deleuze was rather opposed to the idea of the centrality of language. Thinkers within the linguistic turn argued that systems of signs are structured in the same way as the grammar of language is a structure. Where Barthes (1967) looked for a 'grammar' of dress and Metz (1982) for a 'grammar' of film, Michel Foucault (1990 [1976], 2004 [1969]) developed the notion of 'discourse' as a way to analyse relations of power and truth. According to the psychoanalytic theories of Jacques Lacan (1977), even the unconscious is structured like a language.

The linguistic turn strongly puts the central focus on textuality, stretching, however, beyond the written text out towards images, music, architecture or, indeed, fashion. This approach opened up a whole new field of studying popular culture, as semiotics was now applied to all signifying practices, to 'culture as a whole way of life', in the famous words of Raymond Williams (1958). As Barthes showed in *Mythologies* (1973), an advertisement for Italian pasta, a glamorous photo of Greta Garbo or the new Citroën are all sites where meaning is encoded and can therefore be decoded. Popular culture was accorded a complexity previously little discussed. Barthes's project was new in its endeavour to analyse not only high culture but also mass culture, thus shaking the strict boundaries between the two. This is indeed one of the major characteristics of cultural studies (see for historical overviews Grossberg et al., 1992; During, 1993; Storey, 1996).

The Politics of Post-structuralism

Structuralism flowed into post-structuralism, although it is difficult to date or even point to a clear demarcation between the two bodies of thought. Roland Barthes straddles both ways of thinking, more structuralist in *The Fashion System* (1967), but definitely post-structuralist in *The Pleasure of the Text* (1973) and *A Lover's Discourse* (1977).

Post-structuralist thinkers accept the centrality of language, but reject the idea of a stable subject position, the structure of binary pairs and the idea of universal truths (Barker, 2011: 84). Jacques Derrida's (1976) deconstructionism, for example, argues that language and meaning are fundamentally unstable and forever deferred and shifting. François Lyotard (1984) heralds the ending of 'Grand Narratives', proposing that ideologies can no longer authoritatively proclaim a truth nor promise a future of emancipation. Narratives can still present totalizing and unifying 'grand' stories, but we no longer accept their truth. Both Barthes (1967) and Foucault (1969) proclaimed 'the death of the author', marking the end of the author as the authoritative centre of meaning, to make room for multiple pleasures of the reader. The end of the belief in grand narratives and the death of the author coincide with the blossoming of many formerly oppressed or marginalized groups legitimating their particular stories from the 1960s onwards: youth, blacks, women, gays and lesbians, post-colonial groups and the many cross-overs between them (Woods, 1999). As a consequence, people got interested in 'small', fragmented stories of 'partial truths' and 'situated knowledges', as Donna Haraway (1988) would call it. The opportunity – or difficulty, depending on one's viewpoint – of finding modes for the distinct voice of minority groups can be related to the emerging markets in fashion today when 'non-Western' designers find themselves commodified in relation to certain notions of cultural authenticity (Eicher, 1999; Kondo, 1997; Niessen et al., 2003).

Post-structuralism was informed by the left-wing revolution of May 1968 that spread from Paris all over the world. Language-inspired theories like semiotics were developed through radical re-readings of Marx and Freud. The combination of Marxism and psychoanalysis had already inspired thinkers from the Frankfurt School in the 1940s and 1950s like Benjamin, Horkheimer and Adorno, and this happened again after 1968. It is important to realize that many French thinkers were inspired by Marxism, although they – all be it much later – distanced themselves from the dictatorial regimes of communism. The British Birmingham School of Cultural Studies was equally left-wing inspired, which made for a strong focus on the issue of class in the analysis of popular culture (Williams, 1958; Hall, 1997). The post-structuralist project was led by politics to understand 'the cultural logic of capitalism' (to quote the famous subtitle by Jameson, 1991), as well as liberate sexuality from its bourgeois grip. The particular combination of semiotics, Marxism and psychoanalysis also helped to address the dominant meanings and ideologies of popular culture.

The renewed focus on psychoanalysis, mostly inspired by Lacan's (1977) radical rereading of Freud, was applied to the project of putting an end to the idea of the individual as an autonomous, self-knowing subject. A century earlier, Marx had critiqued the idea that human beings are self-determining individuals, asserting instead that they are produced by the forces of labour and capital (Marx, 1990 [1867]; Sturken and Cartwright, 2009: 100). Freud (1964 [1900]) had explained that the subject is more ruled by unconscious desires than rational will. Lacan pushed this even further and claimed that the subject is always already radically split from the moment it comes into being (Lacan, 1977).

While this may sound a rather negative formulation, Marxist and psychoanalytic bodies of thought opened up a new concept of identity as flexible and dynamic, rather than a fixed and unchanging essence that is given at birth by God, nature or chance. If identity is a social construct, that is to say something 'made' in a complex process of negotiation between the individual and society, between nature and culture, then it is also possible to change and transform it. This allowed for politically informed approaches calling for radical change, most notably feminism and black and post-colonial studies (Irigaray, 1985; Trinh, 1989; Gilroy, 1993). Moreover, it produced an intense focus on the vicissitudes of desire in popular culture (Berger, 1995) and a critique of the normativity of bourgeois and heterosexual sexuality (Butler, 1990; Braidotti, 1991). The notion of ideology thus soon encompassed much more than class consciousness, and came to include 'race', ethnicity, gender and sexuality (Hutcheon, 1989; hooks, 1990, 1992). Identity has increasingly come to be considered fluid and flexible without an essential core (Sim, 1998: 367), an idea that is explored in the chapters on Gilles Deleuze and Judith Butler in the present book.

Post-structuralist theory had a significant impact on the social sciences and humanities, with an enthusiastic response in many new fields of study: gender studies, post-colonial studies, cultural studies, media studies and a bit more hesitantly, fashion studies. The idea that identity is now a question of 'fluctuating personality and tastes', as Gilles Lipovetsky writes (1994: 148–49), opens up the importance of dressing and clothing the body as a means of constructing one's identity. As a result of the fragmentation and changing structures of modernity, Lipovetsky argues that in contemporary society the grand narratives of modernity have been replaced by the logic of fashion and consumption (2005: 11–12), an idea that Baudrillard had also engaged with. The post-structuralist concept of identity as characterized by fluidity and flexibility is enhanced by a dynamics of fashion that enables individuals to continuously define their identities anew (2005: 84). As Fred Davis also argues, the meaning of contemporary fashion is characterized by 'awesome, if not overwhelming, ambiguity' (1992: 7). While many fashion theorists, like Davis and Lipovetsky, celebrate fashion's ambiguity and fluidity, sociologist Zygmunt Bauman is more critical of the 'liquidity' of post-modern culture. He deplores the 'intrinsic volatility and unfixity of all or most identities' (2000: 83). Bauman is especially suspicious of the pivotal role that consumption plays in shaping identities within the socio-cultural power structures of fashion, not unlike Barbara Kruger's famous art work *I shop, therefore I am*. The post-modern condition has thus been celebrated as well as criticized for its flexible identities and free floating signifiers; a game that fashion is particularly adept at playing (Baudrillard, 1993 [1976]).

Old and New Materialisms

For Richard Rorty, the linguistic turn signified a paradigmatic shift in Western philosophy. Such a dramatic turn of paradigm does not happen so very often, and Rorty (1967) only signals three in the history of Western philosophy: from *things* in antique and medieval philosophy to *ideas* from the seventeenth till nineteenth century to *words* in the twentieth century. However, we now live in a time where one turn follows the other more quickly than we can keep up reading about them: the visual turn, the experiential turn, the spatial turn, the cultural turn, the performative turn, the affective turn, the material turn, and so on. This not only signifies that the term 'turn' suffers a huge inflation, but also that we live and think in a time of fast change, a period after post-modernism that is not yet clearly defined (Vermeulen and Van den Akker, 2010).

The problem of the linguistic turn was that it put too much emphasis on language. This point has been addressed in fashion studies. Joanne Entwistle, for example, argues that structuralism and post-structuralism have 'effectively displace[d] the idea of embodiment and the individual and can give us no account of experience or agency' (2000: 70). In shaking off the dominant framework of textuality and semiotics, Entwistle and other scholars of fashion enlist different schools of thought, most notably the more sociological approach of Simmel, Goffman, Bourdieu and Latour, who are discussed in *Thinking through Fashion*. In all their differences, such a sociological approach allows us to understand fashion not only as a signifying system, but also as an embodied practice that takes place in a collectively shared social space.

This is where we touch upon the new, or rather revived, concept of materiality, introduced as 'new materialism' or 'the material turn' (Bennett and Joyce, 2010; Coole and Frost, 2010; Dolphijn and Van der Tuin, 2012; Barrett and Bolt, 2013). These authors argue that the post-structuralist focus on language neglected the very matter and materiality of objects and the world. Barbara Bolt emphasizes the relevance of the material turn for the creative arts, including fashion, since its 'very materiality has disappeared into the textual, the linguistic and the discursive' (2013: 4). As Bill Brown argues, this not only holds for art or fashion, but also for our bodies and identities, which are constructed and mediated not only through signs but also *materially* (2010: 60). Identity 'matters'.

The material turn reopens highly relevant issues for fashion studies, such as practice, embodiment and experience. Our agency takes place through material things and objects – such as clothes. As Appadurai argued (2013 [1986]), people's relationship to objects is socially and culturally dependent, which in turn implies that things themselves have a social life. We mediate the social relations to objects, and social systems through which objects become meaningful (or not). Our identities function within a material culture, as we know all too well from our emotional relations to objects, whether it is a chocolate bar that soothes our anxiety, a song that reminds us of a lost love, or a particular dress that makes us feel sexy. Food, music or

clothes have a value. Of course, in high capitalism the value is always financial, but, as Karl Marx demonstrated in *Das Kapital* (1990 [1867]), the value
is mostly a surplus value because of our affective relations to material things.
Matter, objects, have an intrinsic social quality. 'Stuff' – as the title of Daniel
Miller's (2010) book runs – does not merely exist, but is always transformed
by social interaction into a certain value: 'I shop, therefore I am'. Putting
the emphasis on materiality therefore does not preclude an understanding
of matter as symbolic; rather, it shows that there is a constant negotiation
between the material and the symbolic.

New materialism claims to be 'new', which it is in the sense of refocus-
ing on matter and materiality after decades of a dominant focus on text
and textuality. Yet, materialism has a long and prestigious genealogy and
is in fact influenced by several sources and disciplines (Bennett and Joyce,
2010). These theories should not be understood as being completely separated, because many of these theorists have been inspired or even set off
by each other. The first is the historical materialism of Karl Marx with its
emphasis on the praxis of production and labour, as is further explained in
the chapter on Marx in this book. Second, Marxism has inspired a sociological approach to the culture of things as in the work of Thorstein Veblen
and Georg Simmel (Brown, 2010: 62). Marxist Walter Benjamin has understood how the history of production and labour is intimately connected to
circulation and consumption, and thus to 'a history of fascination, apprehension, aspiration' (Brown, 2010: 63). Third, the sociological approach is
closely related to cultural anthropology as the discipline that has put the
'very being of objects' as its central topic (Brown, 2001: 9). Fourth, the
Actor-Network-Theory (ANT) of Bruno Latour (2005) attributes some sort
of agency to non-human actors, which helps to think about the agency of
things and assemblages of human and non-human actors. Fifth, the phenomenology of Maurice Merleau-Ponty has put the focus on the materiality
of the human body, exploring the experience of what he calls 'my-body-in-
the-world' (2002: 167). Sixth, the materialist branch of feminism rethinks
the materiality of the human body and its gendered nature (Braidotti, 2002).
And finally, Gilles Deleuze and Félix Guattari (1987 [1980]) evoke on the
one hand a materialism of the flesh that considers the body as intelligent
matter, and on the other hand add a form of empiricism that rejects the transcendental idea of reason. The convergence of those two strands produces a
vital materialism combining critique with creativity.

The fact that many of these theorists are discussed in *Thinking through Fashion*
signals the importance of materialism for fashion studies. Fashion is not only

a system of signification but also a commercial industry producing and selling material commodities. Fashion, perhaps more conspicuously than other cultural realms, consists of material objects and involves a bodily practice of dressing. This fact has not escaped scholars of fashion. The anthropological perspective has regarded clothes as objects in their own right or as meaningful within practices of dressing (Küchler and Miller, 2005). Daniel Miller (1998) argued for balancing theories to take on the specificity of material cultures. Ethnographic approaches are important methodologies for understanding what people wear and why (Woodward, 2007). Entwistle (2000) has argued for an empirically grounded sociology that takes the embodied practice of dress seriously. Because these diverse approaches have always been vital methodologies for fashion studies, the claim of novelty of 'new materialism' seems a bit singular. In that sense it may be better to speak of 'renewed materialism'.

Fashion studies is then unique in combining many different strands of theory, where the extremes of the linguistic turn have been kept in check by the necessary focus on the very materiality of fashion: its mode of production, but also the textiles, and the clothes in our wardrobe or on our body. As Bill Brown wittily writes, 'culture itself is now appearing not as text but as textile' (2010: 64). *Thinking through Fashion* presents a range of theorists who are carefully chosen and discussed by expert and emergent scholars in the field of fashion studies. The authors of the present volume set up intellectual conversations amongst themselves and amongst the theorists they discuss, opening up new intellectual adventures for the reader. If anything, the book should disclose the particular dynamism of the field of fashion studies and its contribution to thinking through social and cultural theory. It should therefore be invaluable not only to fashion studies students and scholars, but also to those social and cultural theorists less familiar with the field of fashion, introducing a novel field through which to reflect on the strengths and weakness of the thinkers they and their students engage with.

Perhaps we can finish our necessarily brief mapping of theory and theorists by evoking the *pleasure* of studying fashion. Theory has all too often connotations of dry abstraction or high degrees of difficulty. But it can be exciting and exhilarating to think through fashion. As Daniel Miller writes, to study the things and objects of fashion means to enjoy 'luxuriating in the detail: the sensuality of touch, colour and flow. A study of clothing should not be cold; it has to invoke the tactile, emotional, intimate world of feelings' (2010: 41). We hope that *Thinking through Fashion* will help to find a way through the many theories that can induce us to immerse ourselves in the study of fashion, because, ultimately, fashion is not only fun, but it *matters*.

PART II: THE KEY THEORISTS: SUMMARIES

Chapter 2: Karl Marx (1818–1883)

The book opens with a discussion of Karl Marx's original critique of capitalism, which implicitly underpins the critical study of fashion. Anthony Sullivan sets out the rich theoretical resources that Marx offers to understanding fashion culturally and socially. The Communist Manifesto's vivid characterization of capitalism as a society where change, contradiction and obsolescence trump continuity, stability and tradition, locates fashion's emergence in a milieu in which 'all that's solid melts into air' – to quote Marx's famous words. The chapter explains how in a capitalist 'mode of production' our 'species being' is 'estranged' from our labour and its products. As a result our relationships with each other and with nature are objectified. The Marxist approach has informed existing literature on the production of fashion and the psychologically infused, negative dialectics of the Frankfurt School of the 1940s and 1950s in Germany. Sullivan argues that Marx's distinctive approach to human culture as a conscious material transformation has often been overlooked; 'a dress only becomes a dress by being worn', claims Marx. Thus, Marx prefigured material culture approaches to fashion. Discussing the application of Marx specifically to fashion today, the chapter shows how his work enables us to understand how and why fashion remains so powerful and yet contradictory. Without Marx's analysis of 'commodity fetishism' the mystification and re-presentation of the objects of fashion, whether garments, bags or shoes, as magical and fabulous totems, remain incomprehensible. The chapter concludes by examining the strengths and limitations of Marx's work, focusing on one aspect of its legacy post-Marxism, in relation to understanding branded, ethical and slow fashion.

Chapter 3: Sigmund Freud (1856–1939)

Janice Miller examines the ideas of Sigmund Freud and asks how they might help in the analysis of fashion and dress. She looks at Freud's ideas of a therapeutic technique named psychoanalysis, which he developed in the nineteenth century to treat mental illness. The framework of psychoanalytic concepts can be applied to the analysis of culture as instigated by Freud himself and by the Freudian psychoanalyst Jacques Lacan half a century later. The chapter examines how psychoanalytic concepts such as 'fetishism' or 'the gaze' have been used by writers on fashion. Importantly however, Miller is interested in not only how some psychoanalytic ideas have been embraced as a mechanism to understand the cultural significance of fashion and dress, but also why others have been largely ignored. The aim of the chapter is to evaluate the potential of a variety of psychoanalytic ideas to the study of fashion. Miller ultimately argues that though fashion studies has seemed to prefer socio-cultural readings, psychoanalysis has the potential to refresh the frameworks that currently tend to circulate within the discipline.

Chapter 4: Georg Simmel (1858–1918)

Having lived most of his life in Berlin, Georg Simmel was indelibly formed by the fact of his maturing in one of the great fin-de-siècle European cities. As Peter McNeil shows, Simmel's approach to social forms played a major role in creating a model for understanding fashion that has been particularly influential in the United States of America since the 1910s, being revived in the 1950s and again in the 1980s, and continuing to resonate within many different strands of international fashion studies today. Simmel's analysis of the endless differentiation of objects and details in his contemporary society laid a bedrock for later theorists of everyday life including Roland Barthes. He also influenced the development of North American 'sociology of everyday life', or 'ethno-methodological' sociology and social psychology. Simmel's approach to fashion, embedded within his understanding of modernity, has influenced great writers on fashion, no matter their methodological or disciplinary affiliations. His writing style, according to McNeil, is akin to 'Impressionism' or 'Symbolism' in painting or music; he was, in fact, called 'a philosophical Monet' by the Marxist philosopher Georg Lukács.

Chapter 5: Walter Benjamin (1892–1940)

Adam Geczy and Vicky Karaminas argue that the influence of Walter Benjamin on fashion studies lies in his idea of fashion as elaborated in the *Arcades Project*: fashion is inextricably bound up with modern culture and it is the most specific manifestation of capitalism's will-to-change – the influence of Karl Marx is most direct here. Fashion, style and sensibility are, for Benjamin, internal and fundamental to modern culture. Dress is not only an attribute of class recognition and aspiration, but also a pervasive and persistent statement of temporality. This temporality, as Geczy and Karaminas discuss, is connected to the way in which modernity needs to maintain the semblance of change. Such change is not only economic but also narratalogical, because modernity is always both subverting and improving upon history. Thus fashion has to be seen as a tissue of historical references that are avowed yet also repressed in the name of the current and the new. Benjamin's impact on fashion studies also resides in his seminal insights into media and representation. Geczy and Karaminas note that Benjamin's notion of reproducibility and loss of aura in the much-studied essay 'The Work of Art in the Age of Mechanical Reproducibility', can be of considerable profit to fashion studies. One point in particular is the way in which aura is reinvested or redeemed through the proliferation of reproductions, perpetuating presence and desirability. They argue that the representation of fashion in fantasy environments and against the armature of celebrity is one of the drivers of fashion industry. By engaging in a cross-pollination with art and history, in the past two decades high end fashion has engendered a new relation to time.

Chapter 6: Mikhail Bakhtin (1895–1975)

In an endnote to *Rabelais and his World*, the Russian scholar Mikhail M. Bakhtin writes that it would be 'interesting to trace the struggle of the grotesque and the classical concept [of the body] in the history of dress and fashion'. This remained unfortunately an unrealized project during his lifetime. Francesca Granata argues that Bakhtin's cultural history of the grotesque canon is of great relevance to the study of fashion and, more specifically, to the study of the history of the fashionable body. Epitomized by the open-ended collective body of carnival, and characterized by a transgression of borders, the grotesque stands in contrast to the 'sealed', atomized and individualized classical body – a body which has characterized much twentieth-century high fashion. Intersecting with writings in feminism, gender studies, queer theory and disability studies, Bakhtin's work provides the tools to examine fashion's unique position in upholding normality on the one hand, while paradoxically also being the vehicle to exceed, upend or, to use Bakhtinian terminology, carnivalize ideals of norms and deviation. Conversely, the study of fashion, as Bakhtin himself recognized, constitutes a central area for an application of his theory, thanks to fashion's inextricable relation to the body. Through the use of specific examples, circumscribed both historically and geographically, and by placing his work on a continuum with that of other theorists, Granata shows that fashion studies qualifies and better contextualizes his over-celebratory reading of the grotesque.

Chapter 7: Maurice Merleau-Ponty (1908–1961)

Llewellyn Negrin explains that fashion, by dint of the fact that it is designed to be worn, is inextricably linked with the body. Yet much analysis of fashion has tended to neglect the experience of dress as a tactile and embodied form, treating it primarily as a 'text' to be decoded semiotically. As such, it has been viewed as a purely visual phenomenon while the nature of its interaction with the body of the wearer has been overlooked. In the process, what has been ignored is that fashion is not just the creation of a specific 'look', but is also the comportment of the body in space. Particular garments are significant not just for the meanings they communicate or for their aesthetic appearance, but because they produce certain modes of bodily demeanour. In its disassociation of fashion from the body, fashion theory has perpetuated the mind/body distinction, converting the body into a de-materialized surface of inscription, whose corporeal nature is overlooked. Rather than being regarded as integral to our experience of wearing clothes, the body has been treated as a *tabula rasa* onto which sartorial signs are superimposed. Negrin's chapter discusses how the phenomenology of Maurice Merleau-Ponty, which foregrounds the embodied nature of our experience of the world, can be used to address this lacuna. Central to Merleau-Ponty's phenomenology is an awareness of the body not as a passive receptor of outside stimuli, but rather, as the medium through which we experience the world. As Merleau-Ponty has made clear, our bodies are not simply inert objects existing independently of our minds but rather, are the very means through which we come to know the world and articulate our sense of self. Merleau-Ponty's phenomenology, Negrin argues, provides us with the theoretical tools with which to address fashion not simply as an aesthetic or symbolic phenomenon but as a haptic experience.

Chapter 8: Roland Barthes (1915–1980)

Roland Barthes' *The Fashion System* is a much misunderstood and maligned text (Rick Rylance called it his 'bleakest book'), but as the author himself argued, 'it poses the problem of knowing if there is really an object that we call fashion clothing'. At the heart of Barthes's enquiry is the hypothesis that real clothing – what we wear in our everyday existence – is secondary to the ways in which it can be articulated in the verbal and visual rhetoric of fashion editorials and fashion spreads: 'Without discourse there is no total Fashion, no essential Fashion.' In this chapter, therefore, Paul Jobling discusses the dialectic between two key terms that Barthes evinced – written clothing and image clothing – to analyse the repetitive performativity of word and image in fashion texts. At the same time, Jobling mobilizes key works such as 'The Semantics of the Object' and *The Pleasure of the Text* to consider the relevance of Barthes' ideas concerning the status of fashion as a sign and the semiological meanings of garments, photographs and advertisements.

Chapter 9: Erving Goffman (1922–1982)

Goffman's seminal *The Presentation of Self in Everyday Life*, and more specifically his notions of front and back regions, props and performance, offer useful tools for an understanding both of individuals' everyday engagement with fashion and of the division of labour and specialization through space that characterizes the fashion industry. In this chapter Efrat Tseëlon looks at Goffman's analysis of the dramaturgy of the social self to reflect on the role of fashion within it and the idea of fashion as communication. Goffman identified the kernel of social behaviour as a collective endeavour to avoid shame, loss of face and embarrassment. Combining a micro analysis of everyday behaviour together with insights based on a variety of empirical and fictional sources, he distilled the tacit rules and codes that structure Western society, interrogating their boundaries through their breach. The chapter provides empirical evidence to support the thrust of Goffman's dramaturgical thesis with regard to clothes, without falling into a common misconception of attributing authenticity to backstage and manipulation to front stage. Identity is created through performance, and clothes are a key tool in this process of self-construction. Clothes can be seen as 'props' central to the way individuals as performers negotiate their relations to others in various social settings, as Tseëlon discusses in relation to the idea of professional appearance. Although Goffman's study is mostly concerned with individuals' work of self-presentation, Tseëlon argues that it can be extended to organizational and institutional practices such as those at play in the field of fashion.

Chapter 10: Gilles Deleuze (1925–1995)

Gilles Deleuze's philosophy is often situated within the school of French post-structuralism, but his thought does not share the same emphasis on the centrality of language. Deleuze aims to come up with new concepts so as to rethink and revitalize life and he can thus be situated as a vitalist and materialist thinker. Although Deleuze's ideas have hardly yet been applied to fashion, Anneke Smelik argues that concepts such as 'becoming', the 'body-without-organs' and 'the fold' can illuminate the study of contemporary fashion. The continuous process of creative transformations is what Deleuze and co-author Guattari (1987) understand by 'becoming'; for example becoming-woman, becoming-animal, becoming-machine. Becoming implies a different way of thinking about human identity and the way one is dressed: not rigid and fixed from cradle to grave but fluid and flexible throughout life. The process of becoming is connected to the idea of the 'body-without-organs', which refers to re-organizing the way in which the body is given meaning. The notion of the body-without-organs can help to counter normative images of what a body should look like – not unlike much of high fashion's extravagant designs. Deleuze's concept of 'the fold' undoes a binary opposition between inside and outside, between appearance and essence. This insight involves a fundamental critique of the idea that fashion is a superficial game of exteriority covering over a 'deep' self hidden in the interior folds of the soul. Rather, identity can be understood as a set of folds; folding-in and folding-out – much like the folds of the garments we wear in daily life. The Deleuzean notion of the fold helps to see how fashion designs set the body in motion, potentially liberating it from the dominant modes of identity in the consumerist world of fast fashion.

Chapter 11: Michel Foucault (1926–1984)

Jane Tynan examines the practices and discourses of fashion through the work of Michel Foucault. His concern with the body as site of social control has inspired theorists from a range of academic disciplines to apply his ideas to the social practices linked to fashion, beauty, style and regulation clothing. The level of academic interest in Foucault's work is largely due to his theory of modern society, centred on the control of bodies in space, which is clearly applicable to the embodied practices of fashion and dress. Focusing on Foucault's concepts of discourse, governmentality and biopolitics, Tynan demonstrates how fashion and dress are implicated in maintaining collective identities. The discussion goes on to explore how subversive fashion practices challenge the forces that seek to normalize power over bodies. By theorizing the body as target of power in modernity, Foucault has given scholars and students of fashion studies scope to consider how dress can unite communities, but also how it divides them.

Chapter 12: Niklas Luhmann (1927–1998)

The work of German sociologist Niklas Luhmann has been fashionable in the social sciences and humanities since the 1990s. Sociologists, philosophers and literary scholars see the values of his universalistic project to explain all things social. Indeed, his 'super theory' offers a general theory of social systems. Luhmann's project renewed the sociological systems theory tradition through the idea of 'autopoiesis' or self-producing systems, by which he aimed to embrace both constructivism and universalism. Luhmann's thought has been relatively understudied in the field of fashion studies, and Aurélie Van de Peer sets out to show how Luhmann's systems theory can offer a fruitful approach to fashion. Rather than explaining in detail Luhmann's framework, which he has gradually developed in over 50 books, she discusses several key ideas that are central to his thought and can be of particular relevance to the study of fashion. These key ideas refer to modern society as a functionally differentiated social system and the centrality of communication. Van de Peer wonders whether in such a society fashion has become an autonomous and autopoietic subsystem with its own paradoxes. If indeed a subsystem of fashion operates by following its own rationality, this has the potential to re-address what numerous fashion scholars have argued before: that fashion has been unrightfully treated with contempt.

Chapter 13: Jean Baudrillard (1929–2007)

One of the major thinkers of post-modernism, Jean Baudrillard blended neo-Marxist, psychoanalytic and post-semiotic linguistics insights to develop a theory of consumption based not on the fulfilment of needs or desires in objects, but on our relation to objects as a discursive system. In this system, objects function like 'signs' fulfilling insatiable desire for the image as a symbolic object. Efrat Tseëlon's analysis of the meaning of fashion in European history uses Baudrillard's three orders of signification of objects from a referential to a self-referential system. The first order of the pre-modern period is founded on imitation. It presupposes dualism in which appearances *reflect* reality, and clothes index social hierarchy. The second order of modernity is founded on production. Mechanization and urbanization made mass-produced clothes available to all classes simultaneously in fabrics and styles formerly reserved only for nobility. Consequently, people could claim a status which wasn't theirs: that is where appearances *mask* reality. The third order of post-modernity, as Tseëlon discusses, is founded on simulation: appearances no longer connect to underlying reality. They stop signifying and replace communication with seduction. They become a playful spectacle of artifice and signs that no longer signify anything, as when religious or national symbols are appropriated for their aesthetic, not symbolic value. In fact, at this stage, appearances *invent* reality.

Chapter 14: Pierre Bourdieu (1930–2002)

In her chapter on Pierre Bourdieu, Agnès Rocamora shows that the French sociologist's influential work provides invaluable tools for interrogating the topic of fashion. She introduces the readers to his key notions of field, cultural capital and habitus, which she also discusses in relation to Bourdieu's own work on the 1970s French field of high fashion. She then turns to his seminal book *Distinction*, where he insists on the importance of approaching the issue of taste through the lens of class, reminding us of the social and cultural forces at play in judgements of taste, such as tastes in fashion. Like many other thinkers discussed in this book Bourdieu wanted to denaturalize the processes and values which culture has turned into nature. In the remainder of the chapter, Rocamora appropriates Bourdieu's theoretical framework to look at fashion blogging. She discusses the relation between the traditional field of fashion journalism and that of fashion blogging to shed light on the changing nature of the contemporary fashion media.

Chapter 15: Jacques Derrida (1930–2004)

Derrida has been one of the most significant thinkers to have addressed the insights of linguistics for theory in general, while questioning attempts to make definitive systems of these theories. It is this insistence not only on the importance of language to theory, but on the openness of all theory to the ambiguities and undecidable confusions of language which have made him a key *post*-structuralist thinker. Alison Gill takes on the challenge of revealing the relevance of Derrida's thought for fashion studies. Her chapter identifies examples where fashion designers appear to critically dismantle the principles of garment making. She first outlines the key features of deconstruction in philosophy, with a focus on the emergence of concepts such as text, trace and double-thinking. She shows how these can be relevant to an alternative thinking about fashion design, one that courts the expression of failure and acts out instability. In the second part of the chapter Gill identifies instabilities in fashion designs that challenge conventional notions of authorship, innovation and fashion history. Derridean thought about textual construction and deconstruction can help make sense of Maison Martin Margiela's unconventional analysis of fashion's very foundations in the materials, structure, techniques and construction of garments. The chapter discusses how to 'put under erasure' fashion's insistent drive to produce collections in line with a commercial system that prizes the aesthetic idealism of innovation, spectacle and seamlessness at a dizzying seasonal pace and a predictable relationship with time.

Chapter 16: Bruno Latour (1947–)

Joanne Entwistle examines the work of French sociologist Bruno Latour. Latour's work has been influential within science and technology studies (STS) and is responsible for inaugurating actor-network-theory or ANT. His work is a radical critique of the major concepts within sociology, such as 'nature' and 'culture', and challenges the conventional notion of the social 'actor': for ANT actors can be human or non-human by virtue of their ability to impact on the networks within which they are entangled. Latour's attention to these networks or 'assemblages' requires close ethnographic observation to the extent that ANT/STS might be better thought of as a methodology. Although important, his work has been little applied beyond studies of science and laboratories. Emerging out of this ANT approach, Michel Callon's work develops the idea of markets as networks, illuminating how markets come together in particular assemblages. In this chapter, Entwistle analyses how Latour's approach can be applied to the analysis of fashion networks that combine human and non-human actors. This approach provides a useful way into understanding fashion markets as particular sorts of assemblages of actors, and Entwistle gives the example of her own research on fashion models and fashion buyers to illustrate the applications of this approach.

Chapter 17: Judith Butler (1956–)

Elizabeth Wissinger explains how Judith Butler's reading of philosophy and feminism posits a body stylized into existence through cultural practice that, while heavily reliant on discourse, still produce a lived, sexed, body. Troubling assumptions about the body's essential nature, Butler's work highlights how performative processes irrevocably fuse self, body and garment. As such, the body expresses its gender via pre-given codes that are nonetheless subject to constant negotiation. Radically destabilizing gender, and interrogating it through her study of gay subcultures, Butler's work helped a nascent queer studies movement gain momentum. At the same time, her notion that all gender is a performance lent new weight to the role of fashion in understanding feminist debates about embodiment. Butler's radical re-reading of psychology and semiotics, Wissinger argues, is also useful to critique long-standing assumptions about fashion's role in social life. Butler's central contribution is her rethinking of agency as no longer residing in the self-determined subject, but rather in the body's unruly tendency to exceed its boundaries, to 'matter' on its own terms.

NOTES

1 The *International Journal of Fashion Studies*, which one of the co-editors of this book – Agnès
   Rocamora – launched with Emanuela Mora and Paolo Volonté, was created to attend
   to the issue of the English language's domination of Fashion Studies and its internationalization, by allowing for the peer-reviewing of articles in all languages.

REFERENCES

Appadurai, A. (ed.) (2013 [1986]) *The Social Life of Things: Commodities in Cultural Perspective*,
   11th edn, Cambridge: Cambridge University Press.
Barker, C. (2011) *Cultural Studies: Theory and Practice*, London: Sage.
Barrett, E. and Bolt, B. (eds) (2013) *Carnal Knowledge: Towards a 'New Materialism' through the Arts*,
   London and New York: I.B. Tauris.
Barthes, R. (1967) 'Death of the Author', reprinted in (1978) *Image, Music, Text*, S. Heath
   (trans), Glasgow: Fontana Collins.
———(1973) *Mythologies*, A. Lavers (trans), London: Paladin.
———(1973) *The Pleasure of the Text*, R. Miller (trans), New York: Hill and Wang.
———(1977) *A Lover's Discourse: Fragments*, R. Howard (trans), New York: Hill and Wang.
———(1983) *Simulations*, New York: Semiotext(e).
———(1990 [1967]) *The Fashion System*, M. Ward and R. Howard (trans), Berkeley and Los
   Angeles: University of California Press.
———(1993 [1976]) *Symbolic Exchange and Death*, I. Grant (trans), London: Sage.
Baudelaire (1999 [1863]) 'Le Peintre de la Vie Moderne', in *Baudelaire: Ecrits sur L'Art*, Paris:
   Le Livre de Poche.
Baudrillard, J. (1993 [1976]) *Symbolic Exchange and Death*, I. Grant (trans), London: Sage.
Bauman, Z. (2000) *Liquid Modernity*, Cambridge: Polity Press.
———(2011) *Culture in a Liquid Modern World*, Cambridge: Polity.
Bennett, T. and Joyce, P. (eds) (2010) *Material Powers: Cultural Studies, History, and the Material Turn*,
   London and New York: Routledge.
Berger, A.A. (1995) *Manufacturing Desire: Media, Popular Culture, and Everyday Life*, New Brunswick,
   NJ: Transaction Publishers.
Best, S. and Kellner, D. (1991) *Postmodern Theory: Critical Interrogations*, London: Macmillan.
Bolt, B. (2013) 'Introduction' in: E. Barrett and B. Bolt (eds), *Carnal Knowledge: Towards a 'New
   Materialism' through the Arts*, London and New York: I.B. Tauris.
Braidotti, R. (1991) *Patterns of Dissonance: A Study of Women and Contemporary Philosophy*,
   Cambridge: Polity Press.
———(2002) *Metamorphoses: Towards a Materialist Theory of Becoming*, Cambridge: Polity Press.
Breward, C. (1995) *The Culture of Fashion*, Manchester: Manchester University Press.
———(2003) *Fashion*, Oxford: Oxford University Press.
Brown, B. (2001) 'Thing Theory' in *Critical Inquiry*, 28 (1): 1–22.
———(2010) 'The Matter of Materialism' in T. Bennett and P. Joyce (eds), *Material Powers:
   Cultural Studies, History, and the Material Turn*, London and New York: Routledge.
Burman, B. and Turbin, C. (eds) (2003) *Material Strategies: Dress and Gender in Historical Perspective*,
   Oxford: Blackwell.

Butler, J. (1990) *Gender Trouble*, New York and London: Routledge.

Cavallaro, D. (2001) *Critical and Cultural Theory*, London: Athlone Press.

Certeau, M. de (1988) *The Practice of Everyday Life*, Berkeley: University of California Press.

Chakrabarty, D. (2000) *Provincializing Europe: Postcolonial Thought and Historical Difference*, Princeton, NJ: Princeton University Press.

Cole, S. (2009) *The Story of Men's Underwear*, New York: Parkstone.

Coole, D. and Frost, S. (eds) (2010) *New Materialisms: Ontology, Agency, and Politics*, Durham, NC: Duke University Press.

Davis, F. (1992) *Fashion, Culture, and Identity*, Chicago: University of Chicago Press.

Deleuze, G. and Guattari, F. (1987 [1980]) *A Thousand Plateaus: Capitalism and Schizophrenia*, B. Massumi (trans), Minneapolis: University of Minnesota Press.

Derrida, J. (1976) *Of Grammatology*, G.C. Spivak (trans), Baltimore, MD: John Hopkins University Press.

Docherty, T. (ed.) (1993) *Postmodernism: A Reader*, New York: Columbia University Press.

Dolphijn, R. and van der Tuin, I. (2012) *New Materialism: Interviews and Cartographies*, Open Humanities Press.

During, S. (ed.) (1993) *The Cultural Studies Reader*, London: Routledge.

Eagleton, T. (1990) *The Significance of Theory*, Oxford: Blackwell.

Eicher, J.B. (1999) *Dress and Ethnicity: Change across Space and Time*, Oxford: Berg.

Eisenstadt, S.N. (2000) 'Multiple Modernities' in *Daedalus*, 129 (1): 1–29.

Entwistle, J. (2000) *The Fashioned Body: Fashion, Dress and Modern Social Theory*, Cambridge: Polity.

Evans, C. (2000) 'Yesterday's Emblems and Tomorrow's Commodities: The Return of the Repressed in Fashion Imagery Today' in S. Bruzzi and P. Church Gibson (eds), *Fashion Cultures: Theories, Explorations and Analysis*, London: Routledge.

———(2003) *Fashion at the Edge: Spectacle, Modernity and Deathliness*, London: Yale University Press.

———(2013) *The Mechanical Smile: Modernism and the First Fashion Shows in France and America, 1900–1929*, London: Yale University Press.

Foucault, M. (1969) 'What is an Author' reprinted in J.D. Faubion (ed.) (1994) *Aesthetics, Method and Epistemology*, London: Allen Lane.

———(1990 [1976]) *The History of Sexuality*, Vol. 1, R. Hurley (trans), London: Penguin.

———(2004 [1969]) *The Archaeology of Knowledge*, London: Routledge.

Freud, S. (1964 [1900]) 'Interpretation of Dreams' in J. Stratchey (ed.), *Standard Edition*, London: Hogarth.

Gaonkar, D.P. (ed.) (2001) *Alternative Modernities*, Durham, NC: Duke University Press.

Gilroy, P. (1993) *The Black Atlantic: Modernity and Double Consciousness*, London: Verso.

Grossberg, L., Cary, N. and Treichler, P. (eds) (1992) *Cultural Studies*, Routledge: New York.

Hall, S. (1997) *Representation: Cultural Representations and Signifying Practices*, London: Sage.

Haraway, D. (1988) 'Situated Knowledges: The Science Question in Feminism and the Privilege of Partial Perspective', reprinted in (1991) *Simians, Cyborgs and Women: The Reinvention of Nature*, London: Free Association Books.

Hendrickson, H. (ed.) (1996) *Clothing and Difference: Embodied Identities in Colonial and Post-colonial Africa*, London: Duke University Press.

Hills, M. (2005) *How to do Things with Cultural Theory*, London: Bloomsbury.

hooks, b. (1990) *Yearning: Race, Gender, and Cultural Politics*, Boston, MA: South End Press.

———(1992) *Black Looks: Race and Representation*, Boston, MA: South End Press.

Hutcheon, L. (1989) *The Politics of Postmodernism*, London: Routledge.

Irigaray, L. (1985) *This Sex Which Is Not One*, Ithaca, NY: Cornell University Press.

Jameson, F. (1991) *Postmodernism, or the Cultural Logic of Late Capitalism*, London: Verso.

Jary, D. and Jary, J. (1995) *Collins Dictionary of Sociology*, Glasgow: Harper Collins.

Jobling, P. (1999) *Fashion Spreads: Words and Image in Fashion Photography since 1980*, Oxford: Berg.

Kawamura, Y. (2005) *Fashion-ology: An Introduction to Fashion Studies*, New York: Berg.

Kondo, D. (1997) *About Face: Performing Race in Fashion and Theater*, London: Routledge.

Küchler, S. and Miller, D. (2005) *Clothing as Material Culture*, Oxford: Berg.

Lacan, J. (1977) *Écrits: A Selection*, New York: Norton.

Latour, B. (2005) *Reassembling the Social: An Introduction to Actor-Network-Theory*, Oxford: Oxford University Press.

Lehmann, U. (2000) *Tigersprung: Fashion in Modernity*, London: MIT Press.

Lewis, R. (2013) *Modest Fashion: Styling Bodies, Mediating Faith*, London: I.B. Tauris.

Lipovetsky, G. (1994) *The Empire of Fashion: Dressing Modern Democracy*, Princeton, NJ: Princeton University Press.

———(2005) *Hypermodern Times*, London: Polity.

Lyotard, J-F. (1984) *The Postmodern Condition*, Manchester: Manchester University Press.

Marx, K. (1990 [1867]) *Capital Volume One*, B. Fowkes (trans), London: Penguin.

Maynard, M. (2004) *Dress and Globalisation*, Manchester: Manchester University Press.

Merleau-Ponty, M. (2002) *Phenomenology of Perception*, London, New York: Routledge.

Metz, C. (1982) *Psychoanalysis and Cinema: The Imaginary Signifier*, London: MacMillan.

Miller, D. (ed.) (1998) *Material Cultures: Why Some Things Matter*, Chicago: University of Chicago Press.

———(2010) *Stuff*, Cambridge: Polity.

Mills, C.W. (2000 [1959]) *The Sociological Imagination*, Oxford: Oxford University Press.

Mitchell, W. (1994) *Picture Theory: Essays on Verbal and Visual Representation*, Chicago: University of Chicago Press.

Mora, E., Rocamora, A., and Volonté, P. (2014) 'The Internationalization of Fashion Studies: Rethinking the Peer-reviewing Process' in *International Journal of Fashion Studies*, 1 (1): 3–17.

Niessen, S., Leshkowich, A.M., and Jones, C. (2003) *Re-orienting Fashion: The Globalisation of Asian Dress*, Oxford: Berg.

Pine, J. and Gilmore, J. (1999) *The Experience Economy*, Cambridge: Harvard Business School Press.

Rabine, L.W. (2002) *The Global Circulation of African Fashion*, Oxford: Berg.

Rantisi, N. (2004) 'The Designer in the City and the City in the Designer' in D. Power and A.J. Scott (eds), *Cultural Industries and the Production of Culture*, New York: Routledge.

Rocamora, A. (2009) *Fashioning the City: Paris, Fashion and The Media*, London: I.B. Tauris.

———(2012) 'Hypertextuality and Remediation in the Fashion Media: The Case of Fashion Blogs' in *Journalism Pratice*: 92–106.

Root, R. (2013) 'Mapping Latin American Fashion', in S. Black, A. De La Haye, J. Entwistle, A. Rocamora, R. Root and H. Thomas (eds) *The Handbook of Fashion Studies*, London: Bloomsbury.

Rorty, R. (1967) *The Linguistic Turn: Recent Essays in Philosophical Method*, Chicago: University of Chicago Press.

Said, E. (1982) 'Traveling Theory' in *The World, the Text, and the Critic*, Cambridge, MA: Harvard University Press.

Santagata, W. (2004) 'Creativity, Fashion and Market Behavior' in D. Power and A.J. Scott (eds), *Cultural Industries and the Production of Culture*, New York: Routledge.

Saussure, F. de (1996 [1916]) *The Course in General Linguistics*, R. Harris (trans), Chicago and La Salle, IL: Open Court.

Silverman, K. (1983) *The Subject of Semiotics*, New York: Oxford University Press.

Sim, S. (ed.) (1998) *The Icon Critical Dictionary of Postmodern Thought*, Cambridge: Icon Books.

Simmel, G. (1971 [1904]) 'Fashion' in D.N. Levine (ed.), *Georg Simmel*, Chicago: University of Chicago Press.

Stanton, D. (1980) 'Language and Revolution: The Franco-American Dis-Connection' in H. Eistenstein and A. Jardine (eds), *The Future of Difference*, Boston: Hall.

Storey, J. (ed.) (1996) *What is Cultural Studies? A Reader*, London: Arnold.

Sturken, M. and Cartwright, L. (2009) *Practices of Looking: An Introduction to Visual Culture*, Oxford: Oxford University Press.

Trinh, M-H. (1989) *Woman, Native, Other: Writing Postcoloniality and Feminism*, Bloomington: Indiana University Press.

Vermeulen, T. and Van den Akker, R. (2010) 'Notes on Metamodernism' in *Journal of Aesthetics and Culture*, 2: 1–13.

Vinken, B. (2000) *Fashion Zeitgeist: Trends and Cycles in the Fashion System*, Oxford: Berg.

Williams, R. (1958) *Culture and Society: 1780–1950*, Harmondsworth: Penguin.

———(1983) *Key Words*, London: Fontana.

Wilson, E. (2003) *Adorned in Dreams: Fashion and Modernity*, London: I.B. Tauris.

Woods, T. (1999) *Beginning Postmodernism*, Manchester: Manchester University Press.

Woodward, S. (2007) *Why Women Wear What They Wear*, Oxford: Berg.

2

KARL MARX
Fashion and Capitalism

Anthony Sullivan

INTRODUCTION

Given Wilson's comment that 'fashion is the child of capitalism' (2003: 13), this chapter shows how Marx's rich conceptual framework can produce a deeper critical understanding of the origins and dynamics of fashion, socially, culturally and materially. For just like the capitalist system which spawned it, fashion is 'double faced' (Wilson, 2003: 13), a source of both pleasure and pain, expression and exploitation.

A GLIMPSE OF MARX'S LIFE AND A LESSON IN THE SYMBOLIC POWER OF DRESS

In contrast to the grinding poverty which scarred his later life, Marx was born into the relative comfort of a middle class home in the German cathedral town of Trier in the Rhineland in 1818. The son of a Jewish lawyer who converted to Protestantism to escape anti-Semitism, Marx studied law at Bonn in 1835 and philosophy at Berlin University a year later. Despite completing his doctoral thesis on classical Greek philosophy in 1841, aged only 23, Marx dropped his plans to follow an academic career. Instead, he dedicated his life to studying capitalism and to providing the theoretical underpinnings for a grand project: the emancipation of society by ridding it of the suffering caused by the class inequalities and exploitation which prevail under capitalism (Callinicos, 1983). Under this system, or 'mode of production' (Marx, 1976: 3), goods are produced to be sold as commodities to create profit for capitalists, that is, those who own the 'means of production' (the raw materials and manufacturing machinery). For Marx, then, capitalism does not primarily seek to meet the needs of the workers who make these goods. Rather, their 'labour power' is sold to, controlled and exploited by these same capitalists in return for the wages necessary to subsist. Meanwhile, workers themselves are transformed into consumers forced to buy back the things they make at a premium. This exploitative system of production characterizes capitalism and is central to the development of fashion, as we will later see.

Casual journalism, Marx's main source of income after leaving university, was poorly and erratically paid, forcing him to regularly pawn his overcoat to buy food and other essentials for himself and his family. Frequent trips to the pawnbrokers meant he 'knew the value of his coat' (Stallybrass, 1998: 203) as a commodity or means of exchange. However, giving up his coat for cash also brought him face-to-face with one of the most important aspects of fashion: its capacity to signify social status, real or otherwise, 'actual or contrived' (Finkelstein, 1991: 128). Without his coat Marx was unable to study, since 'the reading room [of the British Library] did not accept just anyone off the streets, and a man without an overcoat [...] was just anyone. Without it, Marx was [...] not fit to be seen' (Stallybrass, 1998: 187). Thus, Marx experienced first-hand the symbolic power of dress as a means to create an image or impression of social identity and to 'individuate oneself in the midst of society' (Marx and Engels, 1973: 84).

HEGEL, FEUERBACH AND MARX: THE ROAD TO HISTORICAL MATERIALISM

What made Marx such an exceptional thinker within the history of western thought was his frustration with the cerebral fixation of many of his contemporaries. As he writes, 'philosophers have only interpreted the world in various ways – the point is to change it' (Marx, 1974: 123). As a student Marx was drawn into a bohemian circle of radical thinkers who were heavily influenced by, yet increasingly critical of, the work of Hegel, the most important philosopher of the day. The 'Young Hegelians', as they were known, still basked in the intellectual glow of the eighteenth-century Enlightenment, which stressed that ideas, reason and thought – as opposed to God, nature and supernatural forces – were decisive in understanding history and transforming society. They gathered to drink and discuss ideas at the Berlin Doctors' Club (Gonzalez, 2006), attacking the oppressiveness of the Prussian (now German) society of which they were part.

In Hegel's work Marx found the seeds of his own theory of history: 'historical materialism'. Hegel (1975) had argued that the development of society and the ideas that shaped it, went through distinct stages. Any change from one type of society to another did not come about gradually, but through ruptures and antagonisms rooted in conflicting ideas about how people understood the world. Thus, for Hegel, progress could only come about if this contradiction in ideas was resolved by a move to a new revolutionary way of thinking, a synthesis which provided a more complete and higher level of understanding of the world. He argued that the Prussian state had emerged from such a struggle between those who believed God or supernatural forces shaped history, and enlightenment thinkers for whom everything could be explained rationally.

However, Marx's 'historical materialism' saw social change as arising not from contradictions in the *ideas* in society, but in its *material* conditions of life and the way in which labour was organised. Marx argued that the conflict over ownership, control of production and its product was the central contradiction in capitalist society. It created distinct groups or, in his terms, classes, and resulted in a struggle between them for control of labour power. As he famously put it: 'the history of all hitherto existing society is the history of class struggles. Freeman and slave, patrician and plebeian, lord and serf, guild-master and journeymen, [and worker or proletarian and capitalist], in a word oppressor and oppressed.' (Marx and Engels, 1998: 3). Here he was also influenced by the work of Hegel's biggest critic, Feuerbach, who insisted material life shaped consciousness. Feuerbach's ideas offered an alternative to Hegel's, whose concept of labour as only of the mental kind made him succumb to 'the illusion of conceiving the real as the product of thought' (Marx, 1993: 101). For Marx, who was above all interested in change and how to get it, Feuerbach's materialism was problematic in that it conceived of human nature, thought and behaviour as an unalterable essence.

Thus, it was by both drawing on and critiquing the ideas of these thinkers that Marx developed his 'historical materialist' perspective. He argued that human nature did not remain static, because labour and its effects distinguished our 'species being' from other animals. For Marx, labour changes human nature itself because our active interaction with the material world through labour reshapes our consciousness. At the same time, through our 'material production and intercourse we alter along with the actual world our thinking and its products' (Marx and Engels, 1975: 37). According to Marx, then, it was the contradictions of class relations, the control over labour and its products by a small group or class under capitalism, which prevented the full realisation of our 'species being' or creative labouring powers. This loss of control over our labour is what he termed 'alienation' (1844). The control by the dominant class over labour precluded the establishment of communism, which for Marx and his friend and collaborator Engels was the highest form of society. Under Communism, the production process would be transparent. Labour would be democratically controlled and organized on the basis of social need instead of private profit. In establishing such possibilities, Marx, supported by Engels, became the primary theorist of revolutionary socialism. Via seminal texts like *The Communist Manifesto* (1848) he espoused the belief that only when the working class takes power by destroying the existing capitalist state, will the whole of society be freed from the inequality and suffering caused by class relations, 'alienation', and the exploitation of labour.

CAPITALISM, FROM DRESS TO FASHION

Wilson (2003) links fashion's emergence from tentative beginnings in court society (Elias, 1978) to the rise of capitalism about four or five hundred years ago. She argues that the symbolic use of adornment to indicate group belonging or social identification – be it to a tribe or subculture, gender or class, whether through clothing, jewellery, body paint (make-up) and piercing – is found in all cultures. But that is dress, not fashion. Rather, fashion 'is dress in which the key feature is rapid and continual changing of styles' (Wilson, 2003: 4–5).

Though it does not discuss dress or fashion specifically, Marx's *Manifesto* documents the social milieu in which fashion developed as a wider social practice. It paints a picture of a world in which change and impermanence or ephemerality, continually trump continuity, stability and tradition. This meant, as *The Manifesto* also vividly demonstrates, a transformation from a society in which social life characterised by 'fixed, frozen relations, with their train of ancient and venerable prejudices' was 'swept away' and replaced by capitalism and a modern urban society where, as Marx famously put it, 'all that is solid melts into air' (Marx and Engels, 1998: 38).

Amongst *The Manifesto*'s many memorable vignettes is its portrayal of the collapse of the old certainties derived from a divinely ordained social order, whose social or class relations were determined by a fixed hierarchy from king to noble to peasant. Marx and Engels wrote:

> The bourgeoisie has put an end to all feudal, patriarchal, idyllic relations. It has pitilessly torn asunder the motley feudal ties that bound man to his 'natural superiors', and has left remaining no other nexus between man and man than naked self-interest, than callous 'cash payment'. It has drowned [all of this] in the icy waters of egotistical calculation.
>
> (1998: 37)

The Manifesto thus dramatically depicts 'the shock of the new' (Hughes, 1991) and the impact of modernity; a new form of society in which the possibility of social mobility and the concept of the self and individual identity were ascendant. Moreover, the disturbance of class relations that created the conditions for this mobility was amplified by the fact that the bourgeois class, as Marx and Engels argued, 'subjected the country to the rule of the towns' (Marx and Engels, 1998: 40). Possessed of a surplus income – the profits of labour exploitation – some of which was spent on consumption, the bourgeois class competed on their favoured public urban terrain with the old rural aristocratic noble class. Class leadership was then contested sartorially, as well as economically and politically. As Slater puts it, 'new money buys landed estates, wears the clothes of court and "society", it can indulge in the leisure pursuits of the aristocracy' (1997: 70). According to both Wilson (2003) and Entwistle (2000), a lack of certainty ensued about who was who in class terms. This was felt most keenly as strangers passed strangers on the streets. Such ambiguity about identity in class terms especially fed a heightened sense of the importance of dress as social currency, a means of expressing, and playing with, revealing and concealing, social identity – hence the symbolic weight of Marx's coat. Unsurprisingly, therefore, the early capitalist city was for Wilson the 'crucible of contradiction' (2003: 13), the space where the fashioning of individual identity emerged in a maelstrom of urban encounters set in motion by capitalism's disruption of older social relations.

Only in this new competitive social context could dress become fashion. Its change or endless mutability developed through what has become known as 'trickle down' diffusion, or the spread of fashion from 'superior' to 'inferior' classes (Veblen, 1899). In place of the relative permanence of feudal dress codes established by occupation – whether one was a 'biscuit, knife or stationery seller' (Wilson, 2003: 24–25) and policed by 'sumptuary laws' governing who wore what in terms of fabric and colours (Craik, 2009) – a competitive cycle of fashionable emulation and symbolic 'distinction' developed (Bourdieu, 1984; see also chapter 14 of this book). Entwistle argues that the struggle for dominance between subordinate and superior classes 'was fought out obliquely less with swords than through symbols of which dress was one of the most significant' (2000: 106). Just as the aristocracy attempted to maintain their identity against the new bourgeois class, whose consumption at first mimicked their own, the bourgeoisie in turn developed a more restrained style of dress (for men at least): the sober frock coat and dark coloured suit, which attempted to distinguish them both from the aristocracy and the working class (Breward, 1999). Without understanding the transformation from feudalism to capitalism it is difficult to explain this sartorial class struggle and why both fashion's dynamic of change and the tension between the individual self and the social emerged. Fashion, in class terms especially, as Simmel argues (see also chapter 4), became the means to subjectively negotiate contradictory impulses to fit in and stand out, enabling both 'social adaptation' and 'differentiation' (1971: 296).

PRODUCING AND CONSUMING 'FASHION FOR ALL'?

If we switch our focus to the material dimensions of fashion under capitalism, and more specifically to how clothes came to be produced and consumed under it, the overall picture is one of a significant but uneven and contradictory shift away from a feudal mode of production. Under that slow-moving system, self- and small-scale artisanal provisioning of goods predominated. Cloth and garment manufacture were 'cottage industries' involving shop-based tailors and journeymen and seamstresses or dress makers (Rouse, 1989; Tarrant, 1994; Lemire, 1997). The contrast between this and today's large scale production of fashion as retail commodities – garments which are 'ready to wear' and available off-the-peg in global fashion chains – is both striking and yet, in important respects, misleading.

The era of rapidly changing 'fast fashion' means seductive images of the latest celebrity or catwalk styles, spread virally through internet and social media sites, soon to be picked up by global fashion multiples who quickly turn them into readymade garments for sale to today's consumer. Zara's use of digital technology in design, stock control, buying and logistics processes has cut the lead time between identifying a fashion and getting it into shops to just a few weeks (Edwards, 2011). However, as recently as the mid-1950s, 'it was still normal to make your own clothes or have them made for you' (Rouse, 1989: 244). Surprisingly, then, despite the spread of fashion at first to the bourgeoisie and then to the middle class at the end of the nineteenth and the beginning of the twentieth centuries (Rouse, 1989; Entwistle, 2000; Wilson, 2003), for much of the population a pattern of non-fashionable consumption remained long after the wider demise of feudalism. Unlike today's ecologically damaging culture of throwaway fashion, clothes in the eighteenth and nineteenth centuries were kept for as long as possible, repaired, unpicked, cleaned and reused not just as second hand but as third, fourth, fifth, sixth hand and more (Lemire, 1997). Moreover, right up to the early twentieth century the second hand trade provided the main point of access for readymade clothing for all but the middle, bourgeois and aristocratic classes (Rouse, 1989; Tarrant, 1994).

There was then a contradiction between the emergence and spread of a culture of fashion in the early capitalist period, and the exclusion of the majority of the working class from fashionable ready to wear until the second half of the twentieth century, when fashion genuinely became 'fashion for all' (Rouse, 1989: 278). This was fundamentally an issue of the cost of new readymade garments. A typist who earned 'about £66 per annum in 1910' and had a budget for clothing of about '£5 per annum' could not afford to be fashionably dressed, only 'respectably' so (Rouse, 1989: 278). Marx and Engels argue in *The Manifesto* that the potential productivity of the 'forces of production' was limited or 'fettered' by the class based social relations of capitalism, which created conditions of scarcity in what should have been an era of plenty. This argument is powerfully apposite in the case of fashion. Until the rise of trade unions at the end of the nineteenth and the beginning of the twentieth century forced increases in pay in the developed countries, fashion was simply beyond most working class people's pockets. Fashion is here understood in Barthes' sense of a rapid cycle of stylistic obsolescence where the rate of 'replacement exceeds dilapidation' (Barthes, 1998: 297–298; for more on Barthes, see also chapter 8 in this book). This exclusive history of consumption is mirrored by the reality of fashion production, which has not shaken off its pre-industrial origins because it remains centred on an archaic assembly process known as CMT (Cut, Make and Trim). Indeed, CMT uses technology and techniques that have scarcely changed since the invention of the sewing machine one hundred and seventy years ago.

LABOUR, 'SPECIES BEING' AND THE DUALITY OF ADORNMENT

As indicated earlier, Marx argued that capitalism was a system based on the exploitation of workers by capitalists. Understanding how this exploitation works to extract what he called 'surplus value' can help us to comprehend the contradictions between fashion production and consumption. More specifically, it can explain why fashion in the twenty-first century continues to heavily exploit the labour of the garment workers who produce the clothes most of us wear today. Such toil, little different to the horrific sweated conditions endured by garment workers in Marx's day, persists because if fashion is to continue as a mass consumer phenomenon it must be made and sold cheaply.

Marx's concept of labour as 'species being' is vital to understanding fashion. To take one example, without the social labour involved in each of the 40-plus manufacturing processes from cotton harvest to retail display, off-the-peg cotton chinos – a menswear fashion staple – could not exist (Jarnow and Dickerson, 1997). Some writers have seen Marx's focus on labour as crudely materialistic (Sahlins, 1976; Baudrillard, 1981, 1988), narrowly focused on production, regardless of the quality and aesthetic dimensions of what was produced so long as it had some functionality. This misperception has been reinforced by the fact that 'Communism' produced the infamous Trabant car in East Germany, and the homogenizing uniform of the Mao suit in China. The reasons why these states turned out such 'wonders' are too complex to go into here, except to say they evidence the alienation or lack of democracy and control by workers in both countries, and each state's behaviour was 'state capitalist' rather than communist (Cliff, 1988). As such they would have been anathema to Marx, who argued not for state ownership and the drive for profit, but for workers' democratic control of labour to serve peoples' wants and needs.

At the heart of Marx's work is his richly capacious concept of labour as our active creative 'species being'; the thing which distinguishes human nature from all other species. Though he praises capitalism for developing this productive potential, Marx and Engels attack 'the bourgeois epoch' (1998: 38) as a world in which a fantastic wealth of commodities is created by exploiting the many, whilst their enjoyment is restricted to the few. For Marx, then, consumption is always marred by the fact that under capitalist social relations markets determine access to commodities on the basis of access to money or credit (Fine and Leopold, 1993). For Marx, this contradiction, along with 'alienation' or 'estrangement' (Marx, 1844) from our creative labouring powers, could only be overcome when the limited or 'fettering' role of class relations and the private ownership and control of production was swept away.

Marx's appreciation of the enormous potential of labour to create all manner of stunning things, including dress, emerges strongly across his writing. It is at its clearest when in *Capital Volume One* (1867) he writes: 'spiders conduct operations which resemble weavers', and bees construct honeycomb cells, 'but what distinguishes the worst of architects from the best of bees is that the architect builds the cell in their mind before constructing it in wax' (Marx, 1990: 284). Elsewhere, he writes that unlike animals, who 'produce one-sidedly' to meet 'immediate needs', humans 'produce universally … even when we are free from physical need and truly produce only in freedom from need' (Marx, 1844: n.p.). For Marx, then, labour as our 'species being' involves conscious design and aesthetic creation beyond necessity. It is this quality of the things we create that makes our production uniquely cultural, since, as he puts it, human beings alone 'form objects in accordance with the laws of beauty' (Marx, 1844: n.p.).

Whilst these words jar with assessments of Marx as a crude materialist or 'productivist', they suggest that the very quality of fashion, the thing which makes it such a powerful cultural force, is the duality of adornment. In *Capital Volume One* he defines commodities as things that engage both wants of the 'stomach', that is, bodily or practical needs, and wants of the 'fancy' or the imagination (Marx, 1990: 125). Fashion, then, is a play of form with and over function: we do not just wear shoes for their utility or for protection, but we wear specific styles of shoes, whether loafers, brogues, boots or trainers, for social, symbolic and aesthetic reasons.

Unlike so much writing on fashion, barring a few exceptions (see Braham, 1997; Entwistle, 2000, 2011; Fine and Leopold, 1993; Phizacklea, 1990), Marx's focus was not just on the creative, aesthetic and playful possibilities of things in the abstract. He was resolutely interested in examining how human labour was systematically exploited to produce commodities. He wanted to understand the contradictions this created, especially under capitalism. In the case of fashion, Marx could see its contradictions not just in his personal experience and tribulations with his coat. He focused on something far worse: the question of why the production of fashion took such a cruel, inhuman form. In *Capital Volume One* he examines the textile industry, tailoring and other forms of garment manufacture, to bring home the realities of the exploitation of labour needed to produce fashion's finery. Here, as elsewhere, he argues that 'alienation' meant labour produced what he called 'marvels and beauty beyond necessity', but always at the price of 'deformity' and suffering for the worker (Marx, 1963 cited in Molyneux, 2012: 12–13).

Similarly, Engels, whose father owned a textile mill in Manchester, had already documented the poverty and misery that arose from the production of all kinds of commodities in England's industrial cities in the 1840s. Pointing to the '15,000 mostly young, women seamstresses' who worked, slept and ate in their workshop premises, labouring for 15 to 18 hour days, he wrote: 'it is a curious fact that the production of precisely those articles which serve the personal adornment of the ladies of the bourgeoisie involves the saddest consequences for the health of the workers' (2009: 12). Outraged by the human cost of fashion's cycle of stylistic change, Marx attacked its 'murderous caprices', highlighting the tragedy of Walkley, a 20-year-old milliner who 'worked uninterruptedly for 26.5 hours' and died of overwork (Marx, 1990: 365). Understandably, given these circumstances, Marx hoped that the invention of the 'decisively revolutionary' sewing machine would transform the production of garments through the use of modern industrial methods (Marx, 1990: 443). But Marx's hopes were not fulfilled and the sewing machine intensified the exploitative pressure on garment workers rather than alleviating it. Understanding why this was so, and why no other major advances have been made in the technology used to make clothes in the CMT process, is the key to understanding fashion's contradictory or ambivalent status. Today, we still need a Marxist perspective to understand the Jekyll and Hyde tendency of the fashion industry.

SURPLUS VALUE, SWEATING AND COMPETITION

To explain how 'surplus value' or profit is created through the social relations between capitalist and worker, Marx developed a basic formula for capitalism, or more precisely capitalist exchange: M-C-M (1990: 248–57). It explains how the capitalist or bourgeoisie as the class who owned the means of production made money from the workers, how this dominant class sold them their 'labour power' in exchange for the wages they needed to live. Taking this process step by step, Marx argued that the capitalist advances value in the form of money, M, to purchase the value of 'labour power', C, as a commodity from the worker in the form of wages. But crucially the value created by the worker's total labour in any given time – the second 'M' of the equation – always exceeds that invested or paid out by the capitalist. Thus, the workers receive only a portion of the total value they create, a wage based on what Marx argued was 'socially necessary labour time' or SNLT. For Marx, labour, or more precisely the SNLT taken to make things, is the basis of the value of all commodities. It represents the time needed on average, given socially typical levels of tools and techniques, for workers to create enough value to be paid the wages necessary to live and to return to work fed, rested, clothed and entertained. For Marx, then, the core value of any commodity comes from the amount or measure of SNLT taken to make it. His 'labour theory of value' means that if a worker produces enough value to pay for their subsistence in four hours, for the rest of an eight hour day they worked for nothing, creating four hours 'surplus value' for the capitalist for whom they worked. 'Surplus value', then, is the excess value which the worker creates and the capitalist receives over and above the value of the worker's wages. In money terms this value is realised as profit for the capitalist when the commodity is sold.

This is the general picture. When we turn to examine fashion production in particular, it has specific characteristics ensuring that the amount of wages paid to the garment worker – the value of their SNLT – was and is very low. Historically, the first ready to wear clothes were manufactured using a continuation of the old feudal 'cottage industry' system mentioned above. Known as 'the putting-out system' (Hobsbawm cited in Lemire, 1997: 55), this pre-industrial system of manufacture involved merchants or other middlemen supplying fibres to spinners, thread to weavers or cloth to seamstresses and tailors. They worked these materials respectively up into thread, cloth or garments, for which they were paid a set amount. In this system workers initially had some power, because they sold the product of their labour, not their 'labour power' as a commodity. In the case of artisan hand loom weavers in the late eighteenth and early nineteenth centuries, the control of their labour was lost as large scale mechanization cut the time taken to make cloth. As a result, the value of the 'labour power' which went into textile manufacture quickly collapsed, destroying the livelihood of these weavers who could no longer compete by selling the products of their labour and were forced instead to sell their 'labour power' itself, cheaply.

In the case of garments, Marx argued that the need to raise profitability by cutting the time taken to make clothes so as to reduce the value of 'labour power' took a different form. In *Capital Volume One* Marx quotes 'The Children's Employment Commission' (1864), who reported: 'when work passes through several hands, each takes its share of profits [...], so the pay which reaches the workwoman is miserably disproportioned' (1990: 695).

For Phizacklea (1990) the gradual development of the existing system of 'putting out' or dispersed manufacture by a network of home and small-scale producers, meant there was little incentive to innovate technically. There was no need to invest capital on expensive machines as long as a pool of cheapened women's, child, migrant and later global labour, was readily available for exploitation. This is what Marx termed capital's 'reserve army' (1990: 781).

Crucially, it is Marx who explains how and why 'sweating' was and is central to the garment making chain. He argues it has been shaped by the role of 'parasitic middle men' or 'jobbers' (Leopold, 1992), who profit from 'the difference between the price of labour capitalist "manufacturers" paid and the price workers received' (Marx, 1990: 695). Moreover, the 'interposition' of these middlemen as agents encouraged payment by 'piece wages', as they intervened between stores and larger factory based manufacturers and garment workers themselves, either at home or in smaller workshops and factories (Marx, 1990). Though appearing as a continuation of 'putting out', that is, buying the 'product' of these outworkers' labour and not their actual 'labour power', in reality 'piece rates' and their gradual renegotiation by capitalist merchant middlemen or 'jobbers' (Leopold, 1992) forced wage labour into garment production wherever it took place. 'Fixing the rate', or the amount paid for each garment or piece of garment, Marx contended, removed any meaningful control over the labour process by the producer. It ensured 'the quality and intensity of the work which went into [making clothes] was controlled by its very form' of payment (Marx, 1990: 695). 'Piece wages' therefore raised the level of surplus value extracted, further worsening exploitation. Indeed, whilst pay exceeded the average for some workers who worked flat out to make more garments or pieces, they 'lowered average' pay overall (Marx, 1990: 697), since cutting the time taken to make each garment self-defeatingly reduced the value of the 'labour power' embodied therein.

In general terms, then, agents and subcontractors reduced the value of 'labour power' to the barest minimum, because of the pressure to cut garment production times through 'piece wages'. It not only enhanced the profits of these middle men, but also encouraged further 'sub-letting of labour', subcontracting or 'sweating', to produce enough garments to earn a living wage (Marx, 1990). This meant the home or small producer gave out the work to family members, including children, to try and make more garments to compensate for the fall in the value of each. Finally, Marx argued that the size and cheapness of 'fixed' capital – the sewing machine when it finally arrived in the 1850s (Marx, 1990: 603) – encouraged competition between small producers, since the machines were relatively cheap and small enough to be used anywhere. Thus, he pointed to the competition which 'raged in direct proportion to the number and in inverse proportion to the size of rival capitals' or producers (Marx, 1990: 777). Identified by Marx a century and half ago, these exploitative and competitive dynamics meant, and continue to mean, a constant entry into and exit from the market for fashion manufactures (Leopold, 1992). Today, in Bangladesh and other developing countries, small garment making firms continually underbid each other competing for contracts from the agents who subcontract work for large global retailers such as Walmart, Primark, The Gap, H&M and Arcadia, the home of TopShop. Whilst they have lucratively outsourced and minimized all the risks and costs associated with garment manufacture, clothing workers continue to pay the highest price for inflated corporate profits and 'cheap' clothes.

COMMODITY FETISHISM AND FASHION

Before any other writer, Marx argued in *The Manifesto* that capitalism was fast becoming a world system (Marx and Engels, 1998). This meant that the pool of cheapened labour – the 'reserve army' (Marx, 1990: 792) on which it could draw for intensive manufacturing – was eventually a global one, including countries where the cost of labour as SNLT was at its very lowest. The contradiction between the dazzling light, magical images and excitement which characterise fashion's global retail and consumptive space and the benighted side of its global production, intensifies because of the way clothing as commodities are produced for a profit in a competitive world market. At every step in its production, then, fashion exploits the labour of those involved in its complex and mostly opaque supply chain.

For Marx, separating workers from the means of production negatively affected and distorted our 'species being'. This separation, or 'alienation', as he called it (Marx, 1844), created a new and often damaging relationship with the world of things. This is what he called 'commodity fetishism' (Marx, 1990: 163); a belief in the power of objects in themselves, sold to consumers as goods that can change their lives. In this respect, fashion is exemplary once again. Behind all the hopes and dreams invested in fashion and all the symbolic meanings attached to it in film, marketing and celebrity images (Church-Gibson, 2012; Miller, 2011), lies a single unifying condition of possibility: labour, and what happens when control of it is 'alienated' or 'estranged' (Marx, 1844), separated from and lost to us. In *Capital Volume One* Marx writes that 'the wealth of societies in which the capitalist mode of production prevails appears as an immense collection of commodities' (1990: 165). In essence, he argues, this is an immense collection of labour, a series of largely hidden interrelated co-operative creative acts or 'doings'. It is, he continues, 'nothing but the definite social relation between people themselves assuming for them, the fantastic form of a relation between things' (1990: 165). This argument – the core of Marx's theory of 'commodity fetishism' – captures the gap between fashion's appearance as a visual feast, from catwalk to high street, and its essence or origins in, and continued existence through, productive labour. This separation of production from consumption, and producers from the means of production, created capitalism. Capitalism is then a system based on producing commodities for sale at a profit on the market, exchanging 'labour power' for cash wages, and that money in turn for commodities. It thus subsumes the social labour that goes into making fashion, while hiding its wider social and ecological costs to both people and planet. Moreover, for Marx, who above all argued that our creative 'species being' meant we could change ourselves by changing the world, 'commodity fetishism' threatens our sense of our wider power to make and remake history.

When the Italian political economist Galiani argued that 'value is a relation between persons' (Galiani cited in Marx, 1990: 167), Marx added that it is 'a relation concealed beneath a material shell' (1990: 167). Though mostly hidden from us by the fetishistic effects of branding, markets, distance and routine, occasionally the shell of the fashion commodity cracks.

On 24 April 2013 the Rana Plaza garment factory in Dhaka, Bangladesh, collapsed. It made clothes for Primark and other fashion chains. Over 1,100 died and thousands more were injured as the world caught a glimpse of the global CMT army, the 40 million subcontracted workers who produce fast fashion (Siegle, 2013). Fundamentally, then, it is the combination of class exploitation and inter-firm competition within capitalism that accounts for the persistence of sweated labour in fashion manufacture, in both Marx's day and our own. A century earlier, Bessie Gabrilowich's escape from the Triangle Shirtwaist factory inferno in New York in 1911 involved her 'groping her way through the smoke to the street below'. Many of her co-workers 'leapt from windows on the upper stories'. In half an hour 147 were dead (Anon, 2000). One hundred and one years later on 24 November 2012, Shati Akter Shuchona was amongst 1,000 garment workers in the Tazreen

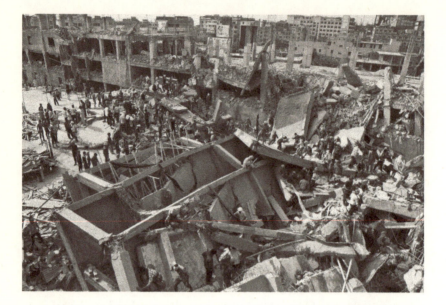

2.1 Photograph of the aftermath of the Rana Plaza garment factory collapse in April 2013. Photograph by: Ismail Ferdous.

Fashions factory near Dhaka, stitching orders for Walmart and C&A. When it suddenly caught fire she was forced to jump from a fourth floor window fleeing a blaze which engulfed a building with no fire certificate, 112 of her colleagues died (Ethirajan, 2013).

CONCLUSION: MARX FASHIONING THE FUTURE

Sixty-five years old at the time of his death in 1883, Marx was laid to rest in Highgate Cemetery in London, his chosen place of political exile since 1849. Though his funeral went unreported in the British press, few would dispute the extent of his influence on twentieth-century history and the world we now live in. Marx's work has inspired workers' struggles and insurrections, such as that of the Bolshevik party in Russia which in 1917 lead the world's first successful workers' revolution, ending both the barbarous tyranny of the Tsars and the pointless butchery of the World War I. Sadly, his work has also been used to justify tyranny and oppression. However, several decades after the revolutions that spread across Eastern Europe and Russia exposed 'actually existing socialism' as a 'state capitalist' sham (Callinicos, 1991), Marx's ideas are today again finding an audience.

Marx's work is re-emerging as a key resource for those who seek an alternative to rapidly deepening global class inequality, exploitation and the threat of environmental catastrophe. His work inspires economists who want to understand the causes of the financial crash of 2008 and the global economic slump that followed it, as well as activists in the global 'Occupy' movement and the revolutionaries of the 'Arab Spring'. As a profoundly ecological thinker, Marx argued that democratic social control of our labour as our 'species being' held the key not just to our emancipation from class society, but also to maintaining what he called our 'metabolism' with nature and to achieving a truly sustainable future (1990: 283). Revisiting Marx's work is relevant for the human species, because we are a species whose wonderful capacity to design and create beauty beyond necessity can be glimpsed in the best of fashion. Such a theoretical investment is surely timely and necessary for fashion scholars, because fashion is 'the child of capitalism'. Rethinking fashion through Marx can only deepen our critical understanding of it.

ACKNOWLEDGEMENTS

With thanks to my colleague in the Department of Cultural and Historical Studies at LCF, Janice Miller, who provided some very useful comments, help and advice with editing previous drafts of this chapter.

REFERENCES

Anon (2000) City life at the Turn of the 20th Century. EyeWitness to History, retrieved from www.eyewitnesstohistory.com on 20 November 2013.

Barthes, R. (1998 [1983]) The Fashion System, M. Ward and R. Howard (trans), London: University of California Press.

Baudrillard, J. (1981) For A Critique of the Political Economy of The Sign, St. Louis, MO: Telos.

———(1988) Selected Writings, London: Polity.

Bourdieu, P. (1984) Distinction: A Social Critique of the Judgment of Taste, Cambridge, MA: Harvard University Press.

Breward, C. (1999) *The Hidden Consumer: Masculinities, Fashion and City Life 1860–1914*, Manchester: Manchester University Press.

Callinicos, A. (1983) *The Revolutionary Ideas of Karl Marx*, London: Bookmarks.

———(1991) *The Revenge of History: Marxism and the Eastern European Revolutions*, Cambridge: Polity.

Church-Gibson, P. (2012) *Fashion and Celebrity Culture*, London: Berg.

Cliff, T. (1988) *State Capitalism in Russia*, London: Bookmarks.

Craik, J. (2009) *Fashion: Key Concepts*, Oxford: Berg.

Edwards, T. (2011) *Fashion in Focus: Concepts, Practices and Politics*, London: Routledge.

Elias, N. (1978) *The Civilizing Process: The History of Manners*, Oxford: Blackwell.

Engels, F. (2009 [1845]) *The Condition of the Working Class in England*, London: Penguin.

Entwistle, J. (2000) *The Fashioned Body: Fashion, Dress and Modern Social Theory*, Cambridge: Polity.

———(2011) *The Aesthetic Economy: Markets and Values in Clothing and Modelling*, Oxford: Berg.

Fine, B. and Leopold, E. (1993) *The World of Consumption*, London: Routledge.

Finkelstein, J. (1991) *The Fashioned Self*, Cambridge: Polity Press.

Gonzalez, M. (2006) *A Rebel's Guide to Marx*, London: Bookmarks.

Hegel, G.W.F. (1975) *Logic, Being Part One of the Encyclopedia of the Philosophical Sciences*, Oxford: Oxford University Press.

Hughes, R. (1991) *The Shock of the New: The Hundred Years of Modern Art, Its Rise, Its Dazzling Achievement, Its Fall*, 2nd edn, New York: McGraw-Hill.

Jarnow, J. and Dickerson, K.G. (1997) *Inside the Fashion Business*, 6th edn, Upper Saddle River, NJ: Prentice-Hall.

Lemire, B. (1997) *Dress, Culture and Commerce: The English Clothing Trade before the Factory*, Basingstoke: Macmillan.

Leopold, E. (1992) 'The Manufacture of the Fashion System' in J. Ash, and E. Wilson (eds), *Chic Thrills: A Fashion Reader*, London: Pandora Press.

Marx, K. (1844) *Economic and Philosophical Manuscripts*, retrieved from https://www.marxists.org/archive/marx/works/1844/manuscripts/labour.htm on 25 November 2013.

———(1963) *Early Writings*, New York: McGraw-Hill.

———(1974) 'Theses on Feuerbach' in *Early Writings*, Harmondsworth: Penguin.

———(1976 [1859]) *Preface to a Contribution to the Critique of Political Economy*, Peking: Foreign Languages Press.

———(1990 [1867]) *Capital Volume One*, London: Penguin.

———(1993 [1857]) *Grundrisse*, London: Penguin.

Marx, K. and Engels, F. (1973) *Selected Works*, Moscow: Foreign Languages Publishing House.

———(1975 [1845]) *The German Ideology*, London: Lawrence and Wishart.

———(1998 [1848]) *The Communist Manifesto*, London: Verso.

Miller, J. (2011) *Fashion and Music*, London: Berg.

Molyneux, J. (2012) *The Point Is to Change It! An Introduction to Marxist Philosophy*, London: Bookmarks.

Phizacklea, A. (1990) *Unpacking the Fashion Industry: Gender, Racism, and Class in Production*, London: Routledge.

Rouse, E. (1989) *Understanding Fashion*, London: BSP Professional Books.

Sahlins, M. (1976) *Culture and Practical Reason*, Chicago: University of Chicago Press.

Siegle, L. (2013) 'Fashion Still Doesn't Give a Damn about the Deaths of Garment Workers' in the *Observer*, Sunday 5 May.

Simmel, G. (1971 [1904]) 'Fashion' in *International Quarterly*, 10: 130–55.

Slater, D. (1997) *Consumer Culture and Modernity*, Cambridge: Polity.

Stallybrass, P. (1998) 'Marx's Coat' in P. Spyer (ed.), *Border Fetishisms: Material Objects in Unstable Spaces*, New York: Routledge.

Tarrant, N. (1994) *The Development of Costume*, London: Routledge.

Veblen, T. (1899) *The Theory of the Leisure Class: An Economic Study of Institutions*, New York: Macmillan.

Wilson, E. (2003 [1985]) *Adorned in Dreams: Fashion and Modernity*, London: I.B. Tauris.

3

SIGMUND FREUD
More than a Fetish: Fashion and Psychoanalysis

Janice Miller

INTRODUCTION

There are few people, in the West at least, who know nothing at all about Sigmund Freud and his ideas, if only in their most synthesised, sensationalized and sometimes distorted form. Freud was born in 1856 in the town of Příbor, now part of the Czech Republic, but then the Austrian Empire, to Jewish parents. He died in London in 1939 at the age of 83, having fled Vienna, where he spent much of his life, when Austria came under the control of the anti-Semitic regime of Nazi Germany. Freud labelled himself 'a Godless Jew' (Simmons, 2006: 111; see also Gay, 1987) and yet his Jewishness would have been fundamental to how he was treated 'in what was a violently anti-Semitic world' (Simmons, 2006: 111) long before the rise of Nazism. Freud qualified as a doctor in Vienna in 1881 and began his private practice in 1886 where he used hypnosis and later 'talk therapy' to treat the symptoms of mental illness. By the late 1890s he had named this technique psychoanalysis.

This chapter will explore various ways that Freudian concepts and ideas have been used to examine and understand fashion, its related imagery and mediation. It argues that whilst useful examples exist, psychoanalysis has been under-estimated as a framework with which to study of fashion. The chapter argues that psychoanalysis should be seen as a means to refresh and complement the theoretical frameworks more commonly used in fashion studies which have tended to rely on more sociological approaches, since there is much that psychoanalysis can reveal about fashion's role in cultural life.

FREUD AND SEXUALITY: PAST AND PRESENT

Freud was a prolific writer of books, articles and letters, some of which were only published after his death. His work looked at a variety of facets of human development and activity. Questions of sexuality and sexual development were important to Freud's work and it is these aspects that have endured the most in the popular imagination. In the period in which Freud was working, sexuality was subject to a variety of prohibitions – particularly for women – and he saw this cultural repression of sexuality as the root cause of many of the neurotic symptoms suffered by his female patients. Despite the sexual revolution of the 1960s, which has arguably allowed for greater sexual expression for both genders, it would seem our interest in such possibilities has not abated. Instead, sexuality remains the focus of excessive amounts of attention, both positive and negative. Indeed as a result of the sexual revolution, in many cultural contexts, individuals are under no less pressure than Freud's patients, but they are now expected to both vehemently express their sexuality in some aspects of their life and to deny it just as vehemently in others. Thus, a system of thought that looks not only at sexuality's fundamental role in constituting the human condition, but also at the ways in which, for various reasons, a culture or an individual might be shaped by the imperative to manage it, continues to have relevance. In turn, this Freudian preoccupation with sexuality suggests a synergy between it and fashion since, as Davis argues, clothing has a 'preoccupation with matters of sexual availability and erotic taste' (1994: 81).

Thanks to this continuing fascination with Freud's work, in popular culture he often features as the archetype of the therapist. Phrases like 'paging Doctor Freud' have become an oft repeated joke in response to any declaration or behaviour that is understood to reveal a less than normative relationship to one's sexuality, one's culture, or even one's own mother. The Freudian slip, where the wrong word inserted into a phrase in the place of another reveals hidden thoughts and feelings, or the notion of the phallic symbol as a description that can be attached to any object that remotely resembles the penis, are just some of the Freudian ideas that have increasingly become part of common parlance. They give away many of the most important tenets of his work, because they are often responses to what culture construes as healthy and unhealthy beliefs, attitudes and desires. Moreover, they suggest that we sometimes hold or reveal attitudes we would prefer to hide or that we may even be unaware of ourselves. Such examples show how common it has become for individuals to recognize the possibility that human beings might be shaped by inner psychical conflicts. This is the central hypothesis of psychoanalysis and its legacy.

THE UNCONSCIOUS

The possibility that human beings might be shaped by inner psychical conflicts, often, but not exclusively in relation to sexuality, is the central hypothesis of psychoanalysis. For Freud inner conflicts resulted in neurotic behaviour. This was brought about by the tensions between the things expected of us, the things that we are conscious of, and the things about ourselves that we or our culture deem so unacceptable or frightening that they must be pushed away or repressed and made unconscious. The concept of the unconscious is fundamental to all of Freud's work. As Rieff writes:

> The unconscious contains not simply what is not conscious or that of which we are at the moment unaware, it contains [...] our forgotten origins. Yet to forget them is not to abolish them. On the contrary, to forget an event or motive is to conserve and even augment its importance.
>
> (1959: 37)

Therefore, Freud understood the unconscious to be a repository of all of the unacceptable feelings, thoughts and urges that because they are unsettling or disturbing, must be hidden away or 'repressed'. He located much of this unsettling information in the early developmental stages of childhood, believing that the conflicts that arose in his 'neurotic' patients came about because of some interruption or stasis of their 'libidinal development'. Throughout his career Freud used many terms to define the different areas of the psyche that could find themselves in conflict. In his later work, for example, he moves away from the use of the terms conscious/unconscious and instead labels the different aspects of the psyche as ego, superego and id. Whatever the language, for Freud neurotic symptoms result when some aspect of the self is overcome by the demands or desires of other aspects and/or when something in the external world brings these aspects of the psyche into a conflict which it fails to properly bring into balance and thus resolve. This perceived struggle between the conscious and unconscious aspects of the individual are fundamental to an understanding of Freud's work.

FREUD ON FASHION

Gay argues 'we all speak Freud whether we know it or not' (1995: xiii). As psychoanalytical principles have clearly become so embedded in the way human psychology is talked about in everyday terms, the key question for this chapter is: did Freud speak fashion? He certainly understood clothing as having a symbolic quality in the experiences of some of his patients. He records his analysis of the dreams of an agoraphobic woman, which feature a hat whose side pieces hang unevenly. He suggests to his patient that this hat signifies the male genitalia. His patient initially resists this interpretation but later seems to confirm it when she asks him 'why it was that one of her husband's testicles was lower than the other, and whether it was the same in all men' (Freud, 1913: 250). For Freud, this particular garment could in some dream contexts connote not only the male genitalia but also the female. It was not the only garment that he felt might symbolize in this way, believing also that 'in dreams of men one often finds the cravat as a symbol for the penis' (Freud, 1913: 247).

What these examples demonstrate is that Freud sometimes tells us something about clothing, but not about fashion if we accept Elizabeth Wilson's definition of it as dress 'in which the key feature is rapid and continual changing of styles' (Wilson, 2005: 3). Though Freud clearly recognizes the potential for garments to symbolise because of their close relationship to the human body, he does not see them as a fluid signifier of social identity as later studies of fashion would (see for example Entwistle, 2000; Wilson, 2005; Kaiser, 2012). References to garments like the cravat, which were once universal and now much less so, act here to root much of this imagery in the aesthetics of the era in which Freud was working. This tells us little about the part that fashionable mores might play in shaping this imagery or how such imagery might change in relation to these mores. It also leaves open the question of what recognising fashion's link to identity might have further revealed about the psyche of Freud's patients, either individually or collectively.

This is a question that the psychoanalyst J.C. Flügel takes up in a little more detail in his 1930 book *The Psychology of Clothes*. It seems that Freud, like many Victorian men, might have felt that fashion had little to do with him and yet he seemed to understand the power of fashion to demarcate the individual: he always dressed in a style befitting the conventional, respectable Victorian man, in 'a well-fitting suit of fine quality, always with a black tie' (Costigan, 1967: 101).

In dressing thus, Freud embodies one of the key ideas offered by Flügel's work – the notion of the 'Great Masculine Renunciation' of the nineteenth century – when, Flügel argued, men turned to sober, restrained and respectable dress and away from decorative and ostentatious display. In making such sartorial statements, men arguably imprinted on their bodies the values of hegemonic Victorian masculinity by disavowing their bodies as a site for the construction and expression of identity or for decoration. Instead, this uniformity of masculine dress served to eschew the body and emphasize the mind and character as at the heart of healthy, 'normal' masculinity. Freudian psychoanalysis itself has been charged in similar vein with privileging the mind over the body. As Joyce McDougall argues: 'Since its inception, psychoanalysis, following Freud, has privileged the role of language in the structuring of the psyche and in psychoanalytic treatment. But not all communication uses language.' (1989: 11). The relationship between language and human experience is a common analytical point for both psychoanalysis and fashion studies and yet the two have been only rarely united in any form of analysis. Flügel is important for this chapter because he was one of the first and few to bring Freud's ideas to bear on the analysis of fashion. In doing so, he offered up the hypothesis that there are three driving factors behind the human activity of dressing: bodily protection, modesty and decoration.

In particular, Flügel set his psychoanalytic sights on the tension between the desire to decorate the body, which, he argues, is driven by an infantile, narcissistic self-regard that wishes to show off the body, and the modesty demanded by a culture which regularly frustrates such desires. The contradictions and confusions that must result from these often un-reconcilable demands creates fashion, since it constantly reformulates the body in line with or as a challenge to notions of decency and modesty in any given period – exposing certain parts of the body to view whilst hiding others. The problem that many later writers have identified with such an approach is that it fails to take full account of the socio-economic factors that impinge upon the individual. As Fred Davis writes:

This is not to say that Flügel is unaware of or indifferent to clothing's sociocultural contexts [...], still his theoretical commitments [...] are clearly towards conceiving of an ambivalence driven fashion in terms of psychically occasioned instabilities rather than culturally derived and symbolically negotiated identity disjunctions.

(1994: 84)

Consequently clothing is, for Flügel, the material manifestation of the internal psychical conflicts that are the object of study for all psychoanalysis.

CASTRATION THEORY

Arguably one of Freud's most examined propositions to focus on the conflicts that he believed shaped the human subject is what has variously come to be labelled as 'castration theory' or 'castration anxiety'. This conflict in particular has proved useful to those examining fashion. Castration anxiety is indelibly tied to the notion of the 'Oedipal complex', where Freud invokes Greek mythology and the story of Oedipus, who unwittingly killed his father and married his mother. The story is used to illustrate Freud's contention that young boys' identification with their father is driven by a desire for their mother and feelings of jealousy and animosity towards the father, whom they see as a rival for their mother's affections. These feelings of jealousy trouble the child and must be repressed and sublimated. Further, the young boy fears that his father will recognize his animosity and retaliate, and that this retaliation will take the form of castration, a possibility instigated by the boy's belief that since his mother lacks a penis, she must have suffered this fate. Such ideas have been criticised for their emphasis on the male phallus as central to the construction of all human subjectivity by feminists (see for example Irigaray, 1985a, 1985b; Silverman, 1988; Braidotti, 1994; Brennan, 2002), who argued that Freud did not allow for female desire or subjectivity in his work. The theory of the Oedipus complex has also been criticised for its inability to account for anything other than a conventional, Western nuclear family (see Spivak, 1998). However, as Anthony Storr writes:

> To allege that all small boys fear castration at the hands of their fathers sounds ridiculous when taken literally. But, if we were to phrase it differently, and affirm that small boys are greatly concerned with establishing their identity as male persons, feel rivalry with their fathers, and are easily made to feel humiliated or threatened by disparaging remarks about their size, weakness, incapacity and lack of experience, most people would concur.
>
> (2001: 34)

The mechanisms via which young boys might sublimate some of this information have indeed proved useful to the study of fashion. In his 1927 essay on fetishism, Freud sees certain objects as acting as a substitution for the penis, which is believed by the young boy to have been removed from his mother. Fetishism acts as an unconscious and symbolic resolution to this fear of castration and becomes 'a token of triumph [...] and a protection against it' (Freud, 1961: 154). The fetish object is thus a way to attempt to represent or make material the lost or fantasy penis of the mother, a mechanism by which:

> Freud believes that the little boy, who becomes a fetishist, recreates the mother as phallic because the horror of imagining her 'castrated' is too great. The little boy disavows the mother as castrated and uses the fetish to fixate on the moment before the horrifying revelation.
>
> (Taylor, 2003: 81)

Fashion and clothing have been drawn into the discussion of fetishism in two ways. First, since clothes are made of fabric, the contention that 'numerous men could only achieve sexual gratification via a specific material object [...] such as fur or velvet' (Mirzoeff, 1999: 157) naturally leads us to think about clothing. Second, there is a natural synergy between clothing and fetishism in Freud's own account, since 'many of the fetish objects are shoes, boots, feet, velvet or pieces of fur because more often than not, the revelation occurred when the little boy was peering up [women's] skirts' (Taylor, 2003: 81).

FASHION AND FETISHISM

Valerie Steele explored the relationship between fetishism and fashion in her 1996 book *Fetish: Fashion, Sex and Power*. Steele's work expands on the connections between clothing and fetishism proposed by Freud's work. She is interested not only in the connection between fashion and sexuality, but also the increasingly fetishistic nature of mainstream fashion. In her analysis she understands fetish garments as something not only to be looked at and engaged with at a distance, but also inhabited and worn. She takes up the notion of the 'phallic woman', who, she argues, can be constituted via many of fashion's most fetishistic objects and symbols from shoes with excessively high, sharp heels to textures and fabrics like leather and fur. The 'phallic woman' is understood by Barbara Creed as a woman who 'either has a phallus or phallic attribute or she herself has retained the male's phallus inside herself' (1993: 153). Steele's phallic woman is one who uses fashion to embody a kind of power that might be understood to threaten conventional masculinity by in turn signifying masculinity through fashion and in relation to the female body. Steele gives the example that women in uniform denote institutional power and can thus be understood as fetish objects. She reminds us of what Freud also recognized, namely that parts of a body, the body itself and thus a person can be a fetishist object too. Since the writing on fashion and popular culture has so keenly adopted the language of fetishism it is important to remember that a true, clinical fetishist would derive pleasure only and purely from the object and 'would probably prefer to remain at home polishing his shoes [rather] than go to the cinema and see Dietrich's black-laced high-heeled wonders' (Weiss, 1994: 5). Such perspectives also act as a reminder that fashion's interpretation of fetishism usually employs symbolism that is a great deal more glamorous than the more mundane examples often found in Freud's work. Importantly then, Steele's work is illustrative of how the initial psychoanalytic definitions of fetishism have been taken up in more ambiguous and fluid ways in cultural analysis. She is interested as much in how a person might choose to embody fetishism as a source of power – particularly women – and fashion's fundamental role in this, as in how objects themselves might be fetishistic. But Freud's work has not only provided a rich conceptual framework with which to understand fetishistic objects in fashion. It has also had significant influence on our understanding of the practices of looking that are so central to our understanding of the role of images in the fashioning of the body.

THE GAZE

It is clear from Freud's own account that it is through looking that the fetishist is formed, and the fundamental role that the visual plays in so many aspects of psychoanalysis goes some way to explain how it moved out of the medical setting of the therapist's office and into the discourses of cultural analysis. As Elliot and Turner argue, Freud's work is entirely concerned with the creative work of the human mind and imagination and yet 'the irony is that while Freud devoted his life to uncovering the creative pathways of the unconscious imagination ... he equally set his face against recognizing the role of the imaginary order in society as such' (2012: 117). It was instead Jacques Lacan who in the twentieth century argued for a return to Freud and in doing so transformed psychoanalytical ideas into a system 'designed for cultural analysis not for use in therapeutic practice' (Mirzoeff, 2009: 169). Like Freud, Lacan (2001) focuses on looking, seeing it as fundamental to the process by which a sense of self or 'subjectivity' is formed – Lacan's notion of the mirror stage describes the moment when the human subject, as a child about six months old, recognises him or herself in the mirror and in doing so also sees a perfected version of him or herself with which the child identifies and yet feels alienated from. For Lacan, the image in the mirror is the child idealized.

Writers on film have, in particular, been interested in the potential of Freudian and Lacanian ideas of looking to explain the relationship between the audience and the image projected on screen. It was Laura Mulvey who in 1975 used the Lacanian concept of the gaze to argue that looking possesses two functions in relation to cinema. First, it produces pleasure when the individual on screen acts as an object of desire – is objectified – functioning as an image which invites us to immerse ourselves in the delights of looking. Second, it plays a fundamental role in identification and thus the formation of identity, echoing the Lacanian mirror stage. Thus Mulvey's work on cinema illustrates how:

> In Lacan's reconceptualization of Freudian analysis, looking has become the gaze [...]. The gaze is not just a look or a glance. It is a means of constituting the identity of the gazer by distinguishing her or him from that which is gazed at. At the same time, the gaze makes us aware that we may be looked at, so that this awareness becomes part of identity itself.
>
> (Mirzoeff, 2009: 171)

As early as 1972, the writer John Berger was making connections between images and the position of women in wider culture and in doing so united the psychoanalytic concept of the gaze with the analysis of gender identities in culture. Berger recognised that across historical European paintings and into the contemporary advertising images of the time he was writing, there existed conventions of representation that objectified women by making them passive objects to be looked at. In such images, women are not shown to be living, breathing or thinking individuals. Nor are they shown to be a complex and diverse group. Instead, they are stereotyped. As we have already seen, the gaze has been argued to be a means of constituting identity and for Berger the core concern is that in terms of these representations and stereotypes women have historically wielded little of the representative power. Thus, how women are shown has been largely out of their hands and has come also to be how they are valued and how they understand their own value. As a result images of women, whatever their form and wherever they are found, have the potential to shape the expectations not only of women as a social group, but also of women of themselves because, Berger argues, this gaze is inherently male and so all encompassing that we are all encouraged to take up this position no matter what our gender.

Concepts of the gaze have been applied to fashion to critique the ways in which it represents the body in imagery and media of all kinds. Leslie Rabine charges fashion images with circulating limited and oppressive images of women, arguing that:

> Associated with the eye of the camera in the domain of film, the gaze functions in the domain of fashion as a framing device of the photograph that invests it with desire and provides the erotic charge in which the image is bathed for the female spectator. Whatever the gender of the gaze in feminist photography or film, in the photography of the Anglo-American fashion magazine it is, with extraordinary exceptions, emphatically male and constitutes its object as heterosexual female. Outside that look, the woman of fashion would not exist.
>
> (1994: 65)

Anneke Smelik (2009) is interested in how bodies on screen reflect and inform the fashionable and often difficult to attain idealized bodies against which the audience measures their own. Her work reminds us of the important point that the body itself is as subject to fashionable change as the clothing that often covers it. For Smelik the contemporary gaze is more neutrally distributed across both genders but it is no less pervasive. As she argues: 'the voyeuristic gaze has been internalized in impossible norms for a thin and yet strong and well-formed body' (Smelik, 2009: 183).

Theories of the gendered gaze have been extended to think of it as homospectorial (see Fuss, 1992) or female (see Gamman and Marshment, 1989). Whilst fashion imagery has often been a space for questioning gender conventions, there is still clear evidence that in much fashion-related imagery women are often (though not always) posed in quite conventional ways. It is also true that men have begun to be similarly objectified at times – see for example the Armani advert featuring David Beckham from 2009. However it is gendered, the psychoanalytic concept of the gaze has proved invaluable to those trying to help us understand how our sense of self and our bodies might be fashioned and refashioned through a process of looking and identification.

GENDER AND THE MASQUERADE

'Fashion is obsessed with gender', writes Elizabeth Wilson, who sees it as fundamental to the way that gender boundaries are maintained and 'redefined' (2005: 117). It has perhaps become clear that much psychoanalytic theory, whether Freudian or Lacanian, is similarly concerned with gender identity. Wilson's statement reflects the now commonly held belief that gender is a construction rather than an unchangeable essence rooted in nature. Freud was much less sure about this, seeing diversions from the fixed binary of masculine/feminine gender identity as evidence of psychic disturbance. Later writers like Judith Butler (1990; see also chapter 17 in this book) have broken apart this sex/gender distinction in order to resist the historical tendency to pathologize any sexual orientation or gender identity that did not fit within the very limited cultural definitions of 'appropriate' behaviour. But as early as 1929 the psychoanalyst Joan Riviere (2011) resisted Freud's tendency to see masculine or feminine behaviours as natural and normal for men and for women respectively, and instead viewed femininity as a 'reaction formation' (see for example McPherson, 2003). In Freudian psychoanalysis reaction formations are defence mechanisms used by individuals to deal with psychical conflict, to maintain a coherent sense of self and to alleviate the anxieties that result from such conflicts. Some are deemed healthier than others. When faced with difficulty we might employ denial and attempt to push a problem away. When we have upset someone we might 'project' our feelings and accuse them of upsetting us instead. Repression itself is a reaction formation. Reaction formations can often be identified because of their excessiveness. For Riviere femininity was employed by one of her female patients to placate the men in her workplace when she felt she had been too strident. Riviere saw femininity as a masquerade in this context, as a kind of camouflage which the woman uses to hide her masculine traits and to adhere instead to the feminine qualities that culture expects from a woman. This allows the woman to compensate or perhaps more accurately *over*-compensate for the fact that by adopting masculine traits she had symbolically 'castrated' her male colleagues. Consequently, using a psychoanalytic framework, Riviere argues that femininity might offer a means for women to compensate for their 'lack' and the anxieties that this might provoke. She also suggests that femininity may not be natural for a woman at all. Consequently, Riviere's work has been compelling for studies of fashion and embodiment (see for example Biddle-Perry and Miller, 2009; Garber, 2012; Miller, 2013;

Tseëlon, 1995), acting as means to explain why fashion has been integral to the lives of women and why it has on many occasions been charged with oppressing them.

PSYCHOANALYSIS AND FASHION

The possibility that fashion might oppress women has been much debated, whether it is the concerns for physical health raised in relation to garments like the corset (see for example Summers, 2001) or others, that, as we have already seen, focus instead on fashion images and use theories of the gaze to think about how such images might place limitations on the groups they also represent. In more contemporary terms writers have grappled with the possibility that fashion might offer women a space of expression. Alison Bancroft (2012) uses Lacanian psychoanalysis to present a more positive reading of fashion as a space of resistance for women. She argues that fashion is a unique cultural product which is always situated within the feminine sphere. She uses the fashion photographer Nick Knight's work to argue that viewing fashion photography as conventional or even malicious in its representations of women is overly simplistic. Instead, Bancroft finds a synergy between Knight's work and surrealist art, arguing that:

> Surrealism's interrogation of the object, its positioning of photography at the boundary between language and the unconscious and most importantly, its demand that the artist represents what is experienced as much as what is seen, all contribute to the location of fashion photography as a representation of the processes of subjectivity.
>
> (2012: 43)

She argues that Lacanian psychoanalysis can help us to see that fashion photography has transgressive potential. Lacan suggested that the human psyche has three aspects to it: the real, the imaginary and the symbolic (see for example Bowie, 1993). It is Lacan's symbolic order that is the most important for Bancroft's analysis of fashion imagery, since the symbolic determines the subject as a part of culture – it is here that the ideological rules and conventions are established. Bancroft argues that Knight's fashion photography fails to adhere to the conventions of representation. Therefore, she argues, it should be seen as resistance and thus in a more positive light in relation to the representation of women.

Bancroft sees not only fashion photography but also haute couture on such terms. She is also interested in how the work of some designers (in particular Alexander McQueen) can present challenging representations of feminine identity that should not be read as oppressive but instead as a form of resistance to the conventions of gender identity, this time in relation to the fashioned body itself. In doing so she invokes the Lacanian notion of 'jouissance', defined by Lacan and later feminist thinkers such as Hélène Cixous (see for example Ives, 2013) as a form of sexual rapture, but one that can, in its excessiveness, be troubling. It is this reading that Bancroft gives to haute couture, arguing that like some fashion photography, it too can create a space for alternative and transgressive versions of femininity. Thus, Bancroft uses psychoanalysis to critique more negative readings of women's relationship to fashion, seeing it as a uniquely female oriented cultural space that we should not be too quick to dismiss as oppressive and devoid of more complex representations of feminine identity.

THE LIMITATIONS OF PSYCHOANALYSIS

Whilst Bancroft's work offers new possibilities for fashion theory and the arguments made in relation to her case studies are compelling, how well they can be applied to the wider field of fashion is less certain. She makes insightful points in relation to haute couture, but fashion is complex both in terms of its imagery and its marketplace and whether psychoanalysis can help us to understand more 'everyday' fashion is yet to be explored. But this is worth exploring, since, as Gillian Rose (2001) reminds us, psychoanalysis itself encompasses a range of ideas which can be used to explore images and objects. As Rose writes, 'Different psychoanalytic concepts brought to bear on the same image' (or other cultural object/artefact) 'can produce very different interpretations of that image' (2001: 150). Psychoanalysis offers many possible ways to think about the significance of images and objects in culture and its relevance to understanding fashion deserves greater exploration.

However, many (see Rose, 2001; Pollock, 2003) have also identified the significant limitations of psychoanalysis as a methodology. These limitations are partly seen to be rooted in the emphasis on sexuality that is so fundamental to the discipline. This has left little room to consider other issues in relation to human subjectivity – race and class for example – within a psychoanalytic framework. This has encouraged those undertaking cultural analysis to turn instead to theorists like Karl Marx and Michel Foucault (see chapters 2 and 11). However, Griselda Pollock has convincingly argued the case for psychoanalysis to be better applied to the study of art and art history, and though psychoanalysis has been critiqued as a mode of cultural analysis because of its inability to take into account the lived experience of those making and consuming cultural products (Rose, 2001), Pollock argues that art is 'not either social or psychic, public or private, historical or semiotic' (2003: xxxvii). Such arguments are equally legitimate in relation to any cultural product, including fashion, which deserves greater exploration on such terms.

CONCLUSION

This chapter has presented some of the ways that writers have used psychoanalytic concepts to understand aspects of fashion and dress. It has hopefully made clear that fashion studies has tended to both turn to and shy away from psychoanalytic frameworks as ways to understand fashion in equal measure. As a result, concepts like fetishism have been embraced, but other aspects of psychoanalytic theory have often proved too individualistic and consequently too much at odds with the socio-cultural readings of fashion which dominate fashion theory. In recent years it has tended to focus a great deal more on the experience of consumers, on the processes of production and on a more 'democratic' idea of fashion diffusion. Bancroft encourages us to return to haute couture fashion and makes a compelling argument for it to be understood as a creative practice rather than merely an economic commodity.

Bancroft's work certainly reminds us that psychoanalysis has much to offer fashion theory and that it has potential to refresh the frameworks that currently tend to circulate within it. Whilst she uses Lacan as the framework for her analysis of fashion, Movahedi and Homayounpour (2013) return to Freud to analyse the Iranian garment the chador. They move beyond Freud's work on sexuality and focus instead on what he perceived as the role of repetition to play out and overcome painful experiences in his work *Beyond the Pleasure Principle* (2003), originally published in 1922. Here Freud focuses on what he sees as his 18-month-old grandson Ernst's attempts to symbolically master the upsetting emotional experience of a parent going away from him by playing a game in which he throws away and then pulls back a cotton reel on a string. Using such concepts, Movahedi and Homayounpour see the relationship between the Iranian garment the chador, the women who wear it and the patriarchal culture that encourages it as embodying a kind of ideologically driven but psychical struggle in their choice to wear or reject a garment that might be understood to oppress themselves and their gender. In their work the chador acts as a second skin that represents the 'lost' body of the mother and it is through the covering and uncovering of the female body that gender identities are constituted and maintained as the woman wearing the chador identifies with the mother and the man is separated from her. In his game of sending away and retrieving Ernst was, in Freud's terms, enacting his unconscious wishes through play. In their novel use of Freudian concepts to analyse traditional forms of dress Movahedi and Homayounpour's work makes some important suggestions for how this approach could be expanded on by those analysing contemporary fashion. There is certainly more that psychoanalysis can say about fashion as object and as image, not least because the writers discussed in this chapter raise as many interesting questions about the possible applications of psychoanalysis to fashion as they answer. After all, if the unconscious reveals itself through play, and fashion like all areas of human activity can be argued to be a form of play (albeit 'necessary play', see for example Bonelli, 2013: 163) then the possibility that psychoanalysis might have more to offer in the study of fashion than current writing suggests, is a compelling one.

REFERENCES

Bancroft, A. (2012) *Fashion and Psychoanalysis: Styling the Self*, London: I.B. Tauris.

Berger, J. (1972) *Ways of Seeing*, London: Penguin.

Biddle-Perry, G. and Miller, J. (2009) '… And If Looks Could Kill: Making Up the Face of Evil' in C. Balmain and L. Drawmer (eds), *Something Wicked This Way Comes: Essays on Evil and Human Wickedness*, New York: Rodopi.

Bonelli, R.M. (2013) *Fashion, Lifestyle and Psychiatry*, London: Bloomsbury.

Bowie, M. (1993) *Lacan*, Cambridge, MA: Harvard University Press.

Braidotti, R. (1994) *Nomadic Subjects: Embodiment and Sexual Difference in Contemporary Feminist Theory*, New York: Columbia University Press.

Brennan, T. (2002) *Between Feminism and Psychoanalysis*, London: Routledge.

Butler, J. (1990) *Gender Trouble: Feminism and the Subversion of Identity*, London: Taylor and Francis.

Costigan, G. (1967) *Sigmund Freud: A Short Biography*, London: Robert Hale.

Creed, B. (1993) *The Monstrous-Feminine: Film, Feminism, Psychoanalysis*, New York: Routledge.

Davis, F. (1994) *Fashion, Culture and Identity*, Chicago: University of Chicago Press.

Elliot, A. and Turner, B.S. (2012) *On Society*, Cambridge: Polity Press.

Entwistle, J. (2000) *The Fashioned Body: Fashion, Dress and Modern Social Theory*, Cambridge: Polity Press.

Flügel, J.C. (1930) *The Psychology of Clothes*, London: Woolf.

Freud, S. (1913) *The Interpretation of Dreams*, A.A. Brill (trans), New York: MacMillan.

————(1961) 'Fetishism' in J. Strachey (ed.), *The Standard Edition of the Complete Works of Sigmund Freud*, Vol. 21, London: Hogarth Press.

————(2003) *Beyond the Pleasure Principle*, London: Routledge.

Fuss, D. (1992) 'Fashion and the Homospectorial Look' in *Critical Inquiry*, 18: 713–737.

Gamman, L. and Marshment, M. (1989) *The Female Gaze: Women as Viewers of Popular Culture*, Seattle: Real Comet Press.

Garber, M. (2012) *Vested Interests: Cross Dressing and Cultural Anxiety*, New York: Routledge.

Gay, P. (1987) *A Godless Jew: Freud, Atheism and the Making of Psychoanalysis*, New Haven, CT: Yale University Press.

————(ed.) (1995) *The Freud Reader*, London: Vintage.

Irigaray, L. (1985a) *Speculum of the Other Woman*, New York: Cornell University Press.

————(1985b) *This Sex Which Is Not One*, New York: Cornell University Press.

Ives, K. (2013) *Cixous, Irigaray, Kristeva: The Jouissance of French Feminism*, Maidstone: Crescent Moon Publishing.

Kaiser, S. (2012) *Fashion and Cultural Studies*, London: Bloomsbury.

Lacan, J. (2001) *Ecrits: A Selection*, London: Routledge.

McDougall, J. (1989) *Theaters of the Body: A Psychoanalytic Approach to Psychosomatic Illness*, New York: Norton.

McPherson, T. (2003) *Reconstructing Dixie: Race, Gender and Nostalgia in the Imagined South*, Durham, NC: Duke University Press.

Miller, J. (2013) 'Heroes and Villains: When Men Wear Makeup' in S. Bruzzi and P. Church Gibson (eds), *Fashion Cultures Revisited: Theories, Explorations and Analysis*, Oxford: Routledge.

Mirzoeff, N. (1999) *An Introduction to Visual Culture*, London: Routledge.

————(2009) *An Introduction to Visual Culture*, 2nd edn, London: Routledge.

Movahedi, S. and Homayounpour, G. (2013) 'Fort!/Da! Through the Chador: The Paradox of the Woman's Invisibility and Visibility' in W. Muller-Funk, I. Scholz-Strasser and H. Westerink (eds), *Psychoanalysis, Monotheism and Morality*, Leuven: Leuven University Press.

Mulvey, L. (1975) 'Visual Pleasure and Narrative Cinema' in *Screen*, 16 (3): 6–18.

Pollock, G. (2003) *Vision and Difference: Feminism, Femininity and the Histories of Art*, Oxford: Routledge.

Rabine, L.W. (1994) 'A Woman's Two Bodies: Fashion Magazines, Consumerism and Feminism' in S. Benstock and S. Ferriss (eds), *On Fashion*, New Brunswick, NJ: Rutgers University Press.

Rieff, P. (1959) *Freud: The Mind of the Moralist*, Chicago: University of Chicago Press.

Riviere, J. (2011) 'Womanliness as Masquerade' in A. Hughes (ed.), *The Inner World and Joan Riviere: Collected Papers, 1929–1958*, London: Karnac.

Rose, G. (2001) *Visual Methodologies: An Introduction to the Interpretation of Visual Materials*, London: Sage.

Silverman, K. (1988) *The Acoustic Mirror: The Female Voice in Psychoanalysis and Cinema*, Bloomington: Indiana University Press.

Simmons, L. (2006) *Freud's Italian Journey*, New York: Rodopi.

Smelik, A. (2009) 'Lara Croft, Kill Bill and Feminist Film Studies' in R. Buikema and I. van der Tuin (eds), *Doing Gender in Media, Art and Culture*, London: Routledge.

Spivak, G. (1998) *In Other Worlds: Essays in Cultural Politics*, Abingdon: Routledge.

Steele, V. (1996) *Fetish: Fashion, Sex and Power*, Oxford: Oxford University Press.

Storr, A. (2001) *Freud: A Very Short Introduction*, Oxford: Oxford University Press.

Summers, L. (2001) *Bound to Please: A History of the Victorian Corset*, Oxford: Berg.

Taylor, C.L. (2003) *Women, Writing and Fetishism, 1890–1950: Female Cross-gendering*, Oxford: Clarendon Press.

Tseëlon, E. (1995) *The Masque of Femininity*, London: Sage.

Weiss, A.S. (1994) *Perverse Desire and the Ambiguous Icon*, Albany, NY: SUNY Press.

Wilson, E. (2005) *Adorned in Dreams: Fashion and Modernity*, London: I.B. Tauris.

4

GEORG SIMMEL
The 'Philosophical Monet'

Peter McNeil

The impressionist philosopher Simmel, who must have known it to be true, once said that there are only fifteen people in the world but these fifteen move about so quickly that we believe there to be many more.

(Bloch cited in Frisby, 1981: 33)

INTRODUCTION

A small clique, always on the move, in the know, creating its own aestheticized existence; sounds like 'fashion'? Yet, this chapter concerns one of the great influences on the development of the sociological interpretation of fashion, Georg Simmel.

Simmel (1858–1918) witnessed the development of modern culture. He lived most of his life in Berlin as a Christianized Jew (someone who probably hasn't converted, but has adopted ways of behaviour and dress characteristic of non-Jews) within an upper-middle class family. He was taken under the wing of a wealthier relative and therefore had a privileged upbringing. Simmel was indelibly formed by his maturing in one of the great *fin-de-siècle* European cities. As one of his pupils from 1910, Albert Salomon (1995: 363) noted in a lecture given in New York in 1963, Simmel 'was and remained the product of a metropolitan civilization, overwhelming through a variety of sensual, intellectual, technological, poetical and artistic impressions'. It was Simmel's attempt to understand the human condition as formed within a modern metropolis of innumerable stimuli that enabled him to generate his particular theory of the intersection of city life and modern fashion, and to influence subsequent thinkers, including Walter Benjamin (see also chapter 5). Although dress fashions were not the main topic of his many enquiries, Simmel's approach to social forms played a major role in creating a model for understanding fashion that has been particularly influential in the United States of America since the 1910s, being revived in the 1950s and again in the 1980s, and continuing to resonate within many different strands of international fashion studies today (see Milà, 2005: 14). Simmel's analysis of the endless differentiation of objects and details in his contemporary society laid a bedrock for later theorists of everyday life, including Roland Barthes. He also influenced the development of North American 'sociology of everyday life', or 'ethnomethodological' sociology and social psychology (Levine et al., 1976: 829). Simmel's approach to fashion, embedded within his understanding of modernity, has influenced many great writers on fashion, no matter their methodological or disciplinary affiliations. They range from the art historian Aileen Ribeiro, who refers to him in her work on nineteenth-century cosmetics *Facing Beauty: Painted Women and Cosmetic Art* (2011) to the cultural theorist Caroline Evans, who makes use of him in her work on the *blasé* air of the modern fashion model, *The Mechanical Smile* (2013). Recent works that attempt to write a philosophy of fashion also consider Simmel to be the foundational writer (Meinhold, 2013). The persistent influence of Simmel can be seen in the work of Gilles Lipovetsky, who crafted a wide-ranging synthesis of fashion in which he argued, now somewhat controversially, that fashion is a mainly Western and post-feudal invention (Lipovetsky, 2002 [1987]).

Simmel's ideas were in the beginning not well received by some parties. He had a challenging time at university and throughout his career, having his first idea for a thesis on musical psychology rejected, and facing many setbacks in his professional career, including being unwaged as a university teacher. Simmel studied the new field of *Völkerpsychologie*, an approach that considered the moulding of a person by a wider whole. Such an approach had been influenced by the philosophy of Nietzsche. In this method, no longer used, society is seen as a form of cultural production rather than having any fixity. He finished his PhD in 1881 and his *Habilitation* (a second, higher degree than the Anglo-Saxon 'Doctorate') in 1885, and although teaching at the University of Berlin, was not made a member of the Faculty there. He was granted a professorship in Strasburg at 65, for which he had to leave his beloved Berlin.

Simmel's learning had an affinity with Charles Darwin, Herbert Spencer, Friedrich Nietszche, Karl Marx, aesthetic and literary Symbolism, the wider movement known as 'art for art's sake' and the philosophy of Henri Bergson. His way of working and writing, across eclectic fields and via the format of the essay, the lecture, journalism and social life, generally without the conventional apparatus of footnotes, led sceptics to judge him as a *dilettante* or lacking in rigour. Simmel's approach did not quite fit in any discipline, even the emerging discipline of sociology that he later disavowed, but nor was he an iconoclast. His independent wealth probably contributed to his lack of concern about following academic conventions. He also had to navigate the very complex and anti-Semitic system which was called by Coser in 1958 'the gelatin of German academic life' (cited in Davis, 1973: 322). As Jürgen Habermas (1996 [1991]) puts it, Simmel's light essay style and his frequent appearances in the press also contributed to the 'informal' sense around his work. We could say that his writing style is akin to 'Impressionism' or 'Symbolism' in painting or music. He was, in fact, called 'a philosophical Monet' by Lukács (cited in Frisby, 1981: vii).

SIMMEL'S SOCIOLOGY

Simmel's sociology is called various things, sometimes 'relational sociology', or he is described as the theorist of social 'relationality' (*Wechselwirkung*). Natàlia Cantó Milà's excellent survey of Simmel's work points to his innovative opinion that everything – people and things – is 'always embedded within a social context' (2005: 31). The area in which Simmel's work was positioned, sociology, also represented a challenge, as this was a newly developed field of study that challenged proponents of conventional disciplines such as literature and history and took as its topic areas of study that had hitherto appeared banal. This is particularly significant for the field of dress fashion research, as previously in the late nineteenth-century the topic had been written about from literary perspectives or as an aspect of historical civilisation in which fashion was a part of aesthetic self-realization (later modernist *Bildung*), as in the writings of Johann Herder and Jacob Burckhardt, for example (McNeil, 2009: xxvi–xxvii).

Simmel's work was particularly influential in the United States in the early twentieth century, where sociology had emerged partly independent of a continental European tradition as a means to understand pressing contemporary issues such as suffrage, race relations and immigration. The rapid changes experienced particularly in women's fashions at this time were both striking and demanded explanation. German sociologists were hardly published in English in prominent academic journals in the United States then, but this was not the case with Simmel, who enjoyed patrons and respect there; many North Americans had attended his Berlin classes and Simmel was listed along with Herbert Spencer and Gabriel Tarde as the most cited sociologist there in a 1927 study (Levine et al., 1976).[1] Simmel's influence never disappeared in the United States, and he underwent a type of renaissance in the 1950s, when he had a major influence on the New School and the Frankfurt School in the United States of America, and then again in the 1980s, when he came to the attention of a new generation via the translations and writings of British figures such as David Frisby. The influence of Simmel on North American scientific research about fashion might therefore be so extensive in part due to his particular role within the formation of American sociology. The United States had a great number of fashion and 'apparel' schools at tertiary level that grew out of the 'Home Economics' movement of the 1890s, and Simmel was frequently used by scholars there to understand taste, trends and the operations of fashion, as we will see below. However, when Frisby (1981: viii) wrote *Sociological Impressionism: A Reassessment of Georg Simmel's Social Theory*, he found that his was the first book in English published on Simmel since 1925. It has also been noted that Simmel's reception in the United States sociological mainstream took place in a 'disjointed manner' over 'seven decades'. This emphasized the fragmentary uptake of the thinker (Levine et al., 1976: 814).

As mentioned earlier, Simmel's work was not primarily about fashion. Rather, he was interested in the inter-linked aesthetic and social aspects of contemporary society. However, Simmel is now famous within the historiography of design for an essay entitled 'The Philosophy of Fashion' (1901, reprinted in English in 1904) as well as a number of essays on style and adornment.[2] Simmel was interested there in what has been called 'sociation' (*Vergesellschaftung*), which has been translated as 'socialisation', and which demands that society is not reducible to the acts of individuals (Milà, 2005: 39). Simmel tried to make sense of the new metropolis of quickening tempos and sensations of people and products that characterized the post-industrial city. Habermas (1996 [1991]: 405) notes, 'In short, for Simmel the membranes of the spirit of the age were wide open.' The clothing that people wore to inhabit these new city spaces intrigued Simmel, and fashion was a useful subject for him to test and also outline his propositions regarding the relationship of aesthetic and social forms. It is incredible that an 18-page essay on dress has had such impact on twentieth-century conceptions of the motive and reasons behind fashionable dressing.

Simmel felt that the middle class and the metropolis had become synonymous with fashion, as the rich and the poor occupied a different cadence of life. Even the rise of travel and the cutting up of the year into segments of time to mark the concept of vacations was, to Simmel, a sign of the heightened neurasthenia of the modern. As with so many things, this was not a completely new position; it was the argument of the poet Stéphane Mallarmé in the fashion journal *La Dernière Mode* in the 1870s. The latter had noted how the invention of the railway demanded a new cadence of day and even created new clothing fashions for that passage of time. Many of the concepts about fashion developed by figures as significant as Charles Baudelaire (1821–1867) and Mallarmé (1842–1898) passed indirectly into the sociology and critical thinking of Simmel and Walter Benjamin (1892–1940) and continue to reverberate in the writings of contemporary fashion theorists including Ulrich Lehmann and Barbara Vinken.[3]

Simmel's writings were very influential on aspects of the 'New Art History' of the late 1970s and 1980s, which had a strong emphasis upon exploring the distinctive visual culture and psychology that grew up alongside nineteenth-century metropolitan life, as depicted by Impressionist and Post-Impressionist artists. It could be argued that a nascent 'fashion studies' as opposed to dress or costume studies emerged in the period circa 1990 from this awakened interest in nineteenth-century visual culture. The women's studies, left criticism and 'Victorian' studies of the 1970s and early 1980s all contributed to the development of 'fashion studies' and the study and rediscovery of Simmel was central to this endeavour.[4] Simmel was more or less compulsory reading for students of art history and cultural anthropology in the 1980s and early 1990s in the Anglophone world. This scholarship built upon the investigation of fashion as a part of *la vie quotidienne* (not yet named 'popular culture') developed by French theorists such as Henri Lefebvre, Georges Perec, Michel de Certeau and Roland Barthes, whose writings in the period from the 1930s until the 1960s explored the socio-politics of everyday life. (For more on Barthes, see chapter 8 in this book.)

SIMMEL'S AESTHETICIZED EXISTENCE

Fashion is a part of human aesthetic experience and this fact Simmel always brought to the fore. Parts of his thinking were strongly coloured by the late nineteenth-century 'art for art's sake' (*l'art pour l'art*) milieu in which he grew up. This literary and artistic movement, of which Oscar Wilde, Walter

Pater and Stéphane Mallarmé were famous proponents, argued for the transcendental horizon of beauty, whether it be a poem, a piece of re-creative criticism or indeed a dress fashion. Simmel's conception of social forms was connected here to his way of living as well as his mode of thinking. Simmel's wife (née Gertrud Kinel), whom he married in 1890, was a portrait painter, and his personal life was heavily aestheticized. His urbane apartment contained collections of Japanese and Chinese ceramics and textiles. Simmel's son Hans wrote that every now and again, the textiles were displayed and select vases filled with roses for a very small number of guests to admire, but only for a matter of hours, 'then everything was cleared away' (Gronert, 2012: 60–61). As German design historian Gronert (2012: 61) notes, this was a type of theatrical performance that shifts 'the narrow boundary between art and reality'. This is also the connoisseurship of late nineteenth-century 'decadence' and J-K. Huysman's *A Rebours* (1884) (*Against Nature*, or *Against the Grain*); Simmel's *milieu* is therefore that of late nineteenth-century aestheticism.

The common thesis that art is a reality independent of life places Simmel within the late nineteenth- and early twentieth-century French and English 'art for art's sake' schools, confirms Davis (1973: 324). A memoir of the period notes: 'it was the culture of the beginning of the century, that Simmel [...] embodied and which only a decade later was to be destroyed in the First World War' (Frisby, 1981: 20). Thus it could be argued that although so influential in the twentieth, Simmel's thought owed its genesis to the previous century.

Simmel enjoyed a high public profile in his time in Berlin. He was famous for his interviews with journalists and his regular literary *salons*. Simmel was in regular contact with many contemporary thinkers, writers, artists and poets, including Rainer Maria Rilke and the sculptor Auguste Rodin. He wrote essays on artists such as Rembrandt van Rijn and Arnold Böcklin. Simmel was interested in the rights of women, writing several essays on suffrage, but also once complained that women should not be allowed to come to his lectures, as their bright dresses distracted him from his particular approach to teaching, which was intense and didactic; 'I prefer it when the auditorium is as colourless and indifferent as possible. The dual form of appearance and the bright clothes disturb me' (Simmel cited in Frisby, 1981: 18). Here Simmel can be placed in a long tradition of male writers who reflected on the fact that a masculine indifference to clothes enabled greater concentration on other activities and allowed other qualities to come to the fore, enabling a reconciliation of nature and artifice. Such thinkers include one of the most celebrated writers of the Enlightenment, Denis Diderot, as well as the famous Johann Wolfgang von Goethe, who dressed very simply.[5]

Simmel would have been aware of these literary precursors, the great range of thinkers who contributed to the possibility of a discourse around fashion emerging slowly over time.

Like most of the major thinkers on fashion who worked in the late nineteenth and first half of the twentieth centuries, Simmel was also attempting to make sense of the environment in which he lived. He contributed thirty articles on decorative arts and design to the Munich-based journal *Jugend*. In these articles he was less judgemental of contemporary taste for the undulating and erotic *Jugendstil* or *Art Nouveau* than his contemporaries such as Thorstein Veblen. Rather than a critique, Simmel attempted to find a theoretical explanation for changes in taste and fashion that characterized his era. His approach can be found in an essay entitled 'Roses: A Social Hypothesis', published in *Jugend*, no. 24, 1897.

Simmel – who clearly liked roses – playfully describes a utopian society in which the right to breed roses was reserved exclusively to a small, privileged group of people. For all other people, it was forbidden by law to breed roses. In this society, the right to breed roses was a pivotal indication of success in life. In the tale, personal striving for success implied that increasingly more people in the society attained the right to breed roses. An agitator wrote a pamphlet stating that everyone had the right to grow roses. To cut a long story short (Simmel goes on in this vein for a bit), after time, turmoil and revolution, all members of the society were allowed to breed roses. Now, as everyone was breeding increasingly more sophisticated and different strains of roses, the people sensed that breeding roses was only of secondary relevance to their lives and no longer a sign of success.[6] This is a classic example of what has come to be called, for the topic of fashion, the 'trickle down theory'. This is also the Achilles heel of Simmel's theory of fashion. The principal shortcoming of Simmel's approach, and one that generally irritates empiricist historians, is that regarding 'class' fashions. As Ruth P. Rubinstein (1995: 149) puts it in *Dress Codes: Meanings and Messages in American Culture*: Simmel 'explained that there is no fashion in a hierarchical society where the boundaries between the social classes are tightly shut and there is no possibility for mobility'. This notion of a rigid pre-industrial society is the principal problem. History demonstrates that although there was certainly not a 'free for all' in the past, there was fluidity between the social orders – at all times.

The paradox of 'individualism' and conformity has also been addressed via the rise of print in the West. Elizabeth Eisenstein proposed in 1979 that 'As an agent of change, printing altered methods of data collection, storage

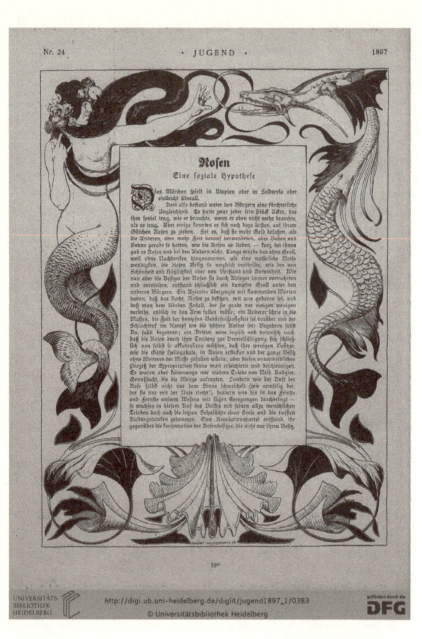

4.1 'Roses: A Social Hypothesis', published in *Jugend*, no. 24, 1897.

and retrieval systems and communications networks used by learned communities throughout Europe. It warrants special attention as it had special effects' (1979: xvi). She goes on to state: 'A fuller recognition of diversity was indeed a concomitant of standardization [...]. In this regard one might consider the emergence of a new sense of individualism as a by-product of the new forms of standardization' (Eisenstein, 1979: 84). Printing, according to Eisenstein's classic account, resulted in effects of dissemination, standardization, organization, preservation, amplification and reinforcement, and began the process from hearing to reading. The dissemination of printed images of fashion undoubtedly transformed its reach. The association of a fashion-image culture with this new individualism was inflected in the formulation famously proposed by Simmel in the first decade of the twentieth century, in which fashion was characterized as a dual action of individualism and conformity (Simmel, 1950 [1905]: 338–44). Such a robust summation of the modern individual who has endless choices but also tends to social conformity has been used in many studies of the paradox of fashion, of belonging and standing out simultaneously via sartorial methods and techniques.

What might, therefore, appear to others to be a 'superficial' topic such as competition in growing rose bushes, is presented by Simmel as a profound social fact. Siegfried Gronert, in 'Simmel's Handle: A Historical and Theoretical Design Study', makes a fascinating case for Simmel's contribution to the theorising of everyday design more generally; Simmel's interests extended beyond sartorial fashions. Although Simmel was not a member of the *Werkbund* like the sociologist Werner Sombart (who wrote a stimulating work on luxury, including fashions), his work was known by the artist-designer members prominent within this movement, such as Henry van de Velde and Peter Behrens. One such essay published in *Jugend* concerned the handles of ceramics. The handle of a jug or teapot can be subject to analysis and the designs of the contemporary designers who were rethinking such vessels can be reframed. To Simmel, the handle might appear 'the most superficial symbol of its category; but precisely because of its superficiality, it reveals the range of the category to the fullest' (Simmel cited in Gronert, 2012: 60). It seems that such an analogy as this might have influenced Roland Barthes decades later, when he wrote that the woman's 'shawl' had 30 elementary categories; whereas the leg, with or without stocking, was not very rich semiologically (Carter, 2003: 162).

Simmel, Gronert concludes, therefore leaves a legacy throughout twentieth-century 'aphoristic' design writing including Giedion's case for the coffee spoon as part of collective history (1948) and Roland Barthes' *Mythologies* (1957). Gronert (2012: 68) points out that Barthes never mentions Simmel, but in his reading of Garbo's face or the Citroën DS 19 he revealed the 'historicism of the quotidian'. Simmel, therefore, was one of the precursors who created the possibility of 'mythologies of the everyday'. Such a claim might be tempered somewhat by considering the way in which the Symbolist poet and fashion writer Stéphane Mallarmé was also able to mythologize the everyday in the 1870s, as indeed had Charles Baudelaire in the 1860s.

SIMMEL AND LATER SOCIOLOGY

Murray S. Davis, in his essay 'Georg Simmel and the Aesthetics of Social Reality' (1973: 320), cites Arthur Salz, one of Simmel's pupils, as stating that Simmel 'conceives of sociology as the study of forms of sociation. But who-ever speaks of forms moves more in the field of aesthetics. Society, in the last analysis, is a work of art.' (Here we are back to l'*art pour l'art* and the ambience of Simmel's youth.) Simmel conceived of art and society as 'atemporal configurations in space', and not in time (Davis, 1973: 320).

> Simmel, like his contemporary Freud, finds the conflict between man and his social and cultural creations to be eternal, and to be a struggle which man is continually losing. Except for the brief moment of creation, man must suffer his own creations, endure his past organisations of his cultural and social worlds.
>
> (Davis, 1973: 321)

Simmel used the analogy of space and geometry frequently, and this has sometimes been elided in translation.[7] In 'Fashion', for example, he talks of the 'circle' of fashion (1957 [1904]: 558). As society becomes more complex, more social circles arise, overlap and form new combinations, making the issue of 'individuation' more intensive. Hence Simmel's tale of the roses. Simmel also, as Sellerberg (1994: 58) notes, used the notion of the curve to suggest *momentum*.[8]

Simmel works in pairings when he approaches fashion: conformity and differentiation; the shallow surface and the deep inner meaning; the personal and the imitation; the superordinate and the subordinate to the forces of fashion, as Sellerberg (1994: 59) usefully set out. These pairings are not static binaries; 'they counteract each other and actually stimulate each other in doing so, creating a kind of circular stimulation and *Eigendynamik*' (Sellerberg, 1994: 60). Sellerberg, who has conducted research on fashions in baby's names, Swedish interiors and American restaurant menus, argues via Simmel that 'the area of fashion seems to be expanding [in our time ...], pairs of dualistic tendencies, presented together, function as motor forces in this respect' (Sellerberg, 1994: 72). In her earlier short essay on food and fashion she argues that 'fashion fixes the attention of the community on an object or process at a certain time and place' (Sellerberg, 1984: 82). This is also the position of Gilles Lipovetsky, who in *The Empire of Fashion* writes of the increased diffusion of all forms of consumer fashions in twentieth-century life, from movie premieres to Coca-Cola types (Lipovetsky, 2002 [1987]).

WHAT DID SIMMEL ARGUE ABOUT FASHION?

Unlike the theorist of conspicuous consumption, Veblen, Georg Simmel did not entertain the possibility that fashion might advance towards an ideal. His sociology studied interpersonal relations rather than quantitative measures in order to conclude how objects attain value.

Observing the historicism of the design culture around him, Simmel (1997: 215–216) theorized how 'the individual constructs his environment of variously stylized objects; by his doing the objects receive a new centre, which is not located in any of them alone'. In a key essay, 'The Problem of Style' (1908), Simmel (1997: 68) argued that objects and surroundings must be stylised in order to make a 'person the main thing'. Frédéric Vandenberghe (1999: 63), in a study of Simmel and Weber as founders of sociology, noted that 'the Simmelian spirit is the "*esprit de finesse*", the spirit of subtlety, refinement, tact, delicacy, and perceptivity [...]. For Simmel nothing is too trivial.'

Simmel is also influential in the field of fashion studies for another essay, 'Adornment' (1905). In the original German the latter had a secondary title (printed much smaller) 'Exkurs über den Schmuck', an expression that has been translated differently as adornment or jewellery, clearly meaning rather different things. To Simmel there can be no fashion in a pre-industrial society. He argues that fashions are always 'class fashions' and have the 'double function of holding a given social circle together and at the same time closing it off from others'. In a fragmented modern life, 'the pace, tempo and rhythm of gestures is fundamentally determined by clothing'. On the so-called 'neurasthenia' of modern life he wrote:

> Changes in fashion reflect the dullness of nervous impulses; the more nervous the age, the more rapidly its fashions change, simply because the desire for differentiation, one of the most important elements of all fashion, goes hand in hand with the weakening of nervous energy. This fact in itself is one of the reasons why the real seat of fashion is found among the upper classes.
>
> (Simmel, 1957 [1904]: 547)

Simmel is here referring to the nature of the bourgeois condition, which had previously been remarked by Marx (for more on Marx, see also chapter 2). He builds on Marx, who also analysed the 'soul movements' of the bourgeoisie and the 'relentless dissolving energy of bourgeois rationality' (Wayland-Smith, 2002: 889).

In 'Adornment' Simmel offers the following significant, because so often repeated, explanation for the female attachment to fashion:

> The fact that fashion expresses and at the same time emphasizes the tendency towards equalization and individualization, and the desire for imitation and conspicuousness, perhaps explains why it is that women, broadly speaking, are its staunchest adherents [...]. The relation and the weakness of her social position, to which woman has been doomed during the far greater portion of history, however, explains her strict regard for custom, for the generally accepted and approved forms of life, for all that is proper [...]. But resting on the firm foundation of custom, of what is generally accepted, woman strives anxiously for all the relative individualization and personal conspicuousness that remains.
>
> (Simmel, 1957 [1904]: 550)

Simmel then goes on to use what we would today call the notion of fashion as a 'voice' or 'agency' for women, a concept that is widely deployed in contemporary historical studies of women and fashion. He writes of the emerging individualism of the late middle ages in Germany: 'Women, however, took no part in this individualistic development: the freedom of personal action and self-improvement were still denied her. She sought redress by adopting the most extravagant and hypertrophic styles in dress' (Simmel,

1957: 551). Simmel's notion that when a woman is silenced she might express herself through clothing has been used by a great many historians interested in fashion and gender. However, it does not explain the etiolation in male dress that also characterized the Middle Ages, unless one were to conclude that courtiers were also without power and therefore used clothing as a form of expression. In Simmel's day it was not uncommon to see *ancien-régime* and post-revolutionary societies analysed in rather more simplistic ways than they actually functioned. This has a major impact on how we might interpret dress – as custom or fashion.

TRICKLING DOWN

Simmel never used the expression 'trickle down', but he has become identified with this notion. Sproles (1981: 119) noted in the context of an essay on marketing that the so-called 'trickle down' theory is almost entirely derived from Simmel, who in the 1904 version of his essay 'Fashion' wrote, 'Naturally the lower classes look and strive towards the upper, and they encounter least resistance in those fields which are subject to the whims of fashion' (Simmel, 1997: 190). Sproles points out that the upper class theory is also connected to Thorstein Veblen's *Theory of the Leisure Class* (1912 [1899]). Simmel had studied the fashion paradox of the opposing urge of wishing to belong or conform and to simultaneously express individuality. He noted that 'the peculiarly piquant and stimulating attraction of fashion lies in the contrast between its extensive, all-embracing distribution and its rapid and complete transitoriness' (Simmel, 1997: 205).

In 'Fashion' (1904) Simmel connects two thoughts – one about class fashions and another that is reminiscent of the poetry and criticism of Baudelaire, that fashion enables something particular to occur:

> The fashions of the upper stratum of society are never identical with those of the lower; in fact, they are abandoned by the former as soon as the latter prepares to appropriate them. Thus fashion represented nothing more than one of the many forms of life by the aid of which we seek to combine in uniform spheres of activity the tendency towards social equalization with the desire for individual differentiation and change.
>
> (Simmel, 1957: 543)

Simmel then goes on to pursue the analogy of fashion and 'death' that has been much repeated in more theoretical explorations of fashion:

> As fashion spreads, it gradually goes to its doom [...]. Fashion always occupies the dividing line between the past and the future, and consequently conveys a stronger feeling of the present, at least while it is at its height, than most other phenomena.
>
> (Simmel, 1957: 547)

Fashion, therefore, has special characteristics that make it particularly worthy of attention, despite the tendency by commentators to dismiss it as the empty-headed pursuit of women and the vain younger men who may be found in any urban society.

Simmel then announces his famous maxim that brings together fashion, individualism and conformity in a special pairing: 'It is peculiarly characteristic of fashion that it renders possible a social obedience, which at the same time is a form of individual differentiation' (1957: 548–549)

Simmel comments in this essay at length on the demi-monde (a difficult to translate concept of the literal 'half-world/society' – upper sex-worker or courtesan and also actress grouping) of mid-to-late nineteenth-century Europe. Here he perhaps recalls the fascination regarding the fine levels of distinction of dress fashions and social caste made possible in a modern city as outlined by Baudelaire and Mallarmé many decades earlier:

> The fact that the demi-monde is so frequently a pioneer in matters of fashion, is due to its peculiarly uprooted form of life. The pariah existence to which society condemns the demi-monde, produces an open or latent hatred against everything that has the sanction of law, of every permanent institution, a hatred that finds its relatively most innocent and aesthetic appearance in the striving for ever new forms of appearance. In this continual striving for new, previously unheard of fashions [...] there lurks an aesthetic expression of the desire for destruction, which seems to be an element peculiar to all that lead this pariah-like existence, so long as they are not completely enslaved within.
>
> (Simmel, 1957: 552)

This would seem to contradict a part of his thesis regarding class fashions, as many courtesans, who were not of the upper echelon, set fashions that were in turn copied by the fashionable women accepted within society. It is this section that Elizabeth Wilson (1985: 138), in her famous work *Adorned in Dreams*, takes to infer that Simmel means that 'the deviant, the dissident and the outsider' create the 'iconoclasm, the outrage and the defiance of fashion' in modern culture, which is perhaps not exactly what he intended, but is an imaginative reading of Simmel and one that illustrates his continuing relevance to fashion studies.

Later in the essay, Simmel talks of the wider dissemination of fashion since the Revolutionary period. He writes (1957: 556):

> The frequent change of fashion represents a tremendous subjugation of the individual and in that respect forms one of the essential complements of the increased social and political freedom [...]. Classes and individuals who demand constant change, because the rapidity of their development gives them the advantage over others, find in fashion something that keeps pace with their own soul movements.

Finally Simmel suggests that fashion is not irrational, which is a major statement about something generally characterized as facile or feminine: 'Thus fashion is shown to be an objective characteristic grouping upon equal terms by social expediency of the antagonistic tendencies of life' (1957: 558). This statement is extremely pertinent for fashion studies, as it suggests that fashion may be studied in these terms.

CONCLUSION: THE AFTER-LIFE OF SIMMEL

Simmel's thought had a major impact on subsequent writers on fashion in the 1950s and 1960s. He also found his critics. Herbert Blumer's 'Fashion: From Class Differentiation to Collective Selection' in *The Sociological Quarterly* commented on the role of sociologists such as Simmel (1904), Sapir (1931) and the Langs (1961) as failing to 'observe and appreciate the wide range of operation of fashion' (Blumer, 1969: 275).[9] He critiqued parts of Simmel's view that fashion's primary aspect concerned class fashions. Blumer (1969: 280) argued that it was not the social power of elites that created fashions, but rather that it was the 'suitability or potential fashionableness of the design which allows the prestige of the elite to be attached to it'. Blumer pointed instead to 'collective taste formations' (Gronow, 1993: 95).

By 1908 Simmel felt he had established the field of sociology and he turned his attention to other matters; 'cultural philosophical ones' (Frisby,

1981: 36). He became influenced by Expressionism, which was darker and more introspective. Simmel died relatively young from cancer in 1918.

Simmel has an enduring legacy within fashion studies. For many beginning readers in the field, his texts are amongst the first that they are asked to tackle. Concepts such as 'trickle down' have become everyday terms in conversation and the media. Simmel's inter-linked view of fashion and style, formed within the milieu of late nineteenth-century aestheticism but also within the nascent forms of sociology, was nuanced and engaging. Blumer, in a passage that would be echoed later by the cultural philosopher Lipovestsky and also by the cultural historian Daniel Roche (1994 [1989]), using very different methods, argues that fashion is a positive good: 'Yet the facts are clear that fashion is an outstanding mark of modern civilization and that its domain is expanding rather than diminishing [...]. *Fashion introduces order in a potentially anarchic and moving present*' (Blumer, 1969: 288–89). Blumer's perceptive last note is: 'The recognition that fashion is continuously at work is, in my judgement, the major although unintended contribution of Simmel's analysis' (1969: 290). The success of Simmel is that he considers fashion to examine another and wider process, and this is an approach that is in fact shared with a great deal of history and social studies around the time, for example Werner Sombart on the topic of 'luxury' (1967 [1913]). In suggesting that fashion was not facile but could be subject to analysis, indeed that fashion revealed critical perspectives concerning the process of becoming a modern subject in a modern society, Simmel's approach was one that permitted a space for a vibrant and growing fashion studies to emerge.

NOTES

1 The first department of Sociology in the United States was established at the University of Chicago in 1892. See Levine et al. (1976): 815–16.
2 There are three different versions of the essay on fashion that are fairly close to each other: 1895, 1904, 1911. See Jukka Gronow (1993) 'Taste and Fashion: The Social Function of Fashion and Style' in *Acta Sociologica*, (1): 99; Georg Simmel, 'Fashion' in *International Quarterly*, X, October 1904: 130–55, reprinted in *The American Journal of Sociology*, LXII (6), May 1957: 541–58.
3 Readers should consult Lehmann's stimulating chapter on Simmel in *Tigersprung* (2002: 125–95), in which he emphasises Simmel's affiliation and also enablement of *modernité* and the fragment/fragmentary characteristics that were so central to the early twentieth-century avant-garde. He suggests that Simmel's use of the essay and the *feuilleton* format was quite deliberate, linking him to the French avant-garde of the 1870s who wrote on fashion.

4   I have argued this point further in the Introduction to my *Fashion: Critical and Primary Sources* (McNeil, 2009).
5   For Diderot's essay see *Rameau's Nephew and Other Works* (1956: 325–33).
6   I thank Emily Brayshaw for bringing this article to my attention and for her summary of the translation.
7   For example, 'the intersection of social circles' becomes 'the web of group-affiliations' (Davis, 1973: 323). Davis argues this has been done to make him more up to date and to use modern sociological terms.
8   See also her 'The Practical! Fashion's Latest Conquest' (Sellerberg, 1984).
9   Sapir was interested in the notion that fashion increased one's attractiveness.

REFERENCES

Blumer, H. (1969) 'Fashion: From Class Differentiation to Collective Selection' in *The Sociological Quarterly*, 10 (3): 275–91.

Carter, M. (2003) *Fashion Classics from Carlyle to Barthes*, Oxford and New York: Berg.

Coser, L. (1958) *Georg Simmel*, Englewood Cliffs, NJ: Prentice Hall.

Davis, M.S. (1973) 'Georg Simmel and the Aesthetics of Social Reality' in *Social Forces*, 51 (3): 320–29.

Diderot, D. (1956) *Rameau's Nephew and Other Works*, J. Barzun and R.H. Bowen (trans), New York: Doubleday.

Eisenstein, E.L. (1979) *The Printing Press as an Agent of Change: Communications and Cultural Transformations in Early-modern Europe. Volumes I and II Complete in one Volume*, Cambridge: Cambridge University Press.

Evans, C. (2013) *The Mechanical Smile: Modernism and the First Fashion Shows in France and America 1900–1929*, New Haven, CT: Yale University Press.

Frisby, D. (1981) *Sociological Impressionism: A Reassessment of Georg Simmel's Social Theory*, London: Heinemann.

Gronert, S. (2012) 'Simmel's Handle: A Historical and Theoretical Design Study' in *Design and Culture*, 4 (1): 55–72.

Gronow, J. (1993) 'Taste and Fashion: The Social Function of Fashion and Style' in *Acta Sociologica*, 36 (2): 89–100.

Habermas, J. (1996 [1991]) 'Georg Simmel on Philosophy and Culture: Postscript to a Collection of Essays', M. Deflem (trans) in *Critical Inquiry*, 22 (3): 403–14.

Lehmann, U. (2002) *Tigersprung*, Cambridge, MA and London: MIT Press.

Levine, D.N., Carter, E.B. and Gorman, E.M. (1976) 'Simmel's Influence on American Sociology. I' in *American Journal of Sociology*, 81 (4): 813–45.

Lipovetsky, G. (2002 [1987]) *The Empire of Fashion: Dressing Modern Democracy*, C. Porter (trans), Princeton, NJ: Princeton University Press.

McNeil, P. (2009) *Fashion: Critical and Primary Sources Volume 1: Late Medieval to Renaissance*, Oxford and New York: Berg.

Meinhold, R. (2013) *Fashion Myths: A Cultural Critique*, J. Irons (trans), Bielefeld: Transcript Verlag.

Milà, N.C. (2005) *A Sociological Theory of Value: Georg Simmel's Sociological Relationism*, Bielefeld: Transcript Verlag (distributed by Transaction Publishers).

Ribeiro, A. (2011) *Facing Beauty: Painted Women and Cosmetic Art*, New Haven, CT: Yale University Press.

Roche, D. (1994 [1989]) *The Culture of Clothing: Dress and Fashion in the Ancient Regime*, J. Birrell (trans), Cambridge: Cambridge University Press.

Rubinstein, R.P. (1995) *Dress Codes: Meanings and Messages in American Culture*, Boulder, CO, San Francisco, CA and Oxford: Westview Press.

Salomon, A. and Kaworski, G.D. (1995) 'Georg Simmel Reconsidered' in *International Journal of Politics, Culture and Society*, 8 (3): 361–378.

Sellerberg, A. (1984) 'The Practical! Fashion's Latest Conquest' in *Free Inquiry in Creative Sociology*, 12 (1): 80–82.

———(1994) *A Blend of Contradictions: Georg Simmel in Theory and Practice*, New Brunswick, NJ and London: Transaction Publishers.

Simmel, G. (1950 [1905]) 'The Philosophy of Fashion and Adornment', K.H. Wolff (trans) in *The Sociology of Georg Simmel*, New York: The Free Press.

———(1957 [1904]) 'Fashion' in *The American Journal of Sociology*, LXII (6): 541–558.

———(1991 [1908]) 'The Problem of Style', M. Ritter (trans) in *Theory, Culture and Society: Explorations in Critical Social Science*, 8 (3): 63–71.

———(1997) D. Frisby and M. Fetherstone (eds), *Simmel on Culture: Selected Writings*, London: Sage Publications.

Sombart, W. (1967 [1913]) *Luxury and Capitalism*, W.R. Dittmar (trans), Ann Arbor: University of Michigan Press.

Sproles, G.B. (1981) 'Analysing Fashion Life Cycles: Principles and Perspectives' in *Journal of Marketing*, 45 (4): 116–124.

Vandenberghe, F. (1999) 'Simmel and Weber as Idealtypical Founders of Sociology' in *Philosophy & Social Criticism*, 25 (57): 57–80.

Veblen, T. (1912 [1899]) *Theory of the Leisure Class*, New York: B.W. Huebsch.

Vinken, B. (2005) *Fashion Zeitgeist: Trends and Cycles in the Fashion System*, Oxford and New York: Berg.

Wayland-Smith, E. (2002) 'Passing Fashion: Mallarmé and the Future of Poetry in the Age of Mechanical Reproduction' in MLN, 117 (4), French Issue: 887–907.

Wilson, E. (1985) *Adorned in Dreams: Fashion and Modernity*, London: Virago.

5

WALTER BENJAMIN
Fashion, Modernity and the City Street

Adam Geczy and Vicki Karaminas

INTRODUCTION

It is perhaps more than a coincidence that the first letters of the word 'modern' are 'mode'. Both words are taken from the Latin *modo* meaning 'just now'. Walter Benjamin was extraordinarily attuned to modernity as a process of constant renewal already anticipated, inscribed in what is already there. For the 'now' is itself the crossroads between what will be and what has been. Fashion therefore has an important place in Benjamin's thought. Yet in a comment on a passage by the nineteenth-century French poet Charles Baudelaire, Benjamin dismisses it swiftly: 'one cannot say there is anything profound about this' (Benjamin, 1969: 89). This does not avert the fact that the shell of shifting appearance is one of the central issues in Benjamin's thought.

Born in Berlin in 1892, Benjamin considered himself a 'man of letters' rather than a philosopher, which was a more illustrious title for a man of his time. He made a living as a literary critic and translator, writing articles for many journals and magazines. When the Nazis took office in 1933, as a Jew and left-wing intellectual Benjamin fled to Paris where he befriended many other intellectuals in the same situation, including Hannah Arendt, Gershon Scholem and Theodore Adorno. In Paris he wrote his most influential essays and articles, as well as the ambitious and unfinished '*Das Passagen-Werk*' (*The Arcades Project*, 1938). In this substantial tome he wrote about fashion's social, cultural and psychological meanings in the context of nineteenth-century capitalism. Here we also find Baudelaire's most explicit influence on Benjamin, not only in his referencing of the poet's writings on fashion, but in a large section of the project dedicated to Baudelaire himself. Drawing on Georg Simmel (see chapter 4), Marcel Proust and Charles Baudelaire, Benjamin critiques fashion in terms of hygiene, social class, gender, political and economic power, biology and so on.

The birth of fashion can be said to occur together with the birth of modernity. This makes fashion more than a consequence or complement of modernity. Rather it is the most specific manifestation of capitalism's will-to-change. Yet while we may note Benjamin's aversion to fashion on the grounds of its collusion with the commodity, he also observes that it holds the key to modernity's relationship to time. Moreover, Benjamin offers many insights into the way fashion is intertwined with representation, a relationship that is even more poignant today with the growth of digital fashion, which has altered the way in which fashion is disseminated and perceived. Thus his essay, 'The Work of Art in the Age of its Technological Reproducibility', while pertaining to works of art and not items of fashion, has been of considerable profit to fashion studies (Evans, 2003 and Lehmann, 2000). The representation of fashion will be discussed later in the chapter. We first examine Benjamin's writings on fashion, the influence of Baudelaire and Proust on his work and the relationship between fashion, history and time.

CHARLES BAUDELAIRE'S INFLUENCE ON WALTER BENJAMIN'S WRITING

Walter Benjamin's concept of fashion is unthinkable without considering the poet Charles Baudelaire. His *Berlin Childhood* through to the essay 'Paris, the Capital of the Nineteenth Century' is heavily tempered by Baudelaire's influence. Baudelaire was one of the most important and tragic figures of his era, not only one of the most outstanding poets of his time, but also a formidable art critic. It is indeed in his art criticism, and particularly his much-cited essay 'Painter of Modern Life', that we begin to see what is later developed by Benjamin, namely what is today known as cultural studies. In this essay, Baudelaire develops the notion of the flâneur, the city wanderer-voyeur who observes the life of the modern city: shop windows, parks, stalls, posters, and, in no small measure, what people wear, and how they wear it. Benjamin develops from Baudelaire's technique of extracting poetic insight from observing the anomalies and juxtapositions that appear in everyday life. In this context it means that fashion is central for Benjamin because it represents a conjunction of past, present and future; it usurps the past, represents the now and anticipates, and is inscribed by, its own overcoming.

As a Marxist thinker of historical materialism, Benjamin develops his idea of the dialectical imagination from the writings of Karl Marx (see chapter 2), especially from *Capital* (1867). Marx devoted a considerable amount of time to recounting victimization of the past and to the importance of its memory in political and economic contexts. It is precisely through this relationship between the memory of the victims of capitalism and the promise of liberation governed by the laws of progress that Benjamin revises the question of history. Rather than examining progress in historical development, Benjamin focuses on a new construction of the past in the present. His resistance to the idea of the linear progress of time in favour of a non-instrumental relationship to the future contains messianic and Kabbalistic notions of time. In other words, the past is always contained in the present, simultaneously inside and outside history. The relevance of Benjamin's idea to the study of fashion is twofold; in the way in which garments contain the past in some form, either in their technological development (for instance, boning, corsetry) or in their aesthetic component which looks to the past for stylistic inspiration. The fashion cycle and the rapid speed by which styles come and go is central to the essence of fashion. In this way, fashion, which exists in the present, contains a dialectical relationship to the past. As Michael Sheringham eloquently writes, 'temporality is at the heart of fashion's unstable – yet strangely permanent – present which is linked existentially both to the past, which it incorporates, and to the future which it anticipates' (2006: 182).

Fashion's place in Benjamin's thinking can be seen to have two phases; the first in his writings on Baudelaire, followed by *The Arcades Project* (1938), in particular the section enigmatically called 'Konvolut B'. Drawing from the cup of Marxism, Benjamin is from the first deeply distrustful of fashion since it is the most persistent agent of capitalism's 'false consciousness'. The latter is the notion espoused by Marx and Engels that institutions of capitalism deceive and betray the proletariat, obfuscating means and ends with the overall effect of setting up false realities and thereby impeding the possibility of effective class struggle. Fashion is the semblance of the new, a room of mirrors in which history is played out as a specular game, for which Benjamin used the term 'phantasmagoria' (Markus, 2001). With fashion, the bourgeoisie can play out its false consciousness, and seek consolation in novelty, to the exclusion of the real signs of utility, that is, the operations of truth. One could say that for Benjamin, the transformation of clothing to fashion enacts a violence on this kind of aesthetic utility since it debases beauty, attraction, allure and aura to base integers of arbitrary vanity, whose qualities are exploited since fashionable beauty must die to make way for what comes next.

Thus fashion bears witness to the bad faith in capitalism's claim to progress, in which advancements are only made for the sake of profit. Fashion is in collusion with capitalism in a way that art is not, because fashion and art occupy different modalities of presentation and reception. The differences are less in the objects of fashion and art, since both are aesthetic creations for which judgement is always subjective, but the places of exchange – social, economic, linguistic – that they occupy. Benjamin was able to show how fashion was one of the principal means by which modernity manifests itself, but also diagnoses its own forever changing identity, its *Zeitgeist*. Fashion is a crystal in which aesthetics, consumption, class, industry and personal identity all meet.

The changes wrought by the fashion industry are changes that occur solely for the sake of the commodity fetish – Karl Marx's term for the endless chain of goods that we desire and then relinquish for another object of desire to be purchased. According to this thesis, the signs within fashion are disingenuous. The signifying value of fashion is subordinated to its ability to be desired and consumed. In this respect its meanings are annulled and made redundant. The inherent gratuitousness of fashion is thus on one hand made more gratuitous still through the subservience to commodity value. Fashion is the assurance of bourgeois society's narcissism, complacency and stagnation. On the other hand, there is also the dissimulation of men's fashion down to the base denominator of the black coat. Benjamin understands fashion as participating in ceremonies of death: for women the death of meaning and direction for the sake of fleeting gratification, for men to be reduced to an awkward cipher, in which equality, if not authentic, is given a uniform, or livery as Baudelaire calls it, which is one that inveigles the dead (Baudelaire, 1954b: 676).

In order to understand Benjamin's reflections on fashion, it may be wise to take a small detour through Baudelaire's thoughts on fashion and the dandy. Benjamin was influenced by the poet's approach to fashion as a conduit that manifested the conditions of the present, apprehended by experiences that blur the subjective and the objective. The eminent foil to the predicament of fashion is the dandy who in Baudelaire's words is 'something modern and keeps to wholly modern causes' (Baudelaire, 1954b: 676). Baudelaire's dandy is the closest thing approaching the notion of anti-fashion, since the dandy embraces an attitude more than a particular garment or circumscribable look. Anti-fashion can best be defined as oppositional dress, an umbrella term that is bandied by designers and the fashion industry to describe dress styles that are contrary to the fashion of the present. Punk and the designs of Vivienne Westwood are labelled anti-fashion because they make a statement at a particular historical moment of anti-establishment.

Dandyism is anti-fashion insofar as it tries to step outside the fashions of its time, thereby the dandy announces himself as solipsistic, self-referential and defiantly autonomous. The English dandy, with its originator, Beau Brummell, was highly self-conscious of fashion and style and held several keys to the origins of modern dress. Although a dandy himself who dressed in black from head to toe and slept on black bed sheets, dandyism for Baudelaire was far less sartorial as he insisted that garments were only symbols of a spiritual aristocracy and far more political. The dandy scorns the bourgeois way of life and its elitism as 'the last spark of heroism against decadence' responding to what he considered to be 'encroachments of bourgeois and even mass vulgarity by reasserting traditional virtues of daring, élan and poise' (Williams, 1982: 111). These were the politics of perverse indifference and self-absorption of the troubled and transitory epoch of the nineteenth century that was characterized by mass production and consumption. If there were to be a *symbol* of the dandy's clothing, it would be the ubiquitous black, so that he may blend in with the crowd, as the *flâneur* or city ambler. Benjamin notes how, unlike his contemporaries, Baudelaire 'found nothing to like about the age he lived in […]. *Flâneur*, apache, dandy and ragpicker were so many roles for him' (Benjamin, 2006: 125). But what Benjamin writes next is intriguing from the point of view of fashion: 'For the modern hero is no hero; he is the portrayer of heroes' (2006: 125). In the carnival that is modernity we all play a particular part, cast for us or chosen. Unlike the bourgeois, the dandy is aware of modernity's decay in his own claim to decadence. Whether dandy or bourgeois, the charms of fashion are but anodyne symptoms of much deeper malaise. Such an out of the ordinary statement could be made too much of, although we might assert from this that fashion and elegance are the outer shell of a system that the bourgeois are happy to maintain and to which the dandy is a self-anointed pariah.

HISTORY, MEMORY, TIME

According to Benjamin, dress is not only an attribution of class, recognition and aspiration, but foremost a pervasive and persistent statement of temporality. This temporality runs deep to the measure of the way in which modernity needs to maintain the semblance of change. This is not only economic but narratological, for modernity is always both subverting and improving upon history. Fashion is as a tissue of historical references that are both avowed and also repressed in the name of the 'just now'. These are ideas he explores in his *The Arcades Project*, a title that comes from the proliferation and charm of mercantile galleries, or arcades, in mid-nineteenth century Paris. In this unfinished book, Benjamin is essentially concerned with the history of Paris, a prehistory of modernity. He looks back at the nineteenth century as the birthplace of modernity that would influence contemporary historicism and a materialist interpretation of society. A number of fragments, theoretical reflections, aphorisms and notes constitute his work on the arcades, 'the matrix from which the image of modernity was cast', as 'the mirror in which the century, self-complacently, reflected its very newest past' (Benjamin cited in Steiner, 2010: 147). He writes:

> These arcades, a new invention of industrial luxury, are glass roofed, marble panelled corridors extending through whole blocks of buildings whose owners have joined together for such enterprises. Lining both sides of these corridors, which get their light from above, are the most elegant shops, so that the passage is a city, a world in miniature.
>
> (Benjamin, 1999: 31)

The allure results from the 'ambiguity of space': the roofed streets change into an interior space and they impart the indeterminacy of the streets of Paris. The streets appear to be the 'abode of the collective' and the arcade turns into the salon (Steiner, 2010: 148). Benjamin focuses on these structures as the organizing metaphor for his study because they are a historically specific artefact of the period in question and the particular visual character of nineteenth-century commodity capitalism. The arcades themselves were a site and apparatus for the vast realms of perception for the people of the modern metropolis. The material amassed included the role of the urban crowd for the strolling *flâneur*; the significance of optical devices such as panoramas, peep shows and magic lanterns in the habitation of city dwellers; and the new conditions of the metropolitan experience, in particular the modern practices of display and advertising that emerged in Paris and would come to shape the representation of the world in such a ubiquitous manner.

One of the prominent topics that manifests in Benjamin's writings is the role of fashion as a visual signifier of aesthetics and as both an economic and political force. To fathom fashion philosophically defines Benjamin's efforts as motivated by his interest to find out 'what this natural and totally irrational measure of the historical process is really all about' (Benjamin cited in Steiner, 2010: 147). According to Benjamin, certain historical moments and forms become legible only at a later moment. As the prehistory of one's own present, the past century, which has claimed the concept of modernity for itself, does not move closer to this present time. Rather it retreats into an infinite, prehistoric distance. The sense of time that characterizes this experience is suggested by the way fashions change. Every generation experiences the fashion that has just elapsed, but fashion is more than merely meretricious; it is a continuous and fickle spectacle that illustrates a dialectic of history, because the latest trend or garment in fashion will set the tone 'only where it emerges in the medium of the oldest, the longest past, the most ingrained' (Benjamin, 1999: 64). It is this experience that Benjamin explains further as the attempt 'to distance itself from all that is antiquated – which means, however, from the most recent past' (Benjamin, 1999: 64). Present time is referred back to the past.

In the section Konvolut B, dedicated solely to fashion, we see fashion as a fluid entity within the life of modernity. Benjamin is particularly interested in the way in which fashion invests in historical references while simultaneously undermining them: 'This spectacle, the unique self-construction of the newest in the medium of what has been, makes for the true dialectical theatre of fashion' (Benjamin, 1999: 64). To bring this insight to fashion today: as head designer and creative director of the House of Chanel since 1983, Karl Lagerfeld continuously mines Gabrielle 'Coco' Chanel's archives containing past designs in order to stay true to the brand. His designs incorporate Chanel details, colours, tweed fabrics, quilt stitched leather, gold chains and the 'CC' logo. In later collections, Lagerfeld 'deconstructed' elements of Chanel's looks such as incorporating her signature jersey fabric into men's T-shirts and briefs. Similarly, in Chanel's comeback collection in 1953 she updated her classic looks by reworking her tweed designs and making the Chanel suit, with slim skirt and collarless jacket trimmed in braid and gold buttons, a status symbol for a new generation of women. Fashion is therefore to be seen not only as part of the carnival of commodities but also a complex fold of the past and what will always-soon-be in the present. As opposed to art, which speaks across time, fashion is inscribed with the inevitability of its own overcoming.

PROUSTIAN MEMORY AND THE FOLD

Benjamin's metaphor of the fold, which he employs to explain the way in which fashion contains the ghost of the past in the present via the recycling of past styles, originated in his engagement with the literary method of realization, of bringing something into the present, that the French author Marcel Proust employed when writing the series of novels *Remembrance of Things Past* (1913–27). Proust lavished considerable attention on fabrics and gowns to evoke memories and the metaphysical value of an object, that is 'the significance that fashion and elegance carry for the perception of past and present time' (Lehmann, 2000: 209). The seductions of fashion in Proust's world are part of a much deeper web of memory, association and imaginative invention, in which the desires of the moment collude, wittingly or not, with the dense strata of personal experience and cultural history.

For Benjamin the dialectical process caused by the folds of past present on the one hand, and the anticipated future on the other, puts the truth of present action to the test. This material-temporal imbrication is what causes the explosive event that is pregnant within the past – whose symbol is fashion – that ultimately blasts away the smooth continuum of history to reveal a clearer understanding of the relationship to time, matter and self. Because this explosion is fashion, 'it becomes apparent', writes Ulrich Lehmann, 'that fashion is the indispensable catalyst for both remembrance and a new political – that is, materialist – concept of history' (Lehmann, 2000: 210). Like a shirt cuff whose fabric folds back on itself embedding memory in its creases as it moves forwards and backwards, folding and unfolding on the precise point on the cloth, so too does the dialectical process of history. (See chapter 10 on Deleuze for a similar yet different understanding of the fold of fashion.) Benjamin conjures up the image of the tiger's leap to explain fashion's effortless ability to leap from one temporal setting to another. 'Fashion,' he writes, 'has the flair for the topical whenever it stirs in the thickets of long ago, it is the tiger's leap into the past' (Benjamin, 1968: 263). It is precisely this historical relay, the 'tiger's leap in the open air of history', that renders fashion a dialectical process shifting between the present and the past, for it challenges the linearity of history and becomes a symbol of modernity's potential for change (Benjamin, s.a., Vol. 1.2: 701).

The significance of Proust's fiction for Benjamin's philosophical inquiry into the Parisian arcades and modernity can thus not be underestimated. The representation of memory in *Remembrance of Things Past* was for Benjamin the expression of the historical character of memory and experience that we would later find embedded in the theoretical fragments that make up *The Arcades Project*: 'What the child (and in a much weaker recollection the man) discovers in the folds of a fabric into which he pressed himself while holding on to the mothers skirt – this has to be part of these pages' (Benjamin cited by Lehmann, 2000: 207). Benjamin's analysis of nineteenth-century Paris is an act of remembrance.

Benjamin developed a new approach to the philosophy of history by drawing on Proust's literary model in its epistemological structure and textual appearance. It is the constant realisation of the past within the present in Proust's novel, brought on most forcefully in the revelations wrought from involuntary memory, that leads Benjamin to the concept of the dialectical image. The dialectical image is what Benjamin described as 'literary montage', analogous to the cinematic montage. Typified by early filmmakers such as Sergei Eisenstein, montage is the filmic equivalent of collage. A series of short shots are edited into a dynamic array so as to expand the perceptual flow of space, time and information. It is less symbolic than organizational, deepening the understanding of temporal *durée*, duration. It is through the alignment of both the arbitrary and the intentional ordering of temporal units, the friction between past and present that a third meaning arises. This is not truth as such, but rather, as Benjamin conceives it, an archetype, and a standard for judging the significance of historical reality. According to Benjamin, the images created by past generations contain the desires of those generations, whose relevance maintain their pertinence across time. As a result, the objects of the past are not important for themselves, but for what they represent. The possibility of recognizing the image of the past further depends on being attuned to a peculiar temporality, a movement within the medium of memory in which the meaning of the past is *realized* in the present. In its first incarnation, the past appears distorted, an alteration that Benjamin compares to dreams. The recognition of the image must then be understood as the traversal of that space of semblance that brings out its truth, as the awakening from the dream. The function served by the dialectical image in the understanding of history is expressed by Benjamin himself, when in *Theses on the Philosophy of History* he affirms that 'the past can be seized only as an image which flashes up at the instant when it can be recognized and is never seen again' (Benjamin, 1968: 263). The dialectical image can best be defined as an image of the past that ushers the desires of earlier generations into the present (Karaminas, 2012).

THE PHANTASMAGORIC MACHINE OF CAPITAL

Benjamin was highly sensitive to the manner in which the art object is always in the cusp of being swallowed by the phantasmagoric machine of the commodity. He was fascinated by the phantasmagoria, a form of theatre that used a magic lantern that contained a candle and a concave mirror to project frightening images of demons, skeletons and ghosts onto a wall. The phantasmagoria became a popular form of entertainment in the nineteenth century, partly because of the fascination with science at the time. As well as the increase in productivity enabled by the Industrial Revolution which created new products and lowered the price of existing commodities, technology made possible the material realisation of fantasies which had up until then existed in the realm of the imagination. The advent of cinematography and electrical power resulted in large-scale city lighting that replaced gas illumination and brightly lit the streets of Paris and London. The speed and motion from which everyday life was altered by technological marvels was frightening for Benjamin, who associated the phantasmagoria with commodity culture and its experience of intellectual and material products.

Expanding on Karl Marx's notion of the phantasmagoric powers of the commodity, Benjamin used the term in his essays to explain the way in which images of the past and present collide in the unfolding of the present. It is this dialectical process embedded in history and time that we see prevalent throughout his work and especially in The Arcades Project, where Benjamin explains how fashion has a significant place in modernity and the everyday, by its link to the unfolding present. Fashion is the more visible promise that pervades modernity, since it embodies both past and future, albeit in the most arbitrary and fleeting way. Modernity is not only a project based on industrialisation and rationalisation and oriented towards the future; it is also a collection of dreams – a historical dream, as Benjamin says, which becomes material in objects and architectural constructions. The modern is internal to the phantasmagoric display form of the market, which can be seen in salons, world exhibitions, collections and arcades. What concerns us here are the different strata of seduction that exist in modernity's spectacle. In Benjamin's words, 'every fashion is to some extent a bitter satire on love' (Benjamin, 1999: 64, 79). The word 'satire' suggests that what fashion traffics is mildly counterfeit. The temporality of fashion is therefore to be distinguished from a far deeper temporality that is less perverse and more detached. This is the 'real' history as opposed to the piecemeal and whimsical staging of history within fashion.

Benjamin's account of the temporal essence of fashion is where past and present are inseparable, and for him the rapid tempo of fashion is essentially erotic. Just as fashion represents modification of historical time, it is also in opposition to the natural world: 'every fashion couples the living body with the inorganic world. To the living, fashion defends the rights of the corpse. The fetishism that succumbs to the inorganic world is its vital nerve' (Benjamin, 1999: 79). Apart from being a remarkable observation in itself, this goes to the root of a difference between fashion and clothing. Clothing is what is worn for the sake of protection and warmth. It also applies to basic ritual modesty of covering one's naked body; but with fashion such modesty is elevated to a fetish in which the body is sexualized, although wilfully and self-consciously covered. In Benjamin's view fashion 'titillates' death, since the fetish is a state of renewal immanent with death. Fashion 'mocks' death, which it acknowledges, by creating its own rhythm and by taking its cue from everything fetishistically enlivening inorganic materials such as cloth or plastic. Fashion is a composite of dead references brought to life by the commodity: 'Fashion prescribes the ritual according to which the commodity fetish is worshipped', states Benjamin (1999: 8). To use his colourful terminology, it is allied to the corpse. Fashion's references are prone to be vapid and grotesque, because these references serve no other purpose than to fill a void temporarily. 'Not the body but the corpse is the perfect object for [fashion's] practice', writes Benjamin:

It protects the right of the corpse in the living. Fashion marries off the living to the inorganic. Hair and nails, midway between the inorganic and the organic, always have been subjected most to its action. Fetishism, succumbing to the sex appeal of the organic, is fashion's vital nerve. It is employed by the cult of the commodity. Fashion is sworn to the inorganic world. Yet, on the other hand, it is fashion alone that overcomes death. It incorporates the isolated [das Abgeschiedene] into the present. Fashion is contemporary to each past.

(Benjamin cited in Lehmann, 2000: 271)

Perhaps for Benjamin that temporariness is never hidden. Indeed it is disturbing that the modern consumer, the bourgeoise, is happy to participate in something of a game of deceit and death. The appearance of fashion in the now is already the register of its demise. Or in Benjamin's words: 'Fashions are a collective medicament for the ravages of oblivion. The more short-lived a period, the more susceptible it is to fashion' (1999: 80).

PRODUCTION, REPRODUCTION AND
REPRESENTATION

The metaphor of the dialectical image as a point where the present and the past meet is for Benjamin a method of understanding culture as history. His abiding interest was the manner of photography's representation, and the way in which it afforded us a relationship to time and history that was altogether new. Its possibilities were to give us a closer, more intimate and challenging grasp of history in which the evidential and the material were intertwined with mendacity and seduction. Photography confronts us with the plenitude of history's possibilities while also reminding us of what we have lost. What, though, does this mean for fashion? For Benjamin the present is what is historically present – digital fashion media and print media photography offer the consumer a lifestyle of commodity seduction that immerses the participant in a dream world manifested by the latest styles in dress, artefacts and conspicuous consumption. The promise, or representation, of a life lived and experienced.

Benjamin had a complex philosophical relationship to photography that is not reducible to his essay 'The Work of Art in the Age of its Technological Reproducibility', the famous piece that he wrote at the end of the 1930s but which got published by Adorno posthumously after World War II. One of Benjamin's many preoccupations with photography was the way it is able to preserve the past for the present by means of the image. This is not as facile as it sounds, for photography allows the past to be captured in an image and that image also belongs to the moment of the time captured. The captured image no longer belongs to the domain of art, but now makes a historical claim. He was interested in how photography brings a new dimension to history and historicity. For him, the photograph has the potential to open up history, allowing us to see the past.

Many of these ideas are further developed in his artwork essay. It is most commonly cited for the observation that photographic reproduction denudes the work of art of its 'aura'. But we want to draw attention to the latter part of the essay, in which Benjamin turns the argument on its head. He suggests that it is also through reproduction that the object is reinvested with auratic power, by endowing it with importance; mass reproduction asserts the need for this to take place and therefore the worth of the object. Benjamin defines the aura by the same movement of sight towards a representation of the unrepresentable: 'To perceive the aura of an object we look at means to invest it with the ability *to look at us in return*' (Benjamin cited in Buci-Glucksmann, 1994: 111).

Whilst Benjamin's essay referred to photography and film, rather than fashion, his use of the manner in which the creative object shifts from tradition to mass can be applied to the production of the garment in the contemporary fashion system. Prior to the establishment of the couture industry in Paris in the second half of the nineteenth century, fashion was regulated by strict sumptuary laws and craft guilds comprising of tailors and dressmakers with core artisan skills such as sewing, drapery, pattern making and illustration. Fashion was the domain of the aristocratic elite who set styles and trends and could afford to attend salons and purchase made-to-measure couture garments. The designer Charles Frederick Worth (1825–1895) prised the industry away from the guilds and located it in the couturier, as a matter of unsurpassable talent and creation. In this case, the couture garment functions as an 'original'. Pushing the envelope of what constituted authorship in an activity for hundreds of years relegated to guild-bound craftspeople, Worth suggested that a couturier was an artist. He asserted tendentiously that the difference between his 'creations' and art was but a mere technicality. Can fashion then claim an auratic status and what did Benjamin mean by the 'aura'?

According to Benjamin, a work of art may be said to have an aura if it claims a unique status based on quality and value rather than its distance from the beholder. This distance is not primarily a space between object and viewer, but the creation of a psychological inapproachability and authority based on its position within a tradition and canon. For Benjamin, integration into a canon is synonymous with integration into cultic practices and rituals. 'Originally, the embeddedness of an artwork in the context of tradition found expression in a cult', he writes, 'the earliest artworks originated in the service of rituals [...] in other words, the unique value of the "authentic" work of art always has its basis in ritual' (Benjamin, 2008: 24).

Benjamin's description of the fetishization of a work of art via the process of transmission rather than creation brings to mind Elizabeth Wilson's seminal article 'Magic Fashion' (2004). Wilson traces the connections between art and fashion through the metaphor of dress as having magical qualities and draws on the work of Benjamin and Karl Marx on commodity fetishism to argue that in secular societies, couture garments are more than a status symbol; they take on imagined symbolic qualities. 'It is because we live in a society dominated by capital and consumption,' writes Wilson, 'that we commandeer material goods for the symbolic expression of values remote from materialism. This includes ideas of superstition, magical and spiritual nature. The objects [garments] expressing or embodying them become something like secular fetishes' (Wilson, 2004: 378). If the work of art remains a fetish, a distanced and distancing object that exerts an irrational power, it attains a sacred cultural position that remains in the hands of the privileged few. In this sense the made-to-measure garment, as a unique and authentic material object, is elevated to the status of haute couture and becomes a symbol of value and status, attaining traits of cultic veneration. When fashion, like Benjamin's artwork, loses its uniqueness in the age of mass reproduction due to industrialisation and the possibilities of technology, fashion emancipates itself from its inception. Fashion becomes democratized.

CONCLUSION

Benjamin's artwork essay has been seminal for art history and media studies, but it has not, as yet, penetrated too deeply into fashion studies. What is for sure is that the same question that haunts media theorists holds as much for fashion theory, namely, had Benjamin been alive today, what would he have made of the dense hyper-real worlds of representations? This is a particularly pertinent question for fashion studies, given the slippages that have occurred in recent decades between art, fashion and popular culture. His unfinished *Arcades Project* emphasises the importance of fashion as a project of modernity whose essence is transitory and contingent and is closely linked to the ephemeral and the present. We know this because the majority of Konvolut B is dedicated to the topic. A closer reading of the manuscript reveals the importance that Benjamin placed on fashion as a philosophical tradition and as an expression and interpretation of the lived experience of everyday city life. In the last two decades or so, we have been faced with the paradoxical situation where the popular image also has the capacity to be 'critical' and where some fashions convey as much as art objects. This is surely a symptom of a new relation we have to time. We now inhabit a present that we ambiguously, unimaginatively, call 'the contemporary'. Yet this permanent present is saturated with the histories whose dialectical relations are the image. The most artful of contemporary fashion reminds us that the historical relations within stylistic inspiration serve to offer us a space where images exist for the sake of what is yet to come.

POSTSCRIPT

Just north of the city of Barcelona along the Catalan coast and overlooking the Mediterranean Sea lies the cemetery of Port Bou. Enclosed by a white wall the cemetery itself runs along the contours of terraces where white tombs are embedded. When Hannah Arendt came looking for Walter Benjamin's grave, she found nothing but 'one of the most fantastic and most beautiful spots [she] had ever seen in her life' (Arendt, cited in Taussig, 2006: 3). This is what Arendt wrote to Gershom Scholem, Benjamin's friend who along with Theodore Adorno revived interest in his work after the war. As the Nazis drew closer to Paris in 1939, Benjamin was forced to flee the capital like previous intellectuals and artists had done before, gaining political asylum in the United States. Lisa Fittko and her partner Hans helped Benjamin escape through the winding mountain routes along a smugglers' path that led to the Spanish border, where the American authorities had arranged for him to board a boat for the USA. Benjamin carried a very heavy black briefcase across the Pyrenees that he refused to abandon, saying that it contained his most important work: 'I cannot risk losing it. It is a manuscript that must be saved', he said to Fittko (Taussig, 2006: 9). Benjamin never made it to the border to board the waiting boat. Upon learning that he required a visa to leave France and fearing being caught by the German Gestapo he committed suicide, swallowing a vial of morphine which he carried tucked away safely in his pocket, just in case. His death certificate was made out on 27 September 1940; his age is listed as 48. The judge recorded his personal effects as: a pocket watch and chain, a passport with a Spanish visa, US currency, six photographs, a Parisian ID card, an amber smoking pipe, a pair of nickel reading glasses and several newspapers and personal letters. No manuscript. No briefcase. No cadaver. Lost and never found. It may be, as many scholars have often wondered, that the lost manuscript, Benjamin's most important work as he claimed, was the finished version of *The Arcades Project*. Perhaps we will never know.

REFERENCES

Baudelaire, C. (1954a) 'De L'Héroisme de la Vie Moderne' in Y.G. Dantec (ed), *Salon de 1846, Œuvres Complètes*, Paris: Pléiade.

———(1954b) 'Le Beau, la Mode et le Bonheur' in Y.G. Dantec (ed), *Le Peintre de la Vie Moderne, Œuvres Complètes*, Paris: Pléiade.

———(1954c) 'Le Public Moderne et la Photographie' in Y.G. Dantec (ed), *Salon de 1859, Œuvres Complètes*, Paris: Pléiade.

Benjamin, W. (1968) *Illuminations*, H. Zohn (trans), London: Fontana/Collins.

———(1969) 'Das Paris des Second Empire bei Baudelaire' in *Charles Baudelaire: Ein Lyriker im Zeitalter des Hochkapitalismus*, Frankfurt am Main: Suhrkamp.

———(1999 [1938]) *The Arcades Project*, H. Eiland and K. McLaughlin (trans), Cambridge, MA: Belknap of Harvard University Press.

————(2006) 'Das Paris des Second Empire bei Baudelaire' in M. Jennings (ed), *Walter Benjamin, The Writer of Modern Life: Essays on Charles Baudelaire*, H. Eiland et al. (trans), Cambridge, MA: Belknap of Harvard University Press.

————(2008) 'The Work of Art in the Age of its Technological Reproducibility' in M.W. Jennings, B. Doherty and Y.L. Thomas (eds), *The Work of Art in the Age of Its Technical Reproducibility and Other Writings on Media*, Cambridge, MA: Belknap of Harvard University Press.

————(s.a.) 'Über den Begriff der Geschichte' in *Gesammelte Schriften*, Frankfurt: Suhrkamp.

Benjamin, W., Eiland, H., and Jennings, M.W. (eds) (2006) *Selected Writings, Volume 3: 1935–1938*, Boston, MA: Harvard University Press.

Buci-Glucksmann, C. (1994) *Baroque Reason: The Aesthetics of Modernity*, London: Sage.

Evans, C. (2003) *Fashion at the Edge: Spectacle, Modernity and Deathliness*, New Haven, CT and London: Yale University Press.

Karaminas, V. (2012) 'Image: Fashionscapes – Notes Toward an Understanding of Media Technologies and their Impact on Contemporary Fashion Imagery' in A. Geczy and V. Karaminas (eds), *Fashion and Art*, London and New York: Bloomsbury.

Lehmann, U. (2000) *Tigersprung, Fashion in Modernity*, Cambridge, MA: MIT Press.

Markus, G. (2001) 'Walter Benjamin or: The Commodity as Phantasmagoria' in *New German Critique*, (83), Special Issue on Walter Benjamin.

Sheringham, M. (2006) *Everyday Life: Theories and Practices from Surrealism to the Present*, Oxford: Oxford University Press.

Steiner, U. (2010) *Walter Benjamin: An Introduction to his Work and Thought*, Michael Winkler (trans), Chicago: University of Chicago Press.

Taussig, M. (2006) *Walter Benjamin's Grave*, Chicago: University of Chicago Press.

Williams, R.H. (1982) *Dream Worlds: Mass Consumption in Late Nineteenth-Century France*, Berkeley: University of California Press.

Wilson, E. (2004) 'Magic Fashion' in *Fashion Theory: The Journal of Dress, Body and Culture*, 8 (4): 375–85.

6

MIKHAIL BAKHTIN
Fashioning the Grotesque Body

Francesca Granata

INTRODUCTION

In *Rabelais and His World*, a study from the 1930s and 1940s of the sixteenth-century French author François Rabelais, the Russian cultural and literary historian and theorist Mikhail M. Bakhtin (1895–1975) describes the open-ended, collective body of carnival as the grotesque body par excellence, in contrast to the 'classical body of official culture': 'an entirely finished, completed, strictly limited body, which is shown from the outside as something individual' (Bakhtin, 1984 [1965]: 320).[1] He theorizes the grotesque as chiefly a phenomenon of reversal and of unsettling ruptures of borders, and in particular bodily borders. A constant transgression, merging and exceeding of borders constitutes the central attribute of the Bakhtinian grotesque:[2]

> The grotesque body [...] is a body in the act of becoming. It is never finished, never completed; it is continually built, created, and builds and creates another body. [...] Thus the artistic logic of the grotesque image ignores the closed, smooth, and impenetrable surface of the body and retains only its excrescences (sprouts, buds) and orifices, only, that which leads beyond the body's limited space or into the body's depths.
>
> (Bakhtin, 1984 [1965]: 317–318)

He isolates the late Renaissance, the period in which Rabelais wrote *Gargantua* and *Pantagruel*, as the one in which the classical model starts to displace a

grotesque understanding of the body (Bakhtin, 1984 [1965]: 320). The ety-
mology of the word 'grotesque' and its use in the visual arts support Bakhtin's
reading. It comes from the Italian word *grotto* (meaning cave) and came into
use in the Renaissance as a result of excavations in Rome and other parts of
Italy, which unveiled ancient forms of ornamental painting. These images,
unlike classical statuary, were characterized by fantastic portrayals, which were
condemned as 'monstrous figures' characterized by 'a lack of respect for proportion, symmetry and faithful reproduction of the animate world' (Kayser,
1963: 20). This 'struggle' between the classical and grotesque concepts of the
body, rather than being confined to the visual arts, can be observed in a number of different areas. These include the 'canon of behaviour', which Bakhtin
sees as an attempt 'to close up and limit the body's confines and to smooth
the bulges', as well as the history of dance and, ultimately, fashion, which
makes for a particularly fertile case study, as Bakhtin himself suggests. In an
endnote, he writes that it would be 'interesting to trace the struggle of the
grotesque and classical concept in the history of dress and fashion' (Bakhtin,
1984 [1965]: 322–323). It is this aspect of Bakhtin's work that represents the
more fruitful application for a study of fashion.

Fashion is intimately connected to the history of the body and, as a result,
the history of manner, decorum, as well as health and hygiene – privileged
sites where bodily norms have been historically negotiated. As the fashion theorist and historian Caroline Evans, quoting Norbert Elias, points out, fashion is 'part of "the civilising process"' (Evans, 2003: 4). Dress was famously
enlisted by nineteenth-century social reformers in their effort to control the
social body, and fashion was partially co-opted in their attempts to contain and
'educate' the lower classes and used towards the promotion of a disciplined
and controlled self (Purdy, 2004). Fashion, however, occupied a contested terrain throughout European history. It was accused of fostering a blurring of
class boundaries (a concern which prompted sumptuary laws beginning in
the fourteenth century) and was also recurrently criticized for promoting garments and styles which could be detrimental to a person's health, particularly
women's health, as is perhaps particularly evident in the polemics surrounding
the corset (Kunzle, 1982; Steele, 2001). Ultimately, fashion remains a deeply
ambiguous and unstable cultural product and thus a contested terrain on to
which norms and deviations are constantly being negotiated.

This chapter contextualizes Bakhtin's theories and explores how the
struggle between the classical and grotesque body is played out in experimental fashion at the turn of the twenty-first century. Starting out by covering the way the Russian scholar's work has been applied – although rarely

to fashion studies – the chapter suggests further areas of study. Finally, it illustrates how, through the use of specific examples, circumscribed both historically and geographically and by placing the Russian scholar's work on a continuum with that of other theorists, fashion studies qualifies and better contextualizes Bakhtin's over-celebratory reading of the grotesque.

POSITIONING BAKHTIN

Bakhtin's theories have influenced a number of different disciplines and fields of study, which are not limited to the ones he engaged with during his lifetime. Although chiefly a work of cultural history and literary criticism, *Rabelais* has entered the fields of art history and aesthetics theory, gender studies, performance study, film studies, disability study and surely many others. As the film scholar Robert Stam points out, Bakhtin's wide relevance is due precisely to his interest in borders, liminality and in-betweenness:

> we should not restrict Bakhtin's relevance to those media and subjects he himself happened to address. The 'rightness' of a Bakhtinian approach to film derives, I would suggest, not only from the nature of the field and the nature of the medium but also from the 'migratory' cross-disciplinary drift of the Bakhtinian method. As a self-defined 'liminal' thinker, Bakhtin moves on the borders, at the junctures and points of intersection of academic disciplines as traditionally defined and institutionally regulated. The most productive interdisciplinary relations, Bakhtin argues, occur at the borders between the diverse sectors, and not when those sectors close themselves within their specificity.
>
> (Stam, 1989: 16–17)

Bakhtin's theories have also anticipated later movements and schools of thought. Some of his work preceded post-structuralism – particularly his work on dialogism, which he developed in *The Problems of Dostoevsky's Poetics* and *The Dialogical Imagination*. This foreshadowed the concept of intertextuality, which the literary theorist and psychoanalyst Julia Kristeva, in part, developed as a response to Bakhtin's work (Stam, 1989: 2). A concept similar to intertextuality, dialogism focuses on the dialogical nature of the utterance and particularly the literary text (above all the novel) as open-ended and deriving its constantly fluctuating meaning from interactions with other utterances and other texts (Bakhtin, 1981 [1975], 1984 [1963]). Dialogism makes indispensable an open-ended and ever-evolving model of subjectivity – something Bakhtin did not fully develop in his lifetime. However, this model was later developed by Julia Kristeva's subject in process – a subject which is heterogeneous, always becoming, and in question – and thus in line with the grotesque body (Kristeva, 1984, 1987, 1991). The subject in process has, in fact, been read as a synthesis of Lacanian theories of the subject and Bakhtin's writing on the classical and the grotesque body, a synthesis which overcomes the dyad of subject and object (Stallybrass and White, 1986: 175). This model of the subject allows for a remapping and reassessment of the self and the relation between self and other: for 'a reconception of identity and difference, without a collapse of processes of signification' (Oliver, 1993: 12). This stands in contrast to Lacan's alienated subject position formed through the mirror stage, which creates an irremediable distance between self and other plagued by misrecognitions (Stam, 1989: 6). Much like the grotesque body, 'a body in the act of becoming', Kristeva's subject in process – an open subject whose boundaries are not sealed – gives a central place to the maternal body. Thus, as I will discuss in more detail later in this chapter, Kristeva's theory of subjectivity, alongside Bakhtin's writing, becomes central to a reading of fashion, gynophobia and the maternal body.[3]

Rabelais's account of the European carnival tradition in its focus on inversions anticipated concepts which were later developed by cultural anthropology and in particular symbolic anthropology (Stam, 1989: 2). In its recuperation of popular culture, it foreshadowed late modernity's questioning of the Enlightenment traditions and of Western science and rationality in favour of the same 'marginal, de-centred, contingent and unofficial' discourses privileged by Bakhtin in his writing on the carnival and the grotesque (Gardiner and Bell, 1998: 2).[4] However, the fact that they preceded a number of by now established disciplines also means that Bakhtin's theories need to be properly qualified. This is particularly evident in relation to their over-celebratory discussions of the revolutionary potential of carnival and carnivalesque cultural expressions. These pitfalls of Bakhtin's thought, in part, can be attributed not only to the historical moment in which he wrote his work, but also to the particular political environment that surrounded him: 1930s and 1940s Stalinist Russia.

Additionally, Bakhtin's writings, particularly Rabelais, have a tendency toward presenting uncritically the relation between women's bodies and the grotesque, thus running the risk of naturalizing these connections (Russo,

1995: 63). Fashion studies, in its relation to the body, the feminine and the decorative, is not only a preferential site for the application of Bakhtin's theories, but, through its close-knit connection with gender studies as well as visual and material culture, is well suited to qualify the overly celebratory and uncritical aspects of Bakhtin's work.

BAKHTIN AND FASHION STUDIES

Despite the richness of a potential application of Bakhtin's theories to fashion studies, the only mentions of the Bakhtinian grotesque in fashion literature occur in a handful of articles, which tend to focus on the relation between fashion and television and film studies. The fashion theorist Patrizia Calefato employs the Bakhtinian grotesque in her article 'Style and Styles between Fashion and the Grotesque' for a reading of an array of subcultural styles (primarily observed through film media). Combining Bakhtin's insights with the work of Roland Barthes (see chapter 8), she explores how the grotesque 'denaturalizes discourse thereby revealing its semiotic status' (Calefato, 2004: 30). More recently, Dirk Gindt used Bakhtinian theories of the grotesque in his analysis of Björk's collaborations with Alexander McQueen and Nick Knight (Gindt, 2011). Another mention of the Bakhtinian grotesque in the literature on fashion can be found in Lorraine Gamman's 'Visual Seduction and Perverse Compliance: Reviewing Food Fantasies, Large Appetites and "Grotesque" Bodies', published in the book *Fashion Cultures*. The article, which engages with the feminist literary scholar Mary Russo's work on the grotesque, makes a compelling argument on the way the 'female grotesque' (which, in the article, is understood primarily as the overweight body of TV personality Vanessa Feltz) represents 'the repressed of normative femininity' and can be thus employed 'to keep the ideal feminine norm in place' (Gamman, 2000: 75).

As Gamman's article starts to point out, the relation between the Bakhtinian grotesque and feminism is problematic and unstraightforward. In fact, Bakhtin's grotesque body has been theorized as both a site of appropriation for feminist theory, which in the words of Mary Russo suggests 'cultural politics for women' or as Gamman, as well as Russo, point out, a deviation from the norm which is used to keep a body (and particularly a woman's body) in its proper place (Russo, 1995: 54).

The fraught relation between Bakhtin's understanding of the grotesque and the carnival and feminism can be partially attributed to the fact that

Rabelais's *Gargantua and Pantagruel* is a problematic text in that regard.[5] The gender specificity of the grotesque is discussed at length in Russo's *The Female Grotesque* – a feminist reading of the topic – which opens up and clarifies those aspects of the grotesque which Bakhtin unproblematically takes for granted. Russo argues that, in his protracted discussions of the associations between the grotesque and the female body, Bakhtin never stops to take into account the gynophobic genealogy of such associations and, while viewing the grotesque in a positive light, he does not unveil the gynophobic implications in understanding the female biological organs as grotesque par excellence; rather, by leaving them under-analysed, he ends up naturalizing these connections:

> Bakhtin, like many other social theorists of the nineteenth and twentieth centuries, fails to acknowledge or incorporate the social relations of gender in his semiotic model of the body politic, and thus his notion of the Female Grotesque remains in all direction repressed and undeveloped.
>
> (Russo, 1995: 63)

However, acknowledging that there are particular risks for women, as well as ethnic and racial 'others', in aligning themselves with the grotesque body, insofar as their bodies are already *marked* by grotesque associations, I would argue that an application of Bakhtin's theories to fashion opens up the possibility for a re-appropriation of these associations. Applied to the study of fashion, the Bakhtinian grotesque can become an especially important tool for negotiating ideas of norms and deviations.

BAKHTIN, FASHION AND THE BODY-OUT-OF-BOUND

One of the most fruitful applications of Bakhtinian thought to fashion is an analysis of the ways fashion practitioners and those figures working at the juncture of fashion and the visual arts have questioned normative bodies and explored bodily borders. As I have written elsewhere, fashion's exploration of bodily boundaries and bodies-out-of-bound was precipitated by feminism and the AIDS epidemic and took on greater force from the 1980s onwards (Granata, 2010: 149–50). This is a particularly fertile period for a study of the Bakhtinian grotesque in fashion as it coincides with a heightened attention and policing of bodily boundaries (ibid.).

Among the designers who explored new shapes and ideals of female bodies in the twentieth century are some seminal figures of the 1980s and 1990s fashion: the Paris-based Japanese designer Rei Kawakubo of *Comme des Garçons*, the British designer Georgina Godley, and the British designer, artist and club figure Leigh Bowery. In keeping with the 1980s, Kawakubo, Godley and Bowery resorted to excessive padding and oversized clothes, yet they subverted these signs and produced a silhouette which seems antithetical to the mainstream 1980s silhouette and to the history of fashion more generally. All three created a silhouette implying the maternal body, which had been palpably avoided by fashion design in the twentieth century.

As early as the mid-1980s Georgina Godley radically altered the female silhouette by adding padding on the hips, the thighs and the belly. As the art critic Mariuccia Casadio writes: '[Georgina Godley's] clothes altered and emphasized the form and volume of the female belly, and buttocks with the aid of spectacular padding.' Her autumn/winter 1986/7 collection, titled 'Bump and Lump', drew inspiration:

> from medical, scientific, orthopedic and gynecological circles, with a series of fabrics and forms reinforced to support specific parts of the body. This 'clinical' aesthetic provided the starting point for her new concept of the silhouette. Her clothes formalized unprecedented possibilities of mutation.
>
> (Casadio, 2004: 344)

As Godley herself suggests, this collection was developed in direct contrast to the ideal fashion body and in particular to the überhealthy, masculinized and contained body of 1980s fashion, which was 'engineered' through a combination of technologies of the self, including dieting and exercising and plastic surgery, in addition to fashion, and, in particular, the powersuit.[6]

In her spring/summer 1997 collection 'Body Meets Dress', Rei Kawakubo rendered a deeply altered female silhouette with protuberance on the hips, the back and the belly, which often made reference to the pregnant body. The collection was comprised of a number of sleeveless and cap-sleeved dresses, as well as shirts and skirts, in stretchable nylon fabric, which were accompanied by nylon slips, to which down pads were sewn. Kawakubo's collection set out to explore and question assumptions of female beauty and notions of what is sexually alluring and what is grotesque within the Western vocabulary. This exploration was, however, not always well received or easily digested by the fashion establishment. While some of the press lauded her work (particularly the art press and newspaper-based journalists), the collection was not unconditionally embraced by the fashion glossies. Both *Vogue* and *Elle* made an indirect critique of the Japanese designer's work by photographing the collection with the pads removed, a practice that was embraced by a number of otherwise adventurous *Comme des Garçons* costumers.[7] This resistance brings further proof to the fact that the designer, by making reference to the pregnant body in the rarified environments of Parisian fashion shows, had tapped into what was, perhaps, one of few remaining taboos in fashion design of the period. As the feminist philosopher Kelly Oliver writes, pregnant bodies did not become glamourized in contemporary visual culture until the new millennium – although primarily through celebrity culture and Hollywood as opposed to high fashion (Oliver, 2012: 22). Notable precedents include the by now tame, but then controversial, photograph of a nude pregnant Demi Moore on the cover of *Vanity Fair* in 1991.

Leigh Bowery explored the boundaries of the body throughout his career. His clothes often over-emphasized the belly region, rendering it extremely pronounced through the use of padding. This counteracted the common understanding of the belly as a region to be suppressed. More generally, his oversized body, which he used as the basis for much of his work, did not conform to the toned body of 1980s urban gay culture. Some of his most iconic looks from the late 1980s make reference to the maternal body as well as being inspired by a book on Transformer robots – the toy robots known for their potential to shapeshift – a point which corroborates his interest in the possible mutations and transformations of the human body. These references to the pregnant body culminated in his performances with Minty, the most prominent one being the band's 1993 performance at Wigstock – New York's annual dragfest in Tompkins Square park. On this occasion Bowery, dressed in female costume, 'gave birth' to his wife, whom he had concealed as his pregnant belly through a complex system of harnesses and tights. Bowery's birthing performance in its graphic and threatening quality externalized and rendered visible the problematic Western understanding of the maternal body (and by extension the female body), with its unstable borders and generative potential, as 'grotesque' and in some way monstrous. Or as *New Yorker* critic Hilton Als insightfully commented, it certainly did not present the side of womanhood which drag culture 'was seeking to emulate' (Als, 1998: 83–84). Bowery's performances, in their references to birth processes and exchanges of bodily fluids, also placed on a continuum the bodies of pregnant women and gay men as grotesque and immunologically problematic, particularly considering their contemporary context and Bowery's untimely death of complications from AIDS in 1994.

It is only by looking at fashion history through the lens of the Bakhtinian grotesque that we can fully appreciate the extent to which these designers problematized demarcations between bodily boundaries and questioned the integrity of the subject via references to bodies that deviated from the norm, and more specifically, to the pregnant body and birth processes. Godley, Bowery and Kawakubo re-appropriated the relation between the grotesque, the feminine and the maternal to create work which challenged the sealed and 'contained' body characteristic of much twentieth-century fashion. This model, which conforms to Bakhtin's definition of the classical body, can, in fact, be read in relation to a latent gynophobia in 'dominant' Western thought and representational tradition.

According to Bakhtin, the grotesque body is a body in process: in a constant state of becoming. In contrast, the twentieth-century fashion body conforms to Bakhtin's notion of the 'classical body' of official culture:

a strictly completed, finished product [which ...] was isolated, alone, fenced off from all other bodies. All signs of its unfinished character, of its growth and proliferation were eliminated; its protuberances and offshoots were removed, its convexities [...] smoothed out, its apertures closed. The ever unfinished nature of the body was hidden, kept secret; conception, pregnancy, childbirth, death throes, were almost never shown. The age represented was as far removed from the mother's womb as from the grave. [...] The accent was placed on the completed, self-sufficient individuality of the given body.

Thus, Bakhtin concludes, 'it is quite obvious that from the point of view of these canons [meaning the classical canons] the body of grotesque realism was hideous and formless. It did not fit the framework of the "aesthetics of the beautiful" as conceived by the Renaissance' (Bakhtin, 1984 [1965]: 9).

Bakhtin's understanding of the grotesque is thus in line with the maternal and with Kristeva's writing on the subject. Maternity, according to Kristeva, poses a model of a subject-in-process, a subject whose boundaries are not sealed (as it indeed contains another within), and thus ultimately represents 'a model of discourse' which, together with psychoanalysis and poetic language, 'admit, even embrace, the alterity within them'. It allows 'the redrawing of the boundaries of the social' and allows for an embracement of alterity within the self and within society (Oliver, 1993: 11–12).[8]

Kristeva's understanding of the maternal subject as a model for a subject-in-process has parallels with later scientific writings. The anthropologist of science Emily Martin comes to a similar conclusion, as she explores the way in which pregnancy, as a case of boundary transgression, does not fit current immunological models based on the concept of the pure self. By tolerating another within, it constitutes an immunological 'problem' as it contains both '"self" and the immunologically "other"' (Martin, 1998: 126). It problematizes the immunological metaphors of warfare in which foreign entities are to be expunged from the body and are most often understood as tumourous enemies: 'From an immunological point of view, the fetus is credibly described as a "tumour", that the woman's body should try furiously to attack' (Martin, 1998: 131). According to Martin, this often translates in the pathologization of birth processes, a fact that was eerily reflected in the disparaging descriptions of the protuberances of Kawakubo's garments as 'tumours'.

Thus, it is through Bakhtin's theories, once properly qualified through feminist theory and science studies and integrated into a theory of subjectivity, that we can begin to re-inscribe the maternal body in particular, and, more generally, bodies and subjects that deviate from classical standards of beauty and atomized understanding of the subject, to the history of fashion.

FASHION, CARNIVAL AND INVERSIONS

Bakhtin's theories also spur an exploration of the relation between humour and fashion – a relation that has remained so far relatively understudied. His concept of the carnivalesque and the centrality of what Bakhtin calls laughter, which he discusses in *Rabelais*, opens up overlooked areas of research. Conversely, fashion helps one qualify the Russian scholar's work and its over-celebratory reading of the carnival and attendant carnivalesque practices as always and a priori politically progressive.[9] Fashion study contextualizes Bakhtin's writing on the carnivalesque within visual and material culture. It situates it in specific time and space and anchors it to specific objects and performances, as opposed to what is often a de-contextualized use of the term by Bakhtin.

Bakhtinian writings on inversion allow for an additional reading of 'deconstruction' of the fashion of the 1980s and 1990s. They allow for a recuperation of the carnivalesque and grotesque element of fashion that has been identified under this rubric, and to read it in relation to humour. This is particularly true of the work of Martin Margiela, the designer for whom the term was coined and who is arguably its most visible exponent (Cunningham, 1989: 246).[10] The Belgian designer employs grotesque and carnivalesque strategies of alterations of scale, garments' inversions and play with functionality, as well as his inversion of and play with temporalities. His clothes' disregard for symmetry and proportionality can be perhaps best observed in a series of oversized collections (spring/summer 2000, autumn/winter 2000/1 and spring/summer 2001), and in collections based on enlarged Barbie clothes (spring/summer 1999, autumn/winter 1994/5 and spring/summer 1995). All of these collections explore clownish proportions, which do not conform to Western ideals of beauty and classical aesthetics, as well as the normative body of fashion. Additionally, Margiela's experimental construction techniques, particularly the use of garments meant for one part of the body to clothe another or unveiling the inside of a garment, retain a close affinity with carnivalesque techniques of inversion, travesty and upset proportions which were central to carnival humour and were often articulated through the participant's apparel:

> This is why in carnivalesque images there is so much turnabout, so many opposite faces and intentionally upset proportions. We see this first of all in the participants' apparel. Men are transvested as women and vice versa, costumes are turned inside out, and outer garments replace underwear. The description of a charivari of the early fourteenth century, in *Roman du Fauvel*, says of its participants, 'They donned all their garments backward'.
>
> (Bakhtin, 1984 [1965]: 410–11)

These humorous inversions were inherent in the spirit of renewal and the temporary disruptions of hierarchies staged throughout 'the varied popular festive life of the Middle Ages and the Renaissance', which Bakhtin groups under the name of carnival (Bakhtin, 1984 [1965]: 218). In its theorization of inversions and the world upside down, Bakhtin's work anticipated that of cultural anthropologists and, in particular, the strand known as 'symbolic anthropology', whose work, like Bakhtin's, shared an interest in cultural negations and symbolic inversions. And, as Stallybrass and White point out, cultural anthropology is instrumental in bringing Bakhtin's theories from the realm of the actual historical carnival to bear on a wide range of artistic and cultural expressions (Stallybrass and White, 1986: 18). As the cultural anthropologist Barbara Babcock explains in *The Reversible World: Symbolic Inversion on Art and Society*, ' "symbolic inversion" may be broadly defined as an act of

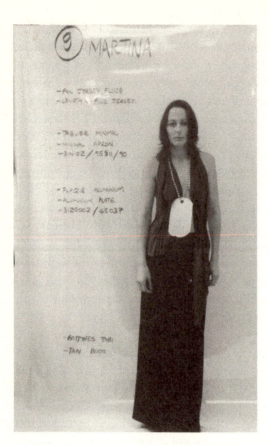

6.1 Martin Margiela, Enlarged Collection, Autumn/Winter 2000–2001, Courtesy of the Maison Martin Margiela.

expressive behaviour which inverts, contradicts, abrogates, or in some fashion presents an alternative to commonly held cultural codes, values, and norms, be they linguistic, literary, or artistic, religious, or social and political' (Babcock, 1978: 14). This definition of symbolic inversion is reflected in common parlance, where the term is used to mean 'a turning upside down', 'a reversal of position, order, sequence, or relation' (*Oxford English Dictionary*, 1991).

Thus, inversion, as Bakhtin also points out, is central to various expressions of the comic, which could be understood as practices of cultural negation (Bakhtin, 1984 [1965]: 410). In their denial of systems and orders and their play with and disruption of category and classificatory systems, they can be read as a critique of closed symbolic systems and fixed categories: 'The essence of such laughter-producing "topsyturvydom" is an attack on control, on closed systems, on, that is, "the irreversibility of the order

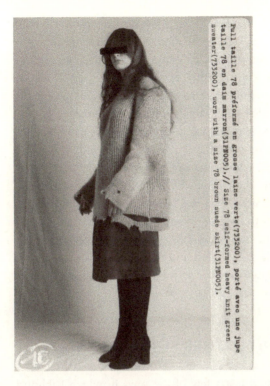

Pull taille 78 préformé en grosse laine verte(733200), porté avec une jupe taille 78 en daim marron(31PM005).// Size 78 self-formed heavy knit green sweater(733200), worn with a size 78 brown suede skirt(31PM005).

6.2 Martin Margiela, Magnified, Doll Clothes Collection, Spring/Summer 1999, Courtesy of the Maison Martin Margiela.

of phenomena, the perfect individuality of a perfectly self-contained series"' (Babcock, 1978: 17).[11] Echoing Bakhtin's theory, cultural anthropology reinforces an understanding of the liberating function of techniques of inversion – or, to use Bakhtin's term, 'carnivalesque' practices – and the attendant 'laughter' they generate. 'Festive laughter', according to Bakhtin, allowed for a dialectical understanding of the world, which could be used as a tool to unmask prevailing truth and orthodoxy. It was through the relativizing lens of humour that (albeit temporarily) a different understanding of the world became possible, one according to which the existing hierarchies were relative and the contemplation of a different social order was possible. And it is through these theories that one can understand Margiela's experiments in fashion as a moment (however circumscribed) of disruption through humour.

This exploration, of course, need not stop at Margiela's work, but could apply to a number of fashion designers, photographers and other fashion practitioners who explore humour and inversion in their work. Bakhtin's writing lends itself particularly well to an exploration of fashion practitioners, like the Belgian designer Walter van Beirendonck and the Paris based German designer Bernhard Willhelm, as well as the aforementioned Leigh Bowery, who explore bodily humour through strategies of inversion, debasement and degradation (Granata, 2008, 2009). Other experimental designers whose work calls for a Bakhtinian reading are Viktor & Rolf, thanks to their focus on inversion and commedia dell'arte characters (Evans and Frankel, 2008). Their spring/summer 2006 collection, titled 'Upside-Down', explored carnivalesque inversion both in its presentation, as well as through the actual garments, the construction of which was inverted. The theme was further explored in their Milan store, their first, where the furniture and mannequins were literally turned upside down and hung from the ceiling. Finally, ripe for exploration is the way the pop performer Lady Gaga has taken up the work of a number of experimental fashion designers. In collaboration with the well-known stylist Nicola Formichetti and the House of Gaga, she has often explored the grotesque canon in her costumes, perhaps most evidently in her various iterations of the meat dress.

CONCLUSION: FURTHER SUGGESTIONS

In this chapter I have discussed just a few of the ways in which Bakhtin's work applies to fashion – particularly contemporary and near contemporary experimental fashion – and, in turn, the ways in which the study of fashion expands and qualifies his thought. Bakhtin's work has much wider potential applications in the field of fashion studies than this chapter could contain, both historically and cross-culturally. His writings are of great relevance to a study of manner and dress throughout fashion history. A particularly poignant period for a further application of Bakhtin's thought to fashion would be the Renaissance, which the Russian scholar identified as an era of drastically shifting bodily norms and canons of behaviour. Another apt application of his thought would be the study of hybrid cultural forms and identities which can be observed in the overlap between fashion and performance. For instance, while teaching on the topic of Bakhtin and fashion, actual carnival costumes and performances in hybrid cultural spaces such as the Caribbean and Brazil, where carnival is still an influential cultural force, quickly became obvious and rich areas of research for students.[12] Another recurrent theme that transpires in my graduate seminars on the topic is how Bakhtinian thought opens a space for the re-inscription of the fat body in fashion, thus pointing to an important link between fashion studies and fat studies.[13]

In his focus on bodily boundaries, Bakhtin's writings also point to the area of intersection between medical history and fashion history and the way these two powerful discourses conceive and visualize the body. As my writings start to address, Bakhtin's thoughts could also be applied to an exploration of medicine, fashion and bodily boundaries. This could be read as explicated historically in the shifting borders between the body, medical devices and clothing as well as, in more contemporary terms, through an exploration of fashion and biomedical science and, in particular, immunology.

In conclusion, Bakhtin's work, particularly his writings on the grotesque and classical canon in *Rabelais*, provides the tools to examine fashion's unique position in upholding normality, while paradoxically also being the vehicle to exceed, upend or, to use Bakhtinian terminology, carnivalize ideals of norms and deviation. Conversely, the study of fashion, as Bakhtin himself recognized, constitutes a central area for an application of his theory, thanks to fashion's inextricable relation to the body and norms of behaviour. As seen in this chapter, through a visual and material culture approach, and by placing his writings on a continuum with a number of other disciplines engaged in discussions of body and the subject (i.e. gender studies, queer theory, disability studies, fat studies), fashion studies has the potential to ground and better-qualify his concepts.

NOTES

1   *Rabelais and His World* remained unpublished in Russia, and elsewhere, until 1965, due to its political charge.
2   The centrality of borders to the Bakhtinian grotesque has been pointed out by a number of scholars. See, for instance, Connelly (2003) as well as Stallybrass and White (1986).
3   I use the term gynophobia, as opposed to the more commonly used term misogyny, because it more aptly describes the fear of the maternal, the prefix *gyno* from the Greek *gyne*, woman, being often associated in the English language with female reproduction. It is also a more pliable term. It has been theorized as allowing for a greater agency on the part of women, and as implying a fear of femininity and of the maternal, which can be experienced regardless of gender or sexual orientation. For a recent assessment of the term, see Apter (1998: 102–22).
4   A number of scholars have pointed out the anticipatory nature of Bakhtin's thought and his relevance to discussions which are often located under the umbrella of post-modernism. On this point, see White (1987–1988: 217–1); Hutcheon (1989: 87–103) and Fiske (1991: 92–93).
5   For a discussion and a rebuke of Rabelais's work, and by extension Bakhtin's, as antifeminist, see respectively Wayne Booth's 'Freedom of Interpretation: Bakhtin

and the Challenge of Feminist Criticism' (1982: 45–76) and Richard M. Berrong's 'Finding Anti-Feminism in Rabelais or, A Response to Wayne Booth's Call for an Ethical Criticism' (1985: 687–97).

6 On the powersuit, see Entwistle (1997: 311–23).

7 For more information on the collection's reception, see Evans (2002–2003: 82–83) as well as Yaeger (1997).

8 Kristeva discusses motherhood as exemplary of the subject-in-process in her essay (originally published in 1977) 'Stabat Mater'. It is also in this piece that she advances her theory of a new ethic based on a new understanding of motherhood, which she calls an 'herethic'. *Strangers to Ourselves* also illustrates the process according to which an understanding and acceptance of ourselves as 'disintegrated' – once again as 'subjects-in-process' – allows for an acceptance of the other (Kristeva, 1991).

9 On this point, see Eagleton (1981) as well as Eco (1984).

10 For a more detailed discussion of the use of the term 'deconstruction' to refer to fashion, both in the journalistic and academic literature, see Granata (2013: 182–98).

11 Here Babcock is referring to Henri Bergson's well-known essay 'Laughter' (Bergson, 1966).

12 The relation between South American and Caribbean carnivals and Bakhtin's theory has been, however, discussed in relation to other cultural practices, as it is the instance in relation to Brazil and cinema with Robert Stam's 'Of Cannibals and Carnivals' (1989).

13 For an introduction to fat studies see Rothblum and Solovay (2009). Among the graduate students in my seminar, who employed Bakhtin to explore the connection of fat studies and fashion studies is Lauren Peters Downing, whose article on the interaction between the two areas of studies is forthcoming in *Fashion Theory*.

REFERENCES

Als, H. (30 March 1998) 'Life as a Look' in *The New Yorker*, 74 (6): 82–86.

Apter, E. (1998) 'Reflections on Gynophobia' in M. Merk et al. (ed), *Coming Out of Feminism*, Oxford: Blackwell Publishing.

Babcock, B.A. (ed) (1978) *The Reversible World: Symbolic Inversion in Art and Society*, Ithaca, NY: Cornell University Press.

Bakhtin, M. (1981 [1975]) *The Dialogical Imagination*, C. Emerson and M. Holquist (trans), Austin: University of Texas Press.

———(1984 [1963]) *The Problems of Dostoyevsky's Poetics*, C. Emerson (trans), Minneapolis: University of Minnesota Press.

———(1984 [1965]) *Rabelais and His World*, H. Iswolsky (trans), Bloomington: Indiana University Press.

Bergson, H. (1966) 'Laughter' in W. Sypher (ed), *Comedy*, New York: Doubleday Anchor Books.

Berrong, R.M. (1985) 'Finding Anti-Feminism in Rabelais: or, A Response to Wayne Booth's Call for an Ethical Criticism' in *Critical Inquiry*, 11 (4): 687–96.

Booth, W. (1982) 'Freedom of Interpretation: Bakhtin and the Challenge of Feminist Criticism' in *Critical Inquiry*, 9 (1): 45–76.

Calefato, P. (2004) 'Style and Styles between Fashion and the Grotesque' in *The Clothed Body*, Oxford: Berg.

Casadio, M. (2004) 'Georgina Godley' in M.L. Frisa and S. Tonchi (eds), *Excess: Fashion and the Underground in the 80s*, Milan: Charta.

Connelly, F. (ed) (2003) *Modern Art and the Grotesque*, Cambridge: Cambridge University Press.

Cunningham, B. (September 1989) 'The Collections' in *Details*.

Eagleton, T. (1981) *Criticism and Ideology: A Study in Marxist Literary Theory*, London: New Left Books.

Eco, U. (1984) 'Frames of Comic Freedom' in U. Eco, V.V. Ivanov and M. Rector, *Carnival!*, New York: Mouton Publishers.

Elias, N. (1994 [1939]) *The Civilizing Process*, Oxford: Blackwell.

Entwistle, J. (1997) '"Power Dressing" and the Construction of the Career Woman' in M. Nava et al. (ed), *Buy this Book: Studies in Advertising and Consumption*, London: Routledge.

Evans, C. (2002–2003) '"Dress becomes Body becomes Dress": Are you an Object or a Subject?' in *032c Magazine*, 4: 82–83.

———(2003) *Fashion at the Edge: Spectacle, Modernity, and Deathliness*, New Haven, CT: Yale University Press.

——— and Frankel, A. (2008) *The House of Viktor & Rolf*, London: Merrell and the Barbican Gallery.

Fiske, J. (1991) 'Offensive Bodies and Carnival Pleasures' in *Understanding Popular Culture*, London: Routledge.

Gamman, L. (2000) 'Visual Seduction and Perverse Compliance: Reviewing Food Fantasies, Large Appetites and "Grotesque" Bodies' in S. Bruzzi and P. Church Gibson (eds), *Fashion Cultures: Theories, Explorations and Analysis*, London: Routledge.

Gardiner, M. and Mayerfeld Bell, M. (eds) (1998) *Bakhtin and the Human Sciences*, London: Sage.

Gindt, D. (2011) 'Björk's Creative Collaborations with the World of Fashion' in *Fashion Theory*, 15 (4): 425–50.

Granata, F. (2008) 'Fashion of Inversions: The Grotesque and the Carnivalesque in Contemporary Belgian Fashion' in *Modus Operandi: State of Affairs in Current Research on Belgian Fashion*, Antwerp: ModeMuseum.

———(2009) 'Fashioning the Grotesque' in F. Granata, H. Ingeborg and S. van der Zijpp, *Bernhard Willhelm and Jutta Kraus*, Amsterdam: NAI Publishers.

———(2010) *The Bakhtinian Grotesque in Fashion at the Turn of the Twenty-First Century* [PhD Thesis], London: University of the Arts.

———(2013) 'Deconstruction Fashion: Carnival and the Grotesque' in *The Journal of Design History*, 26 (2): 182–98.

Hutcheon, L. (1989) 'Modern Parody and Bakhtin' in G.S. Morson and C. Emerson (eds), *Rethinking Bakhtin: Extensions and Challenges*, Evanston, IL: Northwestern University Press.

Kayser, W. (1963) *The Grotesque in Art and Literature*, Bloomington: Indiana University Press.

Kristeva, J. (1984) *Revolution in Poetic Language*, M. Waller (trans), New York: Columbia University Press.

———(1987) *Tales of Love*, L.S. Roudiez (trans), New York: Columbia University Press.

———(1991) *Strangers to Ourselves*, L.S. Roudiez (trans), New York: Columbia University Press.

Kunzle, D. (1982) *Fashion and Fetishism: A Social History of the Corset, Tight-Lacing, and other Forms of Body Sculpture in the West*, Totowo, NJ: Rowman and Littlefield Publishers.

Martin, E. (1998) 'The Fetus as Intruder: Mother's Bodies and Medical Metaphors' in R. Davis-Floyd and J. Dumit (eds), Cyborg Babies: From Techno-sex to Techno-tots, New York: Routledge.

Oliver, K. (1993) Reading Kristeva: Unravelling the Double-Bind, Bloomington: Indiana University Press.

———(2012) Knock Me Up, Knock Me Down: Images of Pregnancy in Hollywood Films, New York: Columbia University Press.

Purdy, D.L. (ed) (2004) The Rise of Fashion, Minneapolis: University of Minnesota Press.

Rothblum, E. and Solovay, S. (ed) (2009) The Fat Studies Reader, New York: New York University Press.

Russo, M. (1995) The Female Grotesque: Risk, Excess, and Modernity, New York: Routledge.

Stallybrass, P. and White, A. (1986) The Politics and Poetics of Transgression, Ithaca, NY: Cornell University Press.

Stam, R. (1989) Subversive Pleasures: Bakhtin, Cultural Criticism, and Film, Baltimore, MD: Johns Hopkins University Press.

Steele, V. (2001) The Corset: A Cultural History, New Haven, CT: Yale University Press.

White, A. (1987–1988) 'The Struggle Over Bakhtin: Fraternal Reply to Robert Young' in Cultural Critique, (8): 217–41.

Yaeger, L. (1 April 1997) 'Material World: Padded Sell' in The Village Voice.

7

MAURICE MERLEAU-PONTY
The Corporeal Experience of Fashion

Llewellyn Negrin

INTRODUCTION

Fashion, by dint of the fact that it is designed to be worn, is inextricably linked with the body. Yet until recently, much analysis of fashion has tended to neglect the experience of dress as a tactile and embodied form, treating it primarily as a 'text' to be decoded semiotically or as an image to be analysed in terms of its aesthetic form. As such, it has been viewed as a purely visual phenomenon while the nature of its interaction with the body of the wearer has been overlooked. In the process, what has been ignored is that fashion is not just about the creation of a specific 'look', but is also about the comportment of the body in space. Particular garments are significant not just for the meanings they communicate or for their aesthetic appearance, but because they produce certain modes of bodily demeanour.

This chapter discusses how the phenomenology of Maurice Merleau-Ponty, which foregrounds the embodied nature of our experience of the world, can be used to address this aspect of fashion. Central to Merleau-Ponty's phenomenology is an awareness of the body not as a passive receptor of outside stimuli, but rather, as the medium through which we experience the world. As Merleau-Ponty has made clear, our bodies are not simply inert objects existing independently of our minds; they are rather the very means through which we come to know the world and articulate our sense of self. His phenomenology, as will be demonstrated, provides us with the theoretical tools with which to address fashion not simply as an aesthetic or symbolic phenomenon but as a haptic experience.

MERLEAU-PONTY'S THEORY OF EMBODIED EXISTENCE

Merleau-Ponty (1908–1961), a French philosopher, developed his theory of embodied existence during the 1940s and 1950s through major works such as The Phenomenology of Perception, The Primacy of Perception, The Prose of the World and The Visible and the Invisible. Building on the phenomenology (i.e. the study of phenomena) of fellow philosophers Edmund Husserl and Martin Heidegger, and Jean-Paul Sartre's existentialism, he emphasized the body as the primary site of knowing the world, grounding our experience of the world in our practical engagement with it. In doing so, he sought to counter the mind–body dualism which has underpinned the tradition of Western philosophy.

For Merleau-Ponty, it is fundamentally mistaken to conceive of the body as a thing that exists apart from us, which can be appraised by us in much the same way as other objects in the world, for, unlike other objects, our bodies never leave us. Rather, they are the medium through which we come to know and experience the world and as such, they are an inextricable part of our being-in-the-world. The idea that we can somehow subject our bodies to scrutiny from an external viewpoint is based on the mistaken premise that the mind can be separated from the body. The mind, however, does not have an existence independently of us as sentient beings, as presupposed by Cartesian dualism, but is always-already embodied. Our sense of ourselves as inhabiting a body is not something that happens after the fact, but is ever-present. As Merleau-Ponty writes:

> The perceiving mind is an incarnated mind. I have tried [...] to re-establish the roots of the mind in its body and in its world, going against doctrines which treat perception as a simple result of the action of external things on our body as well as against those which insist on the autonomy of consciousness.
>
> (Merleau-Ponty, 1964: 3–4) [my emphasis]

When we engage with the world, Merleau-Ponty argues (1962: vii–xxi, 73–89), we do so not on the basis of a purely mental construct in the manner of Descartes' cogito or on the basis of a pre-existing ideational framework as Kantian idealism contends, but rather, by means of implicit forms of practical knowledge that have become concretized into habitual bodily schemas. It is these practical forms of knowledge which are embedded in our corporeal being that direct our interaction with the world. The mind is situated in the body and it is through our corporeal schemas that we come to know the world. Thus, rather than being 'an object in the world', the body forms 'our point of view on the world' (Merleau-Ponty, 1964: 5). External stimuli do not impact on the body in a causal, mechanistic fashion, but are actively mediated by these habitual patterns of behaviour. While in certain circumstances we can become conscious of these to some extent, generally they operate in a largely unconscious and taken-for-granted way, constituting the foundation for our active orientation towards the world.

Even when we appraise ourselves in a more self-conscious way in the mirror, our image of ourselves is never totally disconnected from our haptic experience of the physical body that we inhabit. Rather, the visual and the tactile are always inextricably intertwined. As Merleau-Ponty writes, the image of myself in the mirror:

> refers me back to an original of the body which is not out there among things but in my own province, on this side of all things seen [...]. What prevents its ever being an object is that it is that by which there are objects [...]. The body is not an object in the world but our means of communication with it. It is the horizon latent in all our experience and itself ever-present and anterior to every determining thought.
>
> (Merleau-Ponty, 1962: 91–92)

Thus, we can never totally step outside our bodies and view them as objects apart from ourselves. The awareness we have of our bodies is not just determined by the visual image that we have of ourselves, but more fundamentally, by the kinaesthetic sense that we have of our bodies, acquired through our physical engagement with the world. This for example explains the phenomenon of the phantom limb, where the amputee still experiences the presence of the missing limb despite the visual evidence that attests to its absence. The amputee continues to have a bodily memory of his or her capacities prior to the amputation, which contradicts what he or she sees (Merleau-Ponty 1962: 80–82). This pre-reflective way of experiencing the body is thus more primary than the conscious appraisal of the body as an object of the gaze and is the ground on which the latter is predicated.

Merleau-Ponty argues further that, just as our experience of the world is mediated through the body, so the body cannot be experienced independently of the world. The body exists in relation to the space that it inhabits rather than being totally separate from it. It is always 'emplaced' in a world that is occupied by objects and by other embodied subjects. The space one occupies does not appear as something apart from oneself, but rather, is defined in relation to the practical tasks one is undertaking. Thus, one develops a consciousness of one's body only through one's practical engagement with the world. As he writes:

> my body appears to me as an attitude directed towards a certain existing or possible task. Its spatiality is not, like that of external objects or like that of 'spatial sensations', a spatiality of position, but a spatiality of situation. The word 'here', applied to my body does not refer to a determinate position in relation to other positions or to external coordinates, but the laying down of first coordinates, the anchoring of the active body in an object, the situation of the body in the face of its tasks.
>
> (Merleau-Ponty, 1962: 100)

In our interactions with the world, the objects we encounter do not appear as 'mute' things but have significance insofar as they relate to our practical projects. As such, they cannot be understood apart from us, and our meaningful engagement with them.

This applies not just to our interaction with the physical environment but also to our interchange with other people. In Merleau-Ponty's conception, the body is fundamentally social in nature since we come to an understanding of ourselves through our interaction with others. The body does not exist apart from the social world, which then impinges upon it from the outside but rather, is always-already implicated in the world with which it actively engages. Like the natural world, the social world, argues Merleau-Ponty:

> [does not exist] as an object or sum of objects, but as a permanent field or dimension of existence: I may well turn away from it, but not cease to be situated relatively to it. Our relationship to the social is, like our relationship to the world, deeper than any express perception or any judgement. It is as false to place ourselves in society as an object among other objects, as it is to place society within ourselves as an object of thought, and in both cases the mistake lies in treating the social as an object. We must return to the social with which we are in contact by the mere act of existing, and which we carry about inseparably with us before any objectification.
>
> (Merleau-Ponty, 1962: 362)

No longer conceived as separate from each other, the relation between individuals and the social world they inhabit is one of mutual determination. Individuals cannot be conceived of simply as the passive receptacles of externally imposed cultural codes, or conversely, as entirely free agents who can fashion the world in an autonomous way. Rather, they find themselves already situated in a world that shapes them at the same time as they engage with it.

Our corporeal schemas, then, are not wholly internal to us, but neither are they simply imposed upon us from the outside. Instead, the process is a reciprocal one in which our haptic awareness of ourselves both shapes and is mediated by the situations we encounter. As Merleau-Ponty puts it: 'the body not only flows over into a world whose schema it bears in itself, but possesses this world at a distance rather than being possessed by it' (1973:78). Being fundamentally inter-subjective in nature, our corporeal schemas are always being modified as a result of our interactions with others – a point emphasized by Gail Weiss in her discussion of Merleau-Ponty's phenomenology. As she argues, a central feature of Merleau-Ponty's conception of the body schema is its intercorporeal nature in which body images are 'constructed through a series of corporeal exchanges that take place both within and outside of specific bodies' (Weiss, 1999: 2). One's awareness of one's body is not just influenced by physiological changes in the body or by physical changes in the environment in which one finds oneself but also through one's encounters with others.

The body then, in Merleau-Ponty's phenomenology, can be understood more properly not as an object, which stands over against the world, but as a process, which is forever in a state of becoming, continually being made and re-made. Individuals do not passively internalize cultural systems of meaning, which are imposed upon them from the outside. Rather, there is an active process of mediation between the two in which each is modified by the other. Through our corporeal schema, we engage with the social/cultural world at the same time that we are constituted by it.

MERLEAU-PONTY AND THE NEW MATERIALISM

Merleau-Ponty's phenomenology has gained new currency in contemporary theorizations of the body. One of the most significant features in recent writings on the body has been the emphasis on its material or 'corporeal' nature. While social theorists have paid much attention to the constitution of the body by culture, there has been a tendency to view the body simply as an effect of social systems of signification while its fleshly nature has been neglected. In conceiving of the body as being constructed in and through cultural codes, its materiality has been almost totally subsumed by the textual and the discursive. It is this lacuna that the new materialism seeks to address in highlighting the fact that while the body is mediated by cultural systems of meaning, it is irreducible to these.

In seeking to draw attention to the bodily substrate through which our interaction with cultural systems of meaning is mediated, a number of theorists (for example Crossley, 1995, and Csordas, 1999) have enlisted the insights of Merleau-Ponty's phenomenology. Thus, for instance, Nick Crossley's endeavour to develop a carnal sociology which shifts the focus from an analysis of the various techniques through which the body has been constituted by culture towards an analysis of the active role of the body in social life, is underpinned by Merleau-Ponty's recognition of the fact that 'our body is our way of being-in-the-world, of experiencing and belonging to the world' (Crossley, 1995: 48). As he argues, Merleau-Ponty's acknowledgement of the inescapably embodied nature of existence provides the basis on which we can overcome the reductionistic conception of the body as a passive receptor of culture rather than as an active mediator of it. To quote him:

> [For Merleau-Ponty] perception is based in behavior; that is, in looking, listening and touching, etc. as acquired, cultural, habit-based forms of conduct. The perceiving body constitutes itself as such, [...] by implementing acquired perceptual schemas. It does not passively receive messages from the world but actively interrogates the world, in terms of the cultural schemas which it has acquired.
>
> (Crossley, 1995: 47)

While the body does not exist prior to or independently of its inscription by culture, neither is it simply a product of it. Rather, there is a dialectical relationship between the two in which each presupposes the other while at the same time they are irreducible to each other. As Crossley explains, Merleau-Ponty's phenomenology overcomes the false duality between the body as discursive object on the one hand and fleshly being on the other by conceiving of it as an active agent which engages with the world on the basis of a stock of cultural skills and techniques which it has acquired. 'He allows us to understand that human agent-subjects are bodies and that bodies are sensible-sentient, communicative, practical and intelligent beings' (Crossley, 1995: 60).

Indicative of this new materialist approach to the body, the emphasis has shifted from analyses of cultural representations of the body (i.e. the body as image) to an examination of how the body is experienced in a corporeal way (i.e. the 'felt' body). While in our media-saturated environment where the image reigns supreme, there has been a great emphasis on the construction of the body as visual spectacle, this does not capture the way we experience our bodies as physical beings who move in space. As Mike Featherstone argues, the concept of 'body image' as a purely mental construct in terms of which we fashion ourselves is problematic insofar as it reduces the individual to a disembodied consciousness that views the body as an entity apart from the self. In doing so, it fails to do justice to the fact that we habitually experience our bodies not as objects, which we appraise in a purely cognitive way, but as fleshly entities that are inseparable from us (Featherstone, 2010). To quote him:

> The conception of the reflexive body as our seeing platform and, at the same time, as seen and judged by others, misses the ways in which the body in everyday life is lived in habitual ways and not constantly subjected to the instrumental gaze of the consumer culture technicians [...]. Much of human life is lived in a non-cognitive world in which the body cannot be reduced to a body image, an individual unitary or organic body, the surface for society to fill with signs.
>
> (Featherstone, 2010: 207–8)

He proposes, then, that rather than focusing simply on the visual presentation of the body, more attention needs to be given to the ways in which the body moves in space. Bodily demeanour communicates in powerful ways that can override the surface appearance of the body. In this context, Merleau-Ponty's concept of 'body schema' provides a useful alternative to that of 'body image' as it relates to an embodied repertoire of sensory-motor capacities rather than a set of purely mental constructs as implied by the concept of body image.

TOWARDS A THEORY OF FASHION AS EMBODIED PRACTICE

This materialist turn is also evident in recent fashion theory, where Merleau-Ponty's recognition of the fundamentally embodied nature of existence has been embraced by a number of theorists such as Iris Marion Young, Joanne Entwistle and Paul Sweetman, who have sought to apply his insights to the analysis of the corporeal aspects of dress. In particular, they draw attention to the ways in which body adornment is experienced by its wearers not just as a visual phenomenon, but also as a haptic experience. Their concern is to demonstrate how the adoption of a particular form of attire is not just about the creation of a certain 'look', but is a way of being-in-the-world, which transcends the visual. Clothes, in this view, become a prosthetic extension of the body, mediating our practical interaction with the world through their incorporation into our bodily schemas.

In her application of Merleau-Ponty's phenomenology to the analysis of women's lived experience of dress, Iris Marion Young seeks to highlight the gendered nature of our experience of corporeality – something which Merleau-Ponty neglects in his own account. Thus, in her essay 'Women Recovering our Clothes', she focuses on the sensuous pleasures clothes can provide for women that are not structured around the male gaze but which reside in the tactility of garments. While most attention has been paid to the look of female fashions and how they appear to others, there has been far less focus on the haptic qualities of clothing and how these are experienced by wearers. It has been assumed that women's pleasure in dress is a secondary one which derives from them vicariously placing themselves in the same position as the putative male spectator, that is, they would only experience pleasure through their internalization of the objectifying male gaze, seeing themselves as others see them (Young, 1994).

Young suggests, however, that beyond the ubiquity of idealized images of women in the mass media, there is a female pleasure in dress that is not dependent on the male gaze: the pleasure of touch. This is a pleasure that can be experienced directly by the wearer without the mediation of the male spectator. Unlike sight, which is the most distancing of the senses, in which the subject is separate from the object, with the sense of touch there is no separation between subject and object, since they are in direct proximity to each other. As she describes it:

> Less concerned with identifying things, comparing them, measuring them in their relations to one another, touch immerses the subject in fluid continuity with the object, and for the touching subject the object touched reciprocates the touching, blurring the border between self and other.
>
> (Young, 1994: 204)

Touch encompasses not just the feel of fabric on skin but also 'an orienta-tion to sensuality as such that includes all the senses' (ibid.). Often it is the texture of the material and the cut of a garment, rather than simply its look, which attracts us, such as the warmth and feel of a wool jacket or the volu-minous nature of a skirt that swirls around our bodies as we walk.

Young continues this focus on the gendered nature of corporeal experi-ence in her essay 'Breasted Experience', where she argues that the appraisal of breasts as objects to be judged in terms of idealized media images of what they ought to be, does not adequately account for how women experience their breasts. Ultimately, women do not view their breasts simply as objects separate from themselves, despite their widespread fetishization in our cul-ture, since they cannot totally disconnect themselves from their experience of them as part of their corporeal being (Young, 1990).

As in her essay 'Women Recovering our Clothes', Young proceeds to ana-lyse this embodied experience in terms of the sense of touch rather than sight on the basis that 'from the position of the female subject, what matters most about her breasts is their feeling and sensitivity rather than how they look' (Young, 1990: 194). From this point of view, she criticizes the bra as an item of clothing that serves as a barrier to touch, moulding the breasts in accordance with the patriarchal ideal of them as round and firm in appear-ance. While such breasts may be considered to look more attractive, breasts unrestricted by the bra have a greater sensitivity to touch and are more fluid and malleable, changing in response to the body's position and movements. As such, they are experienced as an integral part of the woman's body rather than as the firm, unyielding objects that phallocentric culture posits as the norm.

Cosmetic surgery is premised on a similar objectification of the breasts where the primary emphasis is on modifying the shape of the breasts in order to attain the desired 'look'. In patriarchal culture, as Young writes, '[w]hat matters most is how breasts look and measure, their conformity with a norm, the impossible aesthetic of round, large and high on the chest. These objectifying constructions are clearly manifest in surgical medicine's angle on the breast' (Young, 1990: 201).

This emphasis on the appearance of breasts, as Young points out, is a male-centric view, which fails to acknowledge the importance of the feeling and sensitivity of breasts for women – factors unrelated to their size or the way they look. Indeed, cosmetic surgery often results in a loss of sensitivity in the breasts and in the sensation of them as 'foreign' objects unrelated to the self, because of their lack of mobility or malleability. Thus, the attainment of a 'sexier' look is at the expense of women's own sensual experience of their breasts.

Like Young, Entwistle's examination of female dress focuses on the corporeal experience of women themselves rather than on visual representations of the idealized body. Her primary concern is to provide an account of women's dress as 'situated bodily practice', analysing how it is lived, experienced and embodied by its wearers (Entwistle, 2000a: 28–35).

Her analysis of the dress of the career woman exemplifies this. Here she draws attention to the different ways in which men and women experience the spaces of work and how this impacts on women's dress practices. As she argues, in entering what was previously a male-dominated arena, the professional woman has to negotiate two contradictory imperatives – on the one hand, she has to dress in such a way as to minimize her sexuality in order to command the respect of her colleagues, while on the other, she needs to maintain her femininity and not appear too masculine (Entwistle, 2000b).

The first of these imperatives is particularly challenging for women since they have traditionally been more closely identified with their bodies than have men. While men are seen to occupy the transcendent realm of the intellect, women remain bound by their carnality. Thus, when women don the 'female' equivalent of the business suit (i.e. the tailored jacket and matching skirt), which is designed to de-eroticize the body, they still continue to be regarded in a more sexual way than their male counterparts. Consequently, they tend to be more self-conscious than men about their dress in the workplace, taking particular care to ensure their appearance is not sexually provocative in any way. For instance, they may wear a jacket to cover their breasts when attending an important business meeting. At the same time, they have to be careful not to appear too masculine, since this could be interpreted as too direct a challenge to male authority. Thus, in their adoption of the business suit, the tailored skirt is preferred to trousers and is frequently teamed with other 'feminine' elements such as a blouse made from soft, silky fabric, scarves, discreet jewellery and high-heeled shoes.

This demonstrates clearly how the gendered nature of the body of the wearer impacts on the clothing that is worn. The body is not a neutral surface onto which signs are imprinted, but has its own materiality, which influences the way clothes are experienced both by the wearer and by those around them. It also makes evident how our sartorial practices are modulated by the spatial and temporal context within which they take place. The decisions about what to wear and how to wear it always occur in relation to a particular situation within which individuals find themselves and cannot be understood in isolation from this.

While Entwistle focuses on women's corporeal experience of dress, Sweetman turns his attention to the practice of tattooing. Critical of the over-emphasis on the semiotic dimension of body adornment in the analysis of youth subcultures, he highlights the significance of the visceral experience of tattooing. As he argues, what is of central importance to the wearers of tattoos is the bodily process of their acquisition rather than the meanings that they convey (Sweetman, 2001a, 2001b). If their primary purpose were simply to communicate a particular message, then a 'fake' tattoo applied to the surface of the skin would be just as effective as a real one. However, this is clearly not the case when one analyses how they function amongst communities of tattooees.

As Sweetman discovered through his study of tattoo wearers, the physical process of their acquisition was just as significant, if not more important, than the finished product. For many, the acquisition of tattoos was considered a cathartic experience, which also served as a means of creating a sense of intercorporeal bonding between fellow wearers (Sweetman, 2001a: 189). Drawing on Michel Maffesoli's analysis of 'neo-tribes' in contemporary society, Sweetman argues that affiliations between individuals are increasingly based on affective ties rather than on shared, cognitively defined goals as in the past (Sweetman, 2001b: 70–71). This is particularly the case amongst youth subcultures where many of the shared activities are centred on the body, such as dancing or riding motorbikes. Tattooing is another of these bodily rituals that gives rise to a sense of affinity between those who have shared this experience. Rather than being simply expressive of such ties, these practices are constitutive of them.

As the analyses of Young, Entwistle and Sweetman clearly demonstrate, the corporeal dimension of our practices of body adornment is central to our experience of fashion. Modes of self-presentation cannot be understood simply in terms of the symbolic meanings they communicate or in purely aesthetic terms, but also need to be considered as an integral aspect of our bodily being-in-the-world.

This is also evident in the work of a number of recent designers of fashion and jewellery such as Issey Miyake, Rei Kawakubo and Naomi Filmer, who are concerned not just with the creation of a new 'look' but with different ways of comporting the body in space. In their investigation of the relation between clothing and the body that inhabits it, their work shows a striking convergence with Merleau-Ponty's conception of embodied being.

PHENOMENOLOGICAL APPROACHES IN RECENT FASHION DESIGN

Miyake's and Kawakubo's concern with the kinaesthetic experience of dress is informed by a Japanese sensibility which conceives of the relation between clothing and the body in a very different manner than the Western tradition. Whereas in Western fashion, the shape of garments is generally fixed by the often elaborate tailoring involved in the making of them, the garments of Miyake and Kawakubo are drawn from the Japanese tradition of wrapping fabric around the body, as Richard Martin points out (Martin, 1995: 215). This allows for a much more fluid and organic relationship between the fabric and the body in which the garment is constantly changing its form in response to the movements of the body. Rather than the body being constricted by the fitted garment as occurs in Western fashion, the designs of Miyake and Kawakubo allow for a greater range of movement. Instead of being constructed around an aesthetic of revelation and concealment, their clothes invoke a kinaesthetic sense of the body in motion, which takes them beyond the Western conception of fashion as a primarily visual art form. Their forms are not conceived of as static, visual representations, but rather as dynamic, three-dimensional sculptures which are constantly being re-formed by the body that inhabits them. Martin describes the difference between the two approaches thus:

> With a layering, cloaking propensity offered as a fundamental alternative to tailored clothing comes as well a completely different body vis-à-vis clothing expression, subverting or at least posing an option for dress beyond the simple erotics and mechanics of underlying and visible body. Wilful scorn of tailoring is also indicative of a nonchalance and preference for the irregular and unconstrained with clothing composed on the body in a kind of informal pastiche.
>
> (Martin, 1995: 215)

In keeping with this, Miyake has commented that his clothes are unfinished since the design isn't completed until someone puts them on (Calloway, 1988: 51). This is encapsulated by the Japanese concept of *fusoku-shugi*, where expressiveness inheres in what is omitted or left out. The incompleteness of Miyake's garments invites the active engagement of the wearers, who re-configure them in ways that suit their own bodies. To quote Miyake: 'My clothes can become part of someone, part of them physically. Maybe I make tools. People buy the clothes and they become tools for the wearer's creativity' (Miyake in Calloway, 1988: 16). Just as for Merleau-Ponty, objects cannot be understood independently of the subject's practical interaction with them, so Miyake's garments are activated by the body of the wearer. Often, Miyake's garments are seamless, hollow forms, which appear as shapeless sacks when not worn. Once inhabited by the body of the wearer, however, their 'personality' emerges. The capacity of Miyake's garments to metamorphose themselves is heightened by such features as the use of pleats, which increases the ability of the garments to expand and contract in concert with the movements of the body (Holborn, 1995: 81–82) and also by the use of soft, lightweight, flexible fabrics such as polyester jersey and Pewlon – an acrylic knit (Holborn, 1995: 30, 36).

Similarly, in Kawakubo's work we see a reciprocal relationship between clothing and the body in which the garment is animated by the body of the wearer at the same time as it influences the wearer's bodily demeanour. This is evident in her 'Body Meets Dress–Dress Meets Body' collection from 1997. In this collection, which consists of a range of outfits made from stretch fabrics with padded protuberances in odd places, the boundaries between the body and dress are blurred such that the garments become a prosthetic extension of the body rather than being separable from it. Clothing and body become indistinguishable from each other as the soft and malleable padded additions filled with goose down change shape in concert with the movement of the wearers. Here, dress is treated not as an object which exists independently of the body and which is subsequently inhabited by it, but as inextricably intertwined with it. Neither can be understood apart from the other as the garments meld imperceptibly with the wearers' bodies.

As with Miyake, Kawakubo's primary concern here is with the ways in which clothing interacts with the body and the corporeal experience of wearing the garments. In an era where prosthetic devices are increasingly being incorporated into our bodily schema as a result of advances in medical technology, Kawakubo's outfits explore new possibilities of embodiment that blur the boundaries between the animate and the inanimate. As Caroline Evans writes, Kawakubo's padded extensions 'sketch new possibilities of subjecthood, a subjecthood which [is] not concerned with containing the body but with extending it, via new networks and new communications' (Evans, 2003: 269).

Contemporary British jewellery designer Naomi Filmer is also interested in exploring the interface between forms of adornment and the body, designing accessories that are integrally related to the contours of the body.

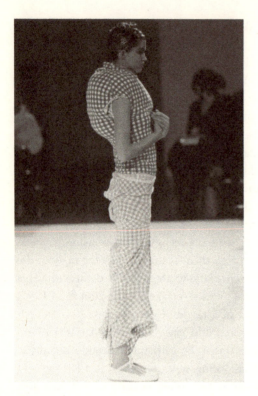

7.1 Rei Kawakubo, outfit from the 'Body Meets Dress–Dress Meets Body' collection, 1997.

Far from being items with their own independent existence, her pieces are an extension of the wearer's body, challenging the clear-cut distinction between self and other.

This is exemplified by her series *Breathing Volume*, 2008, which consists of a series of four items focused on the mouth, chin, and neck areas of the body. Each piece takes as its starting point an imprint of the mouth, chin and neck, and evolves into an organic, oval-like form, which is suggestive of the breath's volume and path through the body. As Filmer explains, the sweeping, linear forms traced by these objects explore the 'balance between interior and exterior, positive and negative space, presence and absence of the body' (Filmer cited in Brüderlin and Lütgens, 2011: 100). Even when not worn on the body, these forms are highly suggestive of the absent body as they circumscribe the negative space of the parts of the body to which they refer. They also describe an association between a volume of space and the body. Just as architecture is interested in the relation between the built environment and the body's interaction with this space, so Filmer's pieces

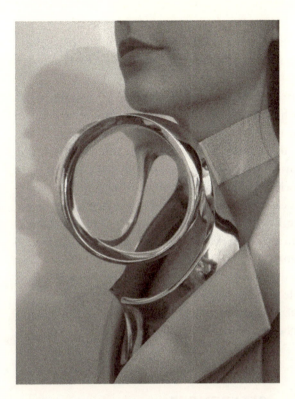

7.2 Naomi Filmer, Orchid Neck Piece, 2008 for Anne Valerie Hash.

explore the relation between the body and the space it occupies, echoing Merleau-Ponty's conception of the body as always-already emplaced. In giving form to the invisible space encompassing those areas where women normally do not wear jewellery, such as under the chin or in the small of the back, Filmer's accessories explore new experiences of embodiment which extend the body's boundaries in a way that is analogous to Kawakubo's padded garments.

CONCLUSION

As the foregoing discussion has demonstrated, fashion designers as well as theorists of fashion are focusing increasingly on dress and adornment not just as a visual phenomenon, but also as a corporeal experience. In this context, Merleau-Ponty's phenomenology, which draws attention to the fundamentally embodied nature of our engagement with the world, provides us with the theoretical tools with which to address our haptic engagement with dress. In doing so, it serves as an effective counter to the objectification of the body in contemporary culture where it is reduced to its outward appearance.

While Merleau-Ponty himself does not specifically address the phenomenon of fashion in his writings, or deal with the ways in which our embodied experience is impacted by such factors as gender, nevertheless his recognition of our fundamentally practical orientation to the world provides a solid basis on which to analyse dress as situated bodily experience. In our image-conscious culture, where the focus is on how we look, Merleau-Ponty's phenomenology reminds us that beyond the body as object of spectacle there is the lived body, which encompasses our kinaesthetic sense of ourselves. From this perspective, it is clear that dress cannot be adequately understood apart from our experience of wearing it. Rather than regarding it as a disembodied form, it can more properly be seen as a second skin, which is inseparable from us. When we act in the world, we do not act just as bodies, but as *clothed* bodies, in which our attire becomes an integral part of our corporeal schema, influencing the ways in which we comport ourselves in space.

REFERENCES

Brüderlin, M. and Lütgens, A. (eds) (2011) *Art & Fashion: Between Skin and Clothing*, Bielefeld: Kerber.

Calloway, N. (ed) (1988) *Issey Miyake: Photographs by Irving Penn*, New York: New York Graphic Society.

Crossley, N. (1995) 'Merleau-Ponty, the Elusive Body and Carnal Sociology' in *Body & Society*, 1 (1): 43–63.

Csordas, T.J. (1999) 'Embodiment and Cultural Phenomenology' in G. Weiss and H.F. Haber (eds), *Perspectives on Embodiment: The Intersections of Nature and Culture*, New York and London: Routledge.

Entwistle, J. (2000a) *The Fashioned Body: Theorizing Fashion and Dress in Modern Society*, Cambridge: Polity.

———(2000b) 'Fashioning the Career Woman: Power Dressing as a Strategy of Consumption' in M. Talbot and M. Andrews (eds), *All the World and Her Husband: Women and Consumption in the Twentieth Century*, London: Cassell.

Evans, C. (2003) *Fashion at the Edge*, New Haven, CT and London: Yale University Press.

Featherstone, M. (2010) 'Body, Image and Affect in Consumer Culture' in *Body & Society*, 16 (1): 193–221.

Holborn, M. (1995) *Issey Miyake*, Cologne: Benedikt Taschen.

Martin, R. (1995) 'Our Kimono Mind: Reflections on "Japanese Design: A Survey since 1950"' in *Journal of Design History*, 8 (3): 215–23.

Merleau-Ponty, M. (1962 [1945]) *The Phenomenology of Perception*, London: Routledge and Kegan Paul.

——(1964) *The Primacy of Perception*, Evanston, IL: Northwestern University Press.

——(1964 [1968]) *The Visible and the Invisible*, A. Lingis (trans), Evanston, IL: Northwestern University Press.

——(1973 [1969]) *The Prose of the World*, Evanston, IL: Northwestern University Press.

Sweetman, P. (2001a) 'Stop Making Sense?: The Problem of the Body in Youth/Sub/Counter-Culture' in S. Cunningham-Burley (ed), *Exploring the Body*, Basingstoke: Palgrave.

——(2001b) 'Shop-Window Dummies?' in J. Entwistle and E. Wilson (eds), *Body Dressing*, Oxford and New York: Berg.

Weiss, G. (1999) *Body Images: Embodiment as Intercorporeality*, London and New York: Routledge.

Young, I.M. (1990) 'Breasted Experience' in I.M. Young (ed), *Throwing Like a Girl and other Essays in Feminist Philosophy and Social Theory*, Bloomington: Indiana University Press.

——(1994) 'Women Recovering our Clothes' in S. Benstock and S. Ferriss (eds), *On Fashion*, New Brunswick, NJ: Rutgers University Press.

8

ROLAND BARTHES
Semiology and the Rhetorical Codes of Fashion

Paul Jobling

[When] we look at image-clothing, we read a described garment.

(Barthes, 1967)

INTRODUCTION

Between 1957 and 1969 Roland Barthes (1915–1980) produced a considerable body of work about the codes of fashion in relation to 'material, photography, language' (Barthes, 2006: 99) for various academic and popular journals, including *Annales*, *Revue Française de Sociologie* and *Marie Claire*.[1] Written under the influence of Berthold Brecht, whom he admired for his ability to fuse Marxist analysis with a reflection 'upon *effects of the sign*: a very rare thing', Barthes' concern is with semiological analysis (Barthes, 1971: 95). At the heart of his inquiry, therefore, is the hypothesis that real clothing – that is, what we wear in our everyday existence – is secondary to the ways in which it can be articulated in the verbal and iconic rhetoric of fashion editorials and fashion spreads: 'Without discourse there is no total Fashion, no essential Fashion' (Barthes, 1990: xi).

The centrepiece of this semiological approach to how garments are translated into language is the book *The Fashion System* (*Système de la Mode*, 1967), where he propounds a particular method for reading or decoding the fashion magazine as a generator of what is fashionable and what is not, an idea which he neatly sums up in the lapidary phrase 'the magazine is a machine that makes Fashion' (Barthes, 1990: 51). Hence, he attempts to uncover why and how it is that apparently trivial phrases like 'This year fuzzy fabrics replace shaggy ones' take on a force that is at once authoritative and mythological.

But there are other essays about fashion by Barthes that, while they do not take an overtly semiological approach, proffer trenchant aperçus about the social and cultural impact of clothes and clothing and echo two of the central ideas he deals with in *The Fashion System*: the transformative potential of the smallest clothing detail and the tension between past and present styles.[2] In 'Dandyism and Fashion' (1962), for instance, he singularly concentrates on male dress as a matter of technique, arguing the crucial role of the detail – what he calls the certain 'je ne sais quoi' (the knot on a cravat or the buttons on a waistcoat) – as the signifiers of the quintessentially individualistic dandy, who 'would *conceive* his outfit exactly like a modern artist might conceive a composition using available materials' (Barthes, 2006: 68). Since the onset of ready-to-wear clothing and the widespread diffusion of fashionable styles, he concludes that such uniqueness is virtually impossible to sustain; that the rise of fashion as a widespread phenomenon, paradoxically, put pay to the radical stance of original dandies like Beau Brummell (Barthes, 2006: 69). And in 'The Contest between Chanel and Courrèges' (1967) he compares the two designers from a similar angle, professing Chanel's garments 'challenge the very idea of fashion' by introducing only subtle variations in any given year, while in contrast, Courrèges always subverts her sense of 'chic' by gravitating each season to the 'absolute new' (Barthes, 2006: 106). By the same measure, in key pieces of writing such as 'Myth Today' (1957, in Barthes 1973a), 'The Photographic Message' (1961, in Barthes 1978), 'The Semantics of the Object' (1964, in Barthes 1994), 'The Advertising Message' (1964, in Barthes 1994) and *The Pleasure of the Text* (1990a [1973]). Barthes is not concerned with fashion at all. Nonetheless, they are useful in illuminating the 'effects of the sign' in the rhetoric of the fashion magazine and advertising. Hence, I want to weave these texts into the argument that follows as both a necessary supplement to the line of semiological inquiry he pursued in *The Fashion System* and a means to redress some of the latter's methodological shortcomings or oversights. In the process, I shall explore the dialectic between two key terms that he evinced – 'written clothing' (*le vêtement écrit*) and 'image clothing' (*le vêtement-image*) – and my intention is to postulate Barthes' writing on the codes of fashion as indispensable for anyone who is interested in the correspondence between words and images, and the idea of repetitive performativity in fashion texts.

THE FASHION SYSTEM AND SEMIOLOGY

The Fashion System emanated from a research scholarship awarded to Barthes by the Centre National de la Recherche Scientifique between 1957 and 1963 and is based chiefly on his paradigmatic exploration of two French women's magazines from June 1958 till June 1959, namely *Elle*, a popular weekly, and *Le Jardin des Modes*, an upmarket monthly.[3] The work was eventually published in 1967 (with the first English translation appearing in 1983), although it was adumbrated by his 1960 essay, 'Blue Is in Fashion This Year', and has been much misunderstood and maligned. Rick Rylance, for instance, called it his 'bleakest book' (Rylance, 1994: 42), while Jonathan Culler found his methodology for distinguishing the fashionable from the unfashionable flawed in the way it centred on a synchronic rather than diachronic reading of fashion magazines (Culler, 1975: 35). But, as Barthes himself argued, selecting only one year's worth of material for analysis was sufficient to reveal how fashion attempts to renew itself through the performative reiteration of archetypal phrases like 'This year, blue is in Fashion' (Barthes, 1990: 77). He concludes: 'The signified Fashion includes only a single pertinent variation, that of the *unfashionable* [...]. Thus, the confusion of Fashion does not stem from its status but from the limits of our memory; the number of Fashion features is high, it is not infinite' (Barthes, 1990: 269 and 299).

As Barthes has it, then, there are three chief ways of defining or conceptualizing fashion: the vestimentary or real code, which deals with the garment itself; the terminological code, or spoken language; and the rhetorical code, concerning how fashion is translated into words and images in magazine spreads – or what he terms 'written clothing' and 'image-clothing'. He posits the vestimentary code belongs to the province of sociology, with the core object acting as a generative mother tongue through which actual garments become instances of speech acts – as with the terminological code, which is based in linguistics, and the rhetorical code, which is rooted in semiology: 'Semiology [...] describes a garment which from beginning to end remains imaginary, or if one prefers, purely intellective; it leads us to recognize not practices but images' (Barthes, 1990: 9–10).[4] Consequently, Barthes makes it plain from the outset of *The Fashion System* that his concern is with clothing as text or sign.

Barthes' interest in semiology arose at a time when the oppositional terms high and low culture were becoming increasingly hard to sustain, witness the reconstitution of mass media images from American comics and advertising in Pop Art collage such as Richard Hamilton's 'Just What Is it that Makes Today's Homes so Different, so Appealing?' (1956). And nor was he alone: this was the start of a fertile period of theoretical and philosophical inquiry in France among intellectuals like Jacques Derrida (chapter 15), Michel Foucault (chapter 11), Pierre Bourdieu (chapter 14) and Julia Kristeva into issues of identity and how and what culture – whether high or low – signifies. Thus Barthes contended in *The Elements of Semiology* (1964): 'There is at present a kind of demand for semiology, stemming not from the fads of a few scholars, but from the very history of the modern world.' (Barthes, 1973: 9). To this end, he inherited and transformed the ideas of Ferdinand de Saussure (1857–1913), who had been involved with analysing the codes of spoken language and paved the way for semiological analysis in the posthumous work *The Course in General Linguistics* (1916), proclaiming: 'The laws which semiology will discover will be laws applicable in linguistics, and linguistics will thus be assigned to a clearly defined place in the field of human knowledge' (Saussure, 1996: 16).[5] In *The Elements of Semiology* Barthes admits his debt to Saussure and other theoreticians, including Charles Sanders Peirce (1834–1914) and Louis Hjelmslev (1899–1965).[6] But building on them, he concludes: 'Semiology [...] aims to take in any system of signs, whatever their substance and limits; images, gestures, musical sounds, objects, and the complex associations of all these, which form the content of ritual, convention or public entertainment' (Barthes, 1973: 9).

The principle dialectic of semiology maintains that every sign is constituted of two elements: a signifier, that is the sensory or material substance from or by which something is made – such as sounds, fabric, painted marks on paper or canvas, written or printed words on paper – and a signified, something conventional or cultural that is inaugurated by or associated with the material signifier. These two entities are indivisible in the sign itself. Thus, if the signifier is changed, then so too is the signified and, by implication, the sign. In the case of clothing, for instance, we can accept a white cotton T-shirt as a cultural sign whose general meaning is understated cool or coolness (whether of temperature or temperament). And yet this somewhat straightforward meaning is altered as soon as something about the material is changed, say a cotton T-shirt that is blue rather than white. While in the hands of Katherine Hamnett the sign 'cool garment' is transformed into an ideological sign of political rebellion when the cotton is emblazoned with slogans in uppercase type like '58% DON'T WANT PERSHING' and 'VOTE TACTICALLY'.

Or, as worn by James Dean and Marlon Brando, the cool T-shirt may also signify the sexual rebelliousness of youth.

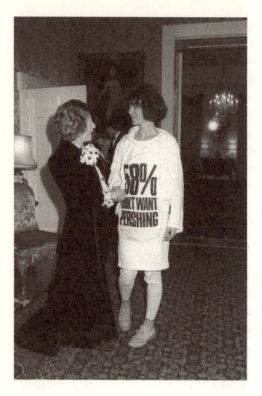

8.1 Mrs Thatcher greets Katherine Hamnett, wearing a T-shirt with an anti-nuclear message, at a reception for British Fashion Week, Downing Street, March 1984.

Semiology, therefore, propounds the very persuasive idea that everything is a text that can be decoded as a sign and, moreover, that the signified object is not like a single word, but rather a sentence in its own right (Barthes, 1994: 186–87). But a sign or sentence on which level? This issue hinges on another semiological dialectic: the concepts of denotation, essentially an act of describing something, and connotation, an open-ended or polysemous interpretation that demands the active engagement of the reader and for which 'There is no "proof" [...] only "probability"' (Barthes, 1990: 233). In regard to the example cited above, the sign at the level of denotation would consequently be expressed as nothing more than 'a white cotton T-shirt'. While this strikes us as a truism, nonetheless it describes a garment and a way of dressing that is a historical and cultural construction. The T-shirt, after all, evolved ca. 1913 from the practice of servicemen in the Royal and US navies shortening the sleeves on their undershirts to perform manual tasks, eventually becoming an item of casualwear after World War II (Sims, 2011: 104). By contrast, at the level of connotation, we begin to decipher the white cotton

T-shirt associatively as an object that either feels or looks cool, or as signified by Hamnett, as an act of political protest.

There is an additional problem we have to address, however, in the case of material objects (or referents in the real world) rather than representations of them.[7] For the cotton T-shirt is not just a cultural sign of coolness (on whatever level) but a functional item that we wear to keep our bodies cool as well. Barthes coined the term *sign-function* in *The Elements of Semiology* to account for this duality (Barthes, 1973: 189), referring to it also as the *function-sign* in *The Fashion System* (Barthes, 1990: 264–65), and it is useful in reconciling the dichotomy he propounds there between the vestimentary (sociological) and rhetorical (semiological) codes of clothing.[8] Hence, the *sign-function* represents a conundrum or paradox that 'always means to struggle with a certain innocence of objects' (Barthes, 1994: 158). The majority of objects exist, then, to serve a function and yet, as he insists in 'The Semantics of the Object', 'a meaning overflows the object's use […]. The function always sustains a meaning […], function gives birth to the sign, but the sign is reconverted into the spectacle of a function' (Barthes, 1994: 182, 189 and 190). To cite another example: a raincoat serves to keep us dry in wet weather, but this functional aspect is imbricated with the emotional meanings we give to rain/rainy days— for some people a sign of melancholy associated with cancelled or ruined events, while for others a token of happy days spent, say, as children playing in puddles.

Furthermore, constituted as a sign Barthes argues that the object 'is at the intersection of two coordinates, two definitions' (Barthes, 1973: 183). The first he terms taxonomic, whereby individual objects are classified according to both their production – in the case of clothing, things like the different weights of fabric and kinds of buttons used in its manufacture – and their consumption, how clothes are displayed hierarchically in museums or which types are collected in archives, for instance. But, of course, consumption also occurs on an everyday level in how we organize, use and wear our own clothes and Barthes deals with this in relation to the Saussurean concepts of *langue*/language, the institutional syntax or rules that govern the use of language, and *parole*/speech, how the individual puts the rules into practice and customizes them. Confusingly, Barthes initially expresses this as the respective distinction between *dress* and *dressing* (Barthes, 2006: 8–10), and then *clothing* and *dress* (Barthes, 1990: 18). In either case, it embraces the conventional grammar of how and when a garment should be worn – for example, breeches and a riding coat as the *dress/clothing* of fox hunting – and how this can be deconstructed through *dressing/dress* by individuals, such as

Beau Brummell's adaption of the same to daywear, as well as by fashion designers, hence Vivienne Westwood's quilted denim hunting jacket for the Anglomania Lee autumn/winter 2012/13 collection.

It is the second, symbolic co-ordinate, however, that preoccupies Barthes in his work on the rhetoric of fashion and in dealing with it he prioritizes written clothing over image-clothing. So, while he maintains that 'Fashion magazines take advantage of the ability to deliver simultaneously messages derived from these two structures – here a dress photographed, there the same dress described', it is the verbal message that he insists has the methodological advantage insofar as it proffers a purer reading of the fashion text:

> Thus, every written word has a function of authority in so far as it chooses – by proxy, so to speak – instead of the eye. The image freezes an endless number of possibilities, words determine a single certainty […]. What language adds to the image is *knowledge*.
>
> (Barthes, 1990: 13, 14 and 17)

Written clothing, therefore, in the form of captions can transmit information that is not necessarily evident in pictorial representation, such as the fabric used in a garment's making, its colour if the image is monochrome, its designer and price tag, or when and why it is being or should be worn. Certainly, all this makes sense when we consider 'Va-va-voom!', a fashion page with photography by Anthony Armstrong-Jones for British *Vogue* (November 1959). Accordingly, we would not be able to glean from the monochrome image alone that the woman's dress was made by Atrima, is black, with a single silk base covered with layers of lace, retailed for 19 guineas (the equivalent of £362 in 2010)[9] and could be worn for dining and dancing.

Furthermore, in such cases we are dealing with *l'écriture*, a form of writing whereby language does not just convey its own meaning(s) but becomes a support for supplementary meanings as well (Barthes, 2006: 47). The caption 'Va-va-voom!' is ostensibly meaningless, for instance, but *Vogue* translates it as 'Let's keep going!'[10] To this end, Barthes argues that written clothing is circumscribed by three rhetorical practices. The first, the poetics of clothing, connotes that 'the garment is sometimes loving, sometimes loved' by suggesting an equivalence between clothing, sensation and mood or by setting up an association between fashion and history, literature or art (Barthes, 1990: 241). The second, the worldly signified, places fashion in the real world of work and leisure – often on location – and may also mobilize topical events, though in such a way that they and life are nothing more than a game per-formed in honour of fashion. Finally, with the reason (or right) of fashion, written clothing is either self-reflexive and speaks about itself by dwelling on the details of garments, or it reinforces exclusivity through phrases like 'This year blue is in Fashion'. Hence, the reason of fashion is a matter of performa-tivity, such that written clothing is a speech act which is reiterated on a cyc-lical basis by 'an exclusive authority' (editors and journalists) to compound and normalize what is fashionable (Barthes, 1990: 215). In my book *Fashion Spreads* (Jobling, 1999) I analyse examples such as 'Amoureuse' (*Elle*, 16 June 1958) to illustrate the above ideas. But I also enlist them to contest Barthes' logocentrism to argue two things about written clothing and image-clothing that are relevant to the period he examined as well our own: often images matter more than words and the meaning of fashion is a matter of intertext-uality between word and image.[11] Coterminously, I assess the intertextual, hyperreal and historicist messages of the poetics of clothing, the worldly sig-nified and the reason of fashion as part of a wider signifying chain or *metalan-guage* that Barthes discusses in 'Myth Today', first written for *Les Nouvelles Lettres* in 1956. With this essay in mind, therefore, I want to illustrate how the poetics of clothing of a 1998 pan-European ad for Yves Saint Laurent Rive Gauche both foregrounds image-clothing and crystallizes his assertion that advertis-ing as mythical speech 'is made of material which has *already* been worked on so as to make it suitable for communication' (Barthes, 1973a: 119).

FASHION, ADVERTISING AND MYTH

Masterminded by French advertising agency Wolkoff et Arnodin, styled by Katie Grand, and photographed by Mario Sorrenti, the ad cribs another sign – Edouard Manet's controversial painting *Olympia* (1863) – but with some significant changes. Hence, Victorine Meurend, the female model whom Manet depicted lying on a divan, naked save for a pair of Japanese slippers, bracelet, earrings and choker, and shielding her genitalia with a flexed left hand, has been transformed into a male model – Scott Barnhill, who had appeared formerly in publicity for Guess jeans – dressed in shirt and trousers designed by Hedi Slimane, but with his feet bare. Similarly, the black female servant appears nude in the ad, whereas in Manet's painting she is fully clothed, and she carries a bouquet of stargazer lilies instead of mixed flowers, while the black cat at the bottom of Olympia's bed has disappeared entirely. Thus the YSL Rive Gauche promotion illuminates what Jean Baudrillard calls post-modern hyperreality, that is, an image based on another image or sign system which results in us no longer being able to distinguish representation from reality (Baudrillard, 1994: 2, see also chapter 13 in this book). Nevertheless, we still need to interrogate whether there are any meaningful correspondences between the form and content of the original artwork and the ad, or whether the YSL campaign is nothing more than a case of vacuous post-modern style raiding.

As Barthes has argued, 'All advertising *says* the product but *tells* something else' (Barthes, 1994: 178). Thus, not only does advertising convey a double-message, converting use value ('buy me') into symbolic value ('buy me because'), it often resorts to a form of myth or metalanguage in the process. If, as he puts it, myth 'is speech stolen and restored' (Barthes, 1973: 136), mythical speech is furthermore dynamic and motivational, its complexity difficult to unravel since it is prone to ambiguous signification whereby 'the reader lives the myth as a story at once true and unreal' (Barthes, 1973: 39). Focusing on the YSL ad in this way, therefore, we end up simultaneously approving and disapproving of the fact that it has bowdlerized an iconic painting for commercial gain in order to connote the myth that French fashion is the art form of the late-twentieth century. More specifically, armed with some knowledge of the debates surrounding the production and reception of Manet's Olympia, we can begin to appreciate better the diffuse photographic style of the ad and the indeterminate sexual status of the male model represented in it.

Crucially, Olympia itself has often been seen as a case of pouring old wine into new bottles insofar as Manet transformed the convention of the female nude in paintings such as Titian's Venus of Urbino (1538) and Goya's Maja Unclothed (1800–1805). In addition, according to Gerald Needham, the relaxed pose and insubordinate gaze of Olympia mimics not so much high art, but rather the brutal and vulgar style of pornographic photographs from the mid-nineteenth century (Needham, 1972: 81–89). Thus, along with the motif of the hissing black cat (according to Champfleury, 1869, a symbol for irresponsible love), and the black woman who delivers a bouquet to Olympia, ostensibly from an 'absent' male client, referred to as 'Monsieur Arthur' by Postwer (Clark, 1985: 87), the painting was regarded both as 'indecipherable' by some critics and attacked by others on the grounds of morality.[12] As Tim Clark argues, however, 'sexuality did appear in the critics' writing but mostly in displaced form: they talked of violence [...] uncleanliness [...] a general air of death and decomposition' (Clark, 1985: 96). Paul de Saint-Victor, for instance, commented in La Presse (28 May 1865) that 'Art sunk so low doesn't even deserve reproach', while Ernest Chesneau stated in *Le Constitutionnel* (16 May 1865) that Manet 'succeeds in provoking almost scandalous laughter' (Hamilton, 1969: 71–72). Critics of the time were likewise opposed to *Olympia* on the grounds of the artist's proto-Impressionist technique; the painting had stirred up a storm at the Salon in 1865 and Thoré remonstrated with Manet for the clumsiness of his brushwork. But, as John A. Smith and Chris Jenks (2006: 59) have been keen to point out, '*Olympia* is [...] a reverberant image'; its meaning hinges on complexity and hence, as they insist, 'Seeing *Olympia* as the first modernist painting does not foreclose other possibilities.'[13]

Taking up this hermeneutic challenge, we can see how the painting invites a series of polysemous responses or interpretations concerning its subject matter and style of representation and how these subtend the form and content of the YSL ad as well. First, in its rejection of high finish, *Olympia* is more often than not regarded as an entirely modern form of painting and yet Manet also owes much to the chiaroscuro style of the seventeenth-century Spanish art he had studied (Tinterow, 2003). Likewise, the YSL ad is technically a liminal image and a rather old-fashioned one as well; a photograph whose muted palette and soft tonalism make it look like a painting, much like Photo-Secessionists such as Alfred Stieglitz had attempted to do with their hand-manipulated photographs in the early-twentieth century (Homer and Johnson, 2002). Even the Yves Saint Laurent Rive Gauche brand name is situated where we would expect to see the artist's signature, while the name of the photographer appears vertically in small print at top left. As Sorrenti himself has admitted about the style of this work, 'I was exploring colour photography and doing a lot of experimentation [...]. These photographs were given a really hard time at the beginning because they were really dark, painterly and rich' (Cotton, 2000: 115). And second, in the way that *Olympia* unashamedly puts the naked female body on public display, staring defiantly at the spectator, we can regard it alternately as the candid portrait of a working class prostitute in 1860s Paris, as Clark has insisted (in his extended and compelling analysis of the work he refers to her as such, rather than relying on the indiscriminate terms *cocotte* or courtesan), or the complex negotiation of a painterly act of seeing between the artist and his model at that point in time, as both Georges Bataille (Hanson, 1977: 52) and Smith and Jenks have proposed: 'the subject, whose meaning was cancelled out, was no more than a pretext for the act – the *gamble* of painting' (Smith and Jenks, 2006: 163). It is the dual sense of focus *Olympia* enacts that Barthes argues is the quintessence of ambiguous signification and that, I feel, is equally the concern of the YSL ad; indeed which helps explain why its producers resorted to such a controversial painting in the first place in order to object-ify the slipperiness of queer masculine identities in the late-1990s. Thus, in comparison to its retro technical style, the Latino-styled male model in the YSL image proffers altogether more contemporary subject matter in simul-taneously representing a fashionable turn-of-the-millennium dandy with his admiring black female partner and a gigolo or rent boy with his slave; the stargazer lilies she holds a tribute from an off-scene client (who may be a woman or a man).[14]

In tracing such parallels between a painting executed in 1863 and an ad in 1998 it has not been my intention to argue that they can simply be traduced as equivalents. To begin with, the painting has only a single author and the ad several – Sorrenti and Yves Saint Laurent, whose names appear in the ad, and Grand and Wolkoff and Arnodin, who are not credited – and by implication the fulcrum of the French avant-garde is transported from the Grands Boulevards, the stamping ground of Manet and the Impressionists, to the Left Bank of Paris, home of the Yves Saint Laurent atelier. But of more significance is the fact that, whether or not Manet objectified Olympia as a prostitute and hence the female body as a commodity, the main focus of the ad is unequivocally commodification – if not of the male body then certainly of male clothing. Accordingly, it connotes both the quality of the product and its nexus to existential factors such as lifestyle and identity. In the final analysis, the publicity represents the excellence and uniqueness of the brand by drawing mythological, poetic associations between it and art. As such, the YSL ad shares much in common with campaigns like Dormeuil's 'Cloth for Men' (1973–1975), which pays homage to late nineteenth-century deca-dent art and literature, and also Levi's 'Settlers Creek' (1994), which mimics the super-realism of Ansel Adams' landscape photography (Jobling, 2014). It is on this level, therefore, that menswear advertising is concerned with the 'great liberation of images' – as much as poetry or narrative is – that Barthes evinces in 'The Advertising Message' and that he insists 'reintroduces the dream into humanity [...] and thereby transforms [...] simple use into an experience of the mind' (Barthes, 1994: 176 and 178).

FASHION AS A TEXT OF BLISS

And yet, the open-endedness of the theory and the idea that signs by their very nature are arbitrary has not been without its critics. In this vein, for example, James Elkins has argued that 'Semiotics makes pictures too easy' (Elkins, 1995: 824), while Stephen Heath has contended that 'Semiology cannot but bring a derangement of sense in its train' (Heath, 1974: 65). Barthes likewise realized as much when he called semiology 'the wildcard of contemporary knowledge' (Barthes, 1982: 474). But nor did he envisage semiology as an analytical free-for-all or a self-contained method that enjoins us to say whatever we like about anything: 'Semiology, once its limits are settled, is not a metaphysical trap, it is a science among others, necessary but not sufficient' (Barthes, 1973a: 121). All signs, therefore, have a historical context and nor does semiology cancel out other methodological modes of inquiry, rather it supplements and co-exists alongside them. Accordingly, I want to suggest that we can build on *The Fashion System* by considering also the phenomenological 'erotics of reading' that Richard Howard argues (in his 'A Note on the Text') is the core of Barthes' *The Pleasure of the Text* (1990) and thereby how it enlists the sign – and *sign-function* – of clothing as a form of embodied experience.

It is interesting, for example, that in *The Fashion System* Barthes states: 'Fashion's *bon ton*, which forbids it to offer anything aesthetically or morally displeasing [...] is the language of a mother who "preserves" her daughter from all evil' (Barthes, 1990: 261). When it comes to sexually charged clothing by designers such as Elsa Schiaparelli or Alexander McQueen, however, this line of argument simply doesn't pass muster (Evans, 1999 and 2003). By extension, it disavows the transgressive messages of connotation in fashion spreads dealing with issues such as heroin chic and the nexus of eroticism to pleasure and pain they often portray (Arnold, 1999).

Rather, we are on the terrain here of *jouissance*, the word Barthes uses in *The Pleasure of the Text* to emphasize sexual bliss and the collisions or breaks through which 'language is redistributed [...] and two edges are created'. One of these edges is the conventional or anticipated use of language, and the other is the unexpected or disruptive edge, which is 'ready to assume any contours' (Barthes, 1990a: 6). What is significant for Barthes, however, is that neither of the two edges is more important than the other; rather it is in the seam between them where the pleasure or erotics of the text resides, and which underscores 'a whole new aesthetics of consumption' (Barthes, 1990a: 58). It is precisely this liminal, disruptive quality that marks out fashion spreads like 'Who says couture is irrelevant?' (*Frank*, October 1997), where Terry Richardson has photographed a female model in a full-length red evening gown by Alexander McQueen ostensibly licking heroin from the top of a console table, and 'Pride and Joy' (*The Face*, April 1997) with photographs by Mario Testino that represent an adolescent boy at home alone, trying on his mother's underwear and masturbating under the bed covers. In such examples, then, bliss literally 'granulates, crackles, caresses, grates, cuts, comes' (Barthes, 1990a: 67). Moreover, the text of bliss challenges us because it does not take sides or criticize (as the YSL ad demonstrates); indeed, it leaves us in the position of the speechless voyeur: 'pleasure can be expressed in words, bliss cannot' (Barthes, 1990a: 17 and 21). The seam, therefore, is very much the province of the reader, and the text of bliss will also designate him/her as a phenomenologically corporeal and singular subject:

> The pleasure of the text is when my body pursues its own ideas – for my body does not have the same ideas as I do [...]. Whenever I attempt to 'analyse' a text which has given me pleasure, it is not my 'subjectivity' I encounter but my 'individuality', the given which makes my body separate from other bodies and appropriates its suffering or its pleasure: it is my body of bliss I encounter.
>
> (Barthes, 1990a: 17 and 62)

Given the exponential sexualization of contemporary fashion and the concomitant representation of sex and pleasure in fashion magazines and advertising across the world, the deconstructive manoeuvre the text of bliss entails is as much our concern today as it was for Barthes in the 1960s and 1970s.

CONCLUSION

Of course, this is not to argue that Barthes' analysis is either faultless or complete. In part, this helps explain the afterlife of much of his writing about both the rhetoric of fashion and the signification of everyday objects and how his ideas have informed the work of several authors as well as being revised or qualified by them. Hence, the tension between an object's utility and its symbolism that he evinced with the *sign-function* has been elaborated by Jean Baudrillard (1996) and Jean-Marie Floch (2001). By contrast, Agnès Rocamora (2009: 65–156) applies the concept of written clothing not just to the captions found in fashion spreads but it also underpins her discursive analysis of reports, interviews and short stories in the French fashion press. Finally, the ideological and mythological purpose of sign systems that Barthes illuminates in 'Myth Today' has been instrumental to Dick Hebdige and his nuanced assessment of the nexus of subculture and style (1979), Judith Williamson's seminal analysis of meaning in advertising (1978), and Patrizia Calefato's socio-linguistic exploration of style, dress, fashionable bodies and the fashion media (2004).

Perhaps the most interesting thing to note is that Barthes' writing is seldom, if at all, illustrated and that, when he does refer to specific examples of images and objects, his analysis – while thick with perceptive ideas – is also selective and not always sustained or subject to citation. This is something Jonathan Culler (1975 and 1983) upbraids him for and that, likewise, I encountered when I set out to interrogate the written clothing he mobilizes in The Fashion System. Thus I could find no trace of prototypical utterances like 'A cardigan sporty or dressy, if the collar is open or closed' in either of the two titles Barthes consulted – Marie Claire and Jardin des Modes – and was left to conclude instead that they are paraphrases, approximating to the kind of statements he would have originally read in them (Jobling, 1999: 86–88). Nonetheless, of huge relevance still is the fact that while objects and images such as the YSL ad or white T-shirt I discussed above are non-verbal signs, as both they and Barthes remind us, any semiological analysis is required 'sooner or later, to find language (in the ordinary sense of the term) in its path, not only as a model, but also as component, relay or signified' (Barthes, 1973: 11). This idea is probably the most enduring legacy of Barthes' semiological inquiry and it reinforces his contention that in an age of mass media and mass-produced items we are now all complicit semioticians, though without necessarily feeling the need to fall back on his methodological or theoretical framework: 'Modern man, urban man, spends his time reading [...]. Signification becomes the mode of thought of the modern world, rather as "fact" previously constituted the unit of reflection of positivist science' (Barthes, 1994: 157 and 159). In this sense, therefore, we are closer to the spontaneous semiotics Barthes himself is also involved with in many of the essays in Mythologies (1973) – 'Soap-powders and detergents', 'Plastic', 'The Face of Garbo' – as well as in his articles about clothing and fashion included in the edited anthology The Language of Fashion (2006).

NOTES

1   Key examples are: 'History and Sociology of Clothing' in Annales 3 (July–September, 1957), 430–41; '"Blue is in Fashion This Year": A Note on Research into Signifying Units in Fashion Clothing' in Revue Française de Sociologie, 1 (2) (1960): 147–62; 'The

Contest between Chanel and Courrèges: Refereed by a Philosopher' in *Marie Claire*, (September, 1967): 42–44.

2 Witness his axiomatic comments, '"nothing" can signify "everything" [...] one detail is enough to transform what is outside meaning into meaning, what is unfashionable into Fashion' and 'In fact, Fashion postulates an achrony, a time which does not exist; here the past is shameful and the present is constantly "eaten up" by the Fashion being heralded' (Barthes, 1990: 243 and 289).

3 Barthes justified his choice of magazines on the socio-economic status of different readerships and to this end he also consulted sporadic copies of *Vogue*, *L'Echo de la Mode* and the weekly fashion features of certain daily newspapers during the proscribed period.

4 In contemporary usage, the terms semiology and semiotics are interchangeable. Semiology, although it has come to be a method for studying all forms of representation – verbal or visual, verbal *and* visual – originates in linguistics and deploys only linguistic theory to decode visual as well as verbal signs. By contrast, semiotics is a broader term that is more popular in English texts and is used to describe verbal and/ or visual sign systems, which either do or do not necessarily have to be interpreted with resort to linguistic theory.

5 Based on course notes and scribblings by de Saussure, *The Course in General Linguistics* was cut and pasted together by Charles Bally and Albert Sechehaye, two of his former students at the University of Geneva.

6 Like de Saussure, C.S. Pierce also used the terms signifier and signified and referred to the process as 'semiosis' in the *Collected Papers*, 8 volumes (1931–58). L. Hjelmslev, *Essais Linguistiques* (1959) argued a correlation between linguistic and non-linguistic languages, while using the terms plane of expression (signifier) and plane of content (signified).

7 The term referent relates to the real thing or person that is represented in any image or text. In regard to photographic images, however, its actuality is crucial and described by Barthes in *Camera Lucida* (1980) thus: 'I call the "photographic referent" not the optionally real thing to which an image or a sign refers but the necessarily real thing which has been placed before the lens, without which there would be no photograph' (Barthes, 1982: 76).

8 The concept of the *sign-function* also informs Baudrillard (1996), Floch (2001) and Jobling (2011).

9 Calculated using 'Measuring Worth', http://www.eh.net/hmit/ppowerbp.

10 Starting in 1998 the same meaning was compounded in a series of ads for the Renault Clio and in 2005 it was defined by the *Oxford English Dictionary* as 'the quality of being excited, vigorous or sexually attractive' (Jobling, 2011: 248).

11 See also Jobling (2002).

12 They included Clément and Gille. See Clark (1985 (49): 287).

13 Another example of the polysemy of Manet's painting and how it can be used, therefore, to connote the ambiguity of sexual identities is George Chakravarthi's performative video, 'Olympia' (2003). In this, the artist poses on a divan as Olympia does, naked and with one hand flexed over his genitalia, but the servant delivering flowers is now male and white.

14 I am thinking here also of the way that footballer David Beckham adopted homo-erotic poses in two fashion shoots – one by Nick Knight for *Arena Homme Plus* (Summer 2000), and 'Captain Fantastic' by David Lachapelle for British *GQ* (June 2002) – and his avowal in the former that he is comfortable with being a gay icon.

REFERENCES

Arnold, R. (1999) 'Heroin Chic' in *Fashion Theory*, 3 (3): 279–95.

Barthes, R. (1971) 'Réponses' [interview] in *Tel Quel*, 47 (autumn): 89–107.

———(1973) *The Elements of Semiology*, A. Lavers and C. Smith (trans), New York: Hill and Wang.

———(1973a) *Mythologies*, A. Lavers (trans), London: Paladin.

———(1978) *Image, Music, Text*, S. Heath (trans), Glasgow: Fontana Collins.

———(1982) *Camera Lucida*, R. Howard (trans), London: Flamingo.

———(1990) [1967]) *The Fashion System*, M. Ward and R. Howard (trans), Berkeley and Los Angeles: University of California Press.

———(1990a [1973]) *The Pleasure of the Text*, R. Miller (trans), Oxford: Basil Blackwell.

———(1994) *The Semiotic Challenge*, R. Howard (trans), Berkeley and Los Angeles: University of California Press.

———(2006) *The Language of Fashion*, A. Stafford (trans), Sydney, Aus: Power Publications.

Baudrillard, J. (1994) *Simulacra and Simulations*, S.F. Glaser (trans), Ann Arbor, MI: University of Michigan Press.

———(1996 [1968]) *The System of Objects*, J. Benedict (trans), London and New York: Verso.

Calefato, P. (2004) *The Clothed Body*, Oxford and New York: Berg.

Champfleury (1869) *Les Chats*, Paris: J. Rothschild.

Clark, T.J. (1985) *The Painting of Modern Life: Paris in the Art of Manet and his Followers*, London: Thames and Hudson.

Cotton, C. (2000) *Imperfect Beauty: The Making of Contemporary Fashion Photographs*, London: Victoria and Albert Museum.

Culler, J. (1975) *Structuralist Poetics: Structuralism, Linguistics and the Study of Literature*, London: Routledge, Kegan and Paul.

———(1983) *Barthes*, London: Fontana.

Elkins, J. (1995) 'Marks, Traces etc.: Nonsemiotic Elements in Pictures' in *Critical Inquiry* (summer): 822–60.

Evans, C. (1999) 'Masks, Mirrors and Mannequins: Elsa Schiaparelli and the Decentered Subject' in *Fashion Theory*, 3 (1): 3–31.

———(2003) *Fashion at the Edge*, New Haven, CT and London: Yale University Press.

Floch, J.M. (2001) *Semiotics, Marketing and Communication: Beneath the Signs, the Strategies*, London: Palgrave.

Hamilton, G.H. (1969) *Manet and his Critics*, New York: Norton.

Hanson, A.C. (1977) *Manet and Modern Tradition*, New Haven, CT and London: Yale University Press.

Heath, S. (1974) *Vertige du Déplacement*, Paris: Fayard.

Hebdige, D. (1979) *Subculture: The Meaning of Style*, London: Methuen.

Homer, W.I. and Johnson, C. (2002) *Stieglitz and the Photo-Secession 1902*, New York: Viking Press.

Jobling, P. (1999) *Fashion Spreads: Word and Image in Fashion Photography since 1980*, Oxford and New York: Berg.

———(2002) 'On the Turn – Millennial Bodies and the Meaning of Time in Andrea Giacobbe's Fashion Photography' in *Fashion Theory*, 6 (1): 3–24.

———(2011) '"Twice the va va voom?": Transitivity, Stereotyping and Differentiation in British Advertising for Renault Clio III' in *Visual Studies*, 26 (3): 244–59.

————(2014) *Advertising Menswear: Masculinity and Fashion in the British Mass Media since 1945*, London and New York: Bloomsbury.

Needham, G. (1972) 'Manet, Olympia, and Pornographic Photography' in T.B. Hess and N. Nochlin (eds), *Woman as Sex Object*, New York: Newsweek.

Rocamora, A. (2009) *Fashioning the City: Paris, Fashion and the Media*, London: I.B. Tauris.

Rylance, R. (1994) *Roland Barthes*, London: Harvester Wheatsheaf.

Saussure, F. de (1996 [1916]) *The Course in General Linguistics*, R. Harris (trans), Chicago and La Salle, IL: Open Court.

Sims, J. (2011) *Icons of Men's Style*, London: Laurence King.

Smith, J.A. and Jenks, C. (2006) 'Manet's Olympia' in *Visual Studies*, 21 (2): 157–66.

Tinterow, G. (2003) *Manet/Velazquez: The French Taste for Spanish Painting*, New York: Metropolitan Museum of Art.

Williamson, J. (1978) *Decoding Advertisements: Ideology and Meaning in Advertising*, London: Marion Boyars.

9

ERVING GOFFMAN
Social Science as an Art of Cultural Observation

Efrat Tseëlon

INTRODUCTION

Erving Goffman (1922–1982) was a Canadian-Jewish academic who became one of the most important sociologists in the twentieth century and whose concepts have become part of the vocabulary of the discipline. Goffman, a controversial figure, was both reviled and revered. An outsider both personally and intellectually, Goffman often refused to play by the rules of social manners. His cynical, skeptical, ironic stance led him to provoke and probe his subjects' responses. He was considered a maverick social scientist: 'an outlaw theorist who came to exemplify the best of the sociological imagination' (Fine and Manning, 2003: 481). A dedicated scholar, he nurtured his talent by vigorous and meticulous reading, thinking, writing and debating. It is difficult to pigeonhole him as he focused neither on deep social structure nor on individual agency, but he did privilege the micro structures of everyday interactions over sociology's more traditional macro structures like the economy, the political system, education or religion.

Goffman received his PhD from the University of Chicago in 1953 with a study of social interactions in the village community on a Shetland Island in Scotland. The Shetlanders' unawareness of the real reason for his coming facilitated his observation of people's behaviour in the company of others, detailing the patterns of personal 'fronts' that individuals enact to convince others of their moral standing. Following a meteoric rise in the academic ranks, he became a full professor with the prestigious Benjamin Franklin Chair in Anthropology and Psychology at the University of Pennsylvania. In

1968 he was elected a Fellow of the American Academy of Arts and Sciences. By the end of the decade he became so popular with the general public that he was profiled in *Time* magazine. His thesis book *The Presentation of Self in Everyday Life* has sold over half a million copies worldwide, and in 1995 featured in *The Times Literary Supplement* as one of the hundred most influential books since World War II. The instant popularity of the subsequent books, *Asylums* (1961) and *Stigma* (1963), illustrated his impact outside his disciplinary field. By the time of his death Goffman's legacy featured in sociology syllabi in American and British universities, in chapters, textbooks, dictionaries and encyclopaedias.

Goffman has carved a new discipline, the study of everyday face-to-face interaction, by blending methodological micro data with conceptual macro insights. In his signature style of fieldwork, he fused statistical data with anecdotal evidence and literary texts like novels, biographies or memoirs. He thus created an original discourse of the individual and the collective. His methodological approach focused on the minutiae of lived experience and thus appealed to the general public. This approach analyses large-scale social forces by means of the systematic investigation of small-scale interactional domains. At the same time, his analyses, classifications and taxonomies that captured the imagination of experts were heuristic. They produced a theoretical framework of the organization of observable, unmarked everyday behaviour, mostly among the unacquainted in urban settings.

In this chapter I explain the most important concepts that Goffman introduced in the study of human behaviour that I can apply to the study of dress and fashion. Goffman's approach, I argue, is unique in focusing neither exclusively on social structure nor on individual behaviour. His analysis of social life is based on cultural observation, that is to say, he takes into account both cultural production and behavioural regularities. He does so by observing individual behaviours. As I show below, his concepts have allowed for what I call *the wardrobe approach*, which studies the unique everyday clothes of individuals whose meaning is part of the individual's set of experiences, interactions and vocabulary. This stands in contrast to the focus on social structure in studies of dress that I call *the stereotype approach*, which involves a study of iconic dress, ritualized dress and over-coded dress (Tseëlon, 1989, 2001). This includes museum pieces, designer dresses, uniforms and clothes that are identified with certain lifestyles or social groups, from gothic style to ball gowns. In terms of fashion research, then, an approach that follows Goffman fits between costume history and materiality, or between consumer behaviour and participant observation.

GOFFMAN'S INTERACTION ORDER

While Goffman had a profound influence on most of the social sciences and he is cited everywhere, he is rarely discussed in detail. Nearly all social scientists can say something about many of his received concepts, but few investigated his ideas on their own terms. Social scientists tended to appropriate parts of his work that bear substantively on their own interests (Fine and Manning, 2003). But as Manning contends: 'Goffman's ideas have been instanced as illustrating this or that theory rather than a brilliant, unique and masterful evocation of the central dilemma – posed as a question – of modern life: what do we owe each other?' (Manning, 2008: 677–78).

Addressing a fundamental sociological question, 'what makes social order possible?', Goffman outlined a system of an interactional order made up of a set of implicit instructions that govern our behaviour. In *Relations in Public* he observed that 'even quite formalized codes, such as the one regulating traffic on roads, leaves many matters tacit' (1971: 126). Take for example how we dress in the privacy of our own home; even then we choose what to wear by taking into consideration social demands and expectations. Those implicit codes and unspoken norms are at work when we unintentionally overdress or underdress. They are grounded in a moral system designed to save the face of all participants in the interaction. This moral system reflects the needs of the self to be recognized and sustained, and is based on mutually binding codes of obligations to self and other. These ground our confidence and trust in the social world by lending to it a quality of predictability, solidity and order. In his 1982 presidential address to the American Sociological Association, delivered shortly before his death, Goffman referred to his project of formalising the grammar rules of interaction order: 'My concern over the years has been to promote acceptance of this face-to-face domain as an analytically viable one – a domain which might be titled, for want of any happy name, the interaction order – a domain whose preferred method of study is microanalysis' (1983: 2).

The laws of the interaction order that Goffman articulated are actually quite visible in the realm of fashion. In *Dress, Law and Naked Truth* (2013), Watt makes an analogy between law and fashion. He notes that the ordering of bodily appearance arranges us for purposes of protection and projection. He then brings an example of a naked rambler who was jailed in Scotland for doing what he thought was his right: walking without clothes along a public path. The rambler defines it as 'the problem to be yourself'. When he chose to come to the hearing naked, he was incarcerated for contempt of

court, 'public indecency' and 'breach of peace'. Watt argues that the underlying attitudes revealed in such cases are that nakedness is indecent, and that
dress is invested with authority to police moral boundaries. This shows how
inseparable dress is from civil order. This aspect of our taken-for-granted
everyday world that we participate in unthinkingly illustrates the idea that
being clothed is expected in polite society in Western cultures. One can find
the strength of this conviction by challenging it, as the naked rambler found
to his misfortune. This example, fundamental and trivial as it may sound,
highlights the working of a basic law of dress. I want to argue that Goffman's
laws of interaction order belong in the same category. By interrogating those
rules through their breach, he was able to identify their boundaries.

THE DRAMATURGICAL MODEL OF PERFORMANCE

Researchers appropriating Goffman's work to the study of clothing and
appearance have mostly drawn on the famous book *The Presentation of Self in
Everyday Life* (1959), in which he introduces the notion of *performance*. Here
he puts forward his notion of self-presentation and the dramaturgical metaphor that guides his analysis of the theatre as a framework for meaningful
human action. Goffman posits that when an individual enters the presence
of others, he or she is trying to influence the definition of the situation, and
the impressions others make of him or her by presenting him- or herself
in a favourable light. The individual 'actor' has two channels of communication about the self: information given intentionally, or information given
off unintentionally – which is where most of Goffman's analysis is focused.
    The social actor lays claim to be a particular kind of person. For such a
claim to have validity 'the individual is expected to possess certain attributes,
capacities, and information which, taken together, fit together into a self that
is at once coherently unified and appropriate for the occasion' (Goffman,
1959: 268). The performance that illustrates the claim is reinforced by
means of visual and material elements from the actor's own environment,
such as props, clothes, grooming and body language. The performance is
sustained by the normative expectations of embodied presentation, ranging
from which body parts can be exposed, or need to be covered, which pos-
ture is not acceptable, the measure of tolerable personal space, style guidelines about formal dress and so on. Such tacit rules of 'situational proprieties'
define the acceptable 'bodily idiom'. For example, Goffman illustrates how
personal appearance and the visible marks of dress are the kind of behaviours

that distinguish normative behaviour from the socially deviant, like the hobo who ignores the social order, or from the mental patient who is unaware of it. Mental patients may slouch in their chair, their clothing disarranged or crumpled, and women may fail to observe the Western expectation of sitting with legs close together when wearing skirts, thereby marking themselves as outsiders. What the mental patient displays goes beyond the specifics of the rules they ignore. The mental patient fails to respect the normative expectations that ground bodily control and appearance. Those expectations concern not just the trappings of adornment, but precisely the kind of 'sustained self-monitoring' that simultaneously fulfils cultural expectations while identifying the actor as having agency.

Both actor and audience are locked into a game designed to save face. Goffman identifies that the prime reason for wanting to manage our impressions is our desire to secure cooperation between participants in an encounter, in order to avoid shame, humiliation, loss of face and embarrassment (Scheff, 2014). These motivators propel people to fit in, to avoid conflict or untoward attention. Embarrassment casts doubt on the credibility of the persona one is trying to claim, and poses a threat for loss of composure. Loss of poise can be expressed in an emotional outburst, in not paying attention to one's grooming, in an involuntary tic. It can also be concealed. Potential loss of face that is due to a momentary *faux pas*, is in essence comparable to becoming discredited with a permanent 'spoiled identity'. Spoiled identity is Goffman's reference to people with actual bodily or mental stigma, that excludes them from full social acceptance.

The conception of embarrassment as a master motivator presupposes the notion of an audience. Indeed, for a public self to be activated by a particular audience, the audience needs not necessarily be present. Research has indicated that imagined audiences are just as effective in influencing people's self-presentations. Goffman (1963a) distinguished different kinds of situation with a different set of involvements and audience: encounters, social occasions and social gatherings. He argued that social expectations achieve different aims with different types of audience. When one is among acquainted people one preserves intimacy, among the unacquainted one achieves trust.

While Goffman did not single out fashion and personal appearance as a topic in its own right, he referred to clothing as part of the elements that constitute the 'personal front' of the actor; these include insignia of office or rank, racial characteristics, size and looks, or body language (1959: 23–24). In his analogy of social life as a theatre Goffman distinguished between back stage, where preparations for a performance take place, and the front stage as a performance. Such distinction can easily lead one to believe that front stage is a public mask, and back stage is where the 'real face' is revealed. In fact, for Goffman one is not more authentic than the other. Both are different kinds of stage, with different expectations, and played to different kinds of audience.

Goffman was also the first to outline the dynamics of the disciplining of the body as a façade of the self. (See also the notion of discipline in chapter 11 on Foucault.) By demonstrating the ground rules of bodily presentation required to make a claim for a certain kind of identity, Goffman put body and appearance centre stage. Frost observed that over the decades following Goffman's pioneering work, much academic scrutiny has been devoted to appearance and image. It rendered appearance as a necessary aspect of identity, and no longer as a mere optional extra (Frost, 2005).

Importantly, Goffman's use of the theatrical metaphor questioned the idea of fixed identity. He articulated a performative perspective by providing a dynamic definition of identity not as a *state of being* but as *acts of doing*. (See in this respect also the concept of performance in chapter 17 on Butler.) Identity is the result of a social product formed and perpetuated through the repetition of behavioural scripts in an interactive social process. As such, it does not 'exist' in individuals: 'it is a dramatic effect arising diffusely from a scene that is presented' (Goffman, 1959: 252–53). Identity is thus located 'in the pattern of social control that is exerted in connection with the person by himself and those around him' (Goffman, 1961b: 168).

In other words, Goffman's actors do not possess an essence behind the performance; they *are* their performance.

THE WARDROBE APPROACH

In fashion studies, Goffman's approach paved the way for the perspective of clothes as 'lived experience'. My own empirical and conceptual research into some of Goffman's main ideas featured in my book *The Masque of Femininity: The Presentation of Woman in Everyday Life* (Tseëlon, 1995), which is an homage to Goffman, and is similarly focused on the mundane details of ordinary experiences. Using individual and group interviews, laboratory, real-life experiments, and questionnaires that covered exhaustively a full range of sartorial behaviours, I created the wardrobe approach. This approach privileges ordinary clothes instead of historical costumes or designer garments. It studies the meaning of clothes and the reasons for choosing which clothes to wear, from the point of view of the wearers. Drawing on 'Symbolic Interactionism' I took on board the notion of meaning as socially constructed and negotiated through interaction. Symbolic Interactionism is a micro-sociological theory that views people as acting toward things based on the meaning those things have for them. These meanings are derived from social interaction.

My approach thus opened the door to a branch of research that was process-based. I developed this approach of looking 'from the inside' at the accounts of users, in contrast to the then prevailing 'stereotype approach', which looked 'from the outside' at the accounts of experts, such as art and costume historians, curators, designers and certain social scientists. The stereotype approach was essentially object-based and attributed meaning to clothes in habitual ways on the basis of some group characteristics, but disregarded use, individual context and interpersonal meaning.

Goffman's distinctions between types of audience, and types of situational rule, provided useful tools for interpreting the data in some of my studies. In these studies participants communicated detailed opinions and practices relating to how and why they choose and wear clothes, and what meanings the clothes have for them. In Goffman's terms, 'Encounters' are situations where dress would be either secondary, or at the forefront, such as in a job interview or a date; in 'Social occasions' behaviour is monitored with clear protocol enforced by either dress code or conformity; and 'Social gatherings' are looser meetings where 'generalised others' are present and dress has no consequence as long as it is within an acceptable range. The first two situations, encounters and social occasions, are a source of higher appearance awareness than social gatherings.

For example, the atmosphere of trust and security versus being judged and exposed explained the amount of effort and attention women devoted to their appearances. Women cared more about their appearance in the company of strangers than with family or friends, although they also cared when alone. Typically, situational anxiety was a function of the formality of the rules, influencing the relationship between the women and others in the situation they were dressing for. In general, the dimension of on-show/off-show was more important than any other factor in isolation. On-show refers to a feeling of being observed, scrutinized and judged. Off-show refers to a sense of being unmarked, safe and invisible. (See also Erlich's ethnography of personal care products, 1987.) Thus, being in a stressful situation or with unfamiliar people whose judgement has consequences elicited more clothing consciousness than being in a relaxed context, such as exists in situations with few rules, when surrounded by one's friends or by strangers who don't care. Clothes were used to bolster confidence in contexts where women felt they were being judged or evaluated. These sometimes coincided with being in the company of unfamiliar people, generalized others or significant others. In the company of a familiar audience where women felt accepted and relaxed, they were not as concerned with their appearance, but even willing to experiment and be daring. Other factors appeared to be related to the reciprocity inherent in relationships. For example, women would be adjusting their dress to not offend an elderly relative or to not embarrass a guest by overdressing.

Woodward (2007) complemented the wardrobe approach by adding an ethnographic dimension to clothing choice. Having observed women making their clothing choices from their wardrobes, she specifically focused on the decisions that go on behind the scenes of public presentations. Her findings confirmed that one cannot fully understand what people wear without looking at the process of selection, and what is rejected is as illuminating as what is selected in the 'back stage'. More recently, Miller and Woodward's research on blue jeans (2012) lent support to my conclusions about the dimension of visibility being the key dimension in dressing for the world, and to my notion of *semiotics fatigue*: that eager researchers and popular culture observers are attributing more meaning to dress than the wearers' themselves (Tseëlon, 1989, 2012). In their global study of denim jeans they found that the ordinariness of blue jeans represented a semiotics-free refuge: a space free from pigeonholing, interpretations, judgements or notice. It was a default position that provided security and comfort, just like the back stage in Goffman's multi-stage model.

AUTHENTIC OR DECEPTIVE?

The essence of self-presentation according to Goffman (1959: 81) is that 'to be a given kind of person is not merely to possess the required attributes, but also to sustain the standard of conduct and appearance that one's social grouping attaches thereto'. This applies to verbal and non-verbal forms of self-presentation. It can be seen in the expectation, in professional contexts, that people who claim certain credentials (e.g. professional competence) would dress the part (with a smart suit, or designer outfit) and would avoid dressing in certain ways (unkempt, scruffy).

Goffman's theorizing has been interpreted as depicting a manipulative view of human nature. The 'manipulative view' was advanced by 'impression-management' researchers (Bolino et al., 2008; Durr and Harvey Wingfield, 2011; Kumra and Vinnicombe, 2010). It relates partly to how Goffman's notion of 'controlling the definition of the situation' is interpreted. If persons attempt to present themselves in the best light, is it deceptive or is it just preventing doing oneself a disservice? 'impression-management' view (Schlenker, 2003: 499) would imply that the terms 'self-presentation' and 'mis-presentation' are used interchangeably (Tseëlon, 1992a, 1992b).

There are some reasons that could have facilitated the mis-presentation interpretation, for example, Goffman's early (1952) study of conmen, which illuminates the identification of mechanisms involved in pure presentation. Generalized as 'a portrait of the human as conman', it could be seen to cast *people* in the role of imperfect conmen. Instead, it reveals Goffman's process of theory-building where he examines extreme cases in order to unearth the mundane assumptions they rely on.

Additionally, a close reading of Goffman shows that according to the dramaturgical account, every individual has a repertoire of possible coherent self-displays. For the most part custom, convention and habit, coupled with context and audience bring out an appropriate pattern of displays from the repertoire. The discrepancy between different performances on different stages serves the needs of depicting oneself in a way that sustains the face of self and other. For example, Cain (2012) applied the front stage/back stage division to the work of health professionals in a hospice who practice compassion in front of patients, and detachment back stage.

In his essay on 'Role Distance' Goffman clarifies that he does not endorse an ideological judgement about the authenticity of behaviour encompassed by the:

> vulgar tendency in social thought to divide the conduct of the individual into a profane and sacred part [...]. The profane part is attributed to the obligatory world of social roles; it is formal, stiff, and dead; it is exacted by society. The sacred part has to do with 'personal' matters and 'personal' relationships — with what an individual is 'really' like underneath it all when he relaxes and breaks through to those in his presence.
>
> (Goffman, 1961a: 152)

In contrast, Goffman argues that managed behaviour is not necessarily deceptive, and off stage is not the same as 'lack of stage'. It means 'a different kind of stage'. In fact, all behaviour is staged: to a present or imagined audience.

Most of this scholarly work, whether by Goffman or by his impression-management spin-off, did not deal with clothes as such, except as aids in face-to-face interaction. For Goffman, 'the disciplined management of personal appearance' or 'personal front' (clothing, make-up, hairdo and other surface decorations) is a mechanism to signal various aspects of the self (Goffman, 1959: 25).

Part of my own research addressed Goffman's theory as a whole as an original unique theory, and looked at its validity on its own terms through clothing research data. The question I addressed was ontological. Seen via clothes, is the Goffmanesque actor an honest person trying not to lose face, or a deliberate manipulator? My research was designed to compare Goffman's original model with impression management. I translated the issue of behavioural self-presentation to clothing self-presentation, in particular the role of sincerity and effort. Specifically, I looked at the following hypotheses:

1) Efforts in presentation in front of a familiar audience would suggest insincerity.
2) Efforts to present an improved image towards a less familiar audience would suggest duplicity.
3) Consciously paying attention to appearance would suggest intentions to present or conceal a false image.

The first hypothesis showed that in general women paid most attention to appearance when with unfamiliar others than when alone, or with family. But a closer inspection of the results shows that the mediating variable is comfort (psychological and physical) versus exposure (see Table 9.1). Attention to appearance is not limited just to those who do not know us well. Making an effort with appearance was seen as a currency in intimate interaction. In fact, respondents may make more effort when around people they know well as they feel secure in this situation, and have the confidence to do so.

The second hypothesis showed women's desire was not to dress in a way that departs dramatically from what they 'are' as exemplified by 'I wouldn't want to pretend to be something I wasn't' (Tseëlon, 1992a: 510). They want to project a *summary image* rather than a *false image* to unfamiliar people.

The third hypothesis showed that conscious attention to appearance is a function of insecurity. In situations of visibility, women used clothes to boost their confidence, whether dressing the part, or in expensive clothes.

I argue that Goffman provides the rhetoric of self-presentation in *amoral* terms while impression-management interprets self-presentation in *immoral*

Table 9.1

How important is your appearance when:Group	A) on your own?	B) with people you don't know well?	C) with your immediate family?
Tseëlon, 1989, 1992a (N=160)	3.5	7.7	4.5
Phillips, 2014 (N=74)	3.7	7.7	4.7

Note: The results indicate a mark on a scale from one to ten.

terms. For Goffman the term 'public' refers to a condition of visibility. For impression-management it signals a potential for duplicity. In fact, the dramaturgical framework does not imply that sincere behaviour needs to be 'spontaneous'. For Goffman it can be stage-managed and planned. As Goffman himself put it: 'While people usually are what they appear to be, such appearances could still have been managed' (Goffman, 1959: 77). Concerned with the mechanics of creating an appearance more than with the relationship between appearance and reality, Goffman stressed that while all dishonest behaviour is 'staged', not all 'staged' behaviour is dishonest. In other words, Goffman's account is not of the *psychology of deception* but rather the *semiotics of drama*.

More recent self-presentation work using Goffman's model found that even on Facebook people do not just present an 'improved self'. Even in a culture of digital self-portraits ('selfies'), people lack total control of the images that can be snapped and displayed online (e.g. being tagged in somebody else's pictures on Facebook). Further, Birnbaum (2008) and Wong (2012) reported that seeking social support was the main motivator of Facebook users. In fact, high disclosure can reveal highly personal, sensitive and potentially stigmatising information (Nosko et al., 2010).

THE UNCANNY METHOD

To uncover the dynamics that sustain social interaction, and reveal its unexamined assumptions and expectations, Goffman used an untraditional mixture of ethnographic work and observations, but also borrowed literary techniques like the use of metaphors, extreme examples, humour and irony. He used them as a critical perspective to deconstruct common sense categories, or strongly held beliefs, that would allow him to reconstruct the underlying order.

I refer to Goffman's method as 'the uncanny method' to deconstruct the working of institutions. I borrow this term from Freud's article by that name which describes a phenomenon when the familiar becomes strange (1955 [1919]). Employed strategically, such a method can be used to approach the banality of the everyday with the curiosity reserved for the rare of the exotic and the dramatic. Such a mind-set enables the researcher to see things with fresh eyes free from pre-conceptions. In the same way that Freud used encounters with pathology of mind in order to understand how the healthy mind works (see also chapter 3 on Freud), Goffman examines deviations from normative expectations, as well as body language and unintended communications (information 'given off' as opposed to 'information given') in order to reconstruct, like an archaeologist, a piecemeal picture of the dynamics of human interaction.

Clifford Geertz (1980) highlights Goffman's work as representing the importance of the 'game analogy' in the social sciences. His strict adherence to a game model of social interaction distances him from emphasis on meaning. By focusing on the detailed accounts of (observed, spoken, written or photographed) behaviour, not on 'why' questions, the assumptions informing behaviours are laid bare. Goffman's method of investigation was to challenge taken-for-granted rules. Geertz makes the point that what is considered common sense is culturally constructed, and thus may differ from one culture to another. Goffman would engineer a clash between the prevailing taken-for-granted assumptions and their incongruous metaphors and propositions. In the course of doing that, he laid down a blueprint for reflexive social science which challenges a system of institutions that make up everyday reality. In one of his early statements, Goffman reveals:

> In our Anglo-American society at least, there seems to be no social encounter which cannot become embarrassing to one or more of its participants, giving rise to what is sometimes called an incident or false note. By listening for this dissonance, the sociologist can generalize about the ways in which interaction can go awry and, by implication the conditions necessary for interaction to be right.
>
> (Goffman, 1967: 99)

Also: 'events which lead to embarrassment and the methods for avoiding and dispelling it may provide a cross-cultural framework of sociological analysis' (Goffman, 1959: 266).

A good example of his innovative methodological approach is the dynamic concept of stigma as a 'spoiled identity' (say, a visible disability) or a *potentially* spoiled one. In *Stigma* (1963b) Goffman elaborated the view that we are all stigmatized, at least potentially, so 'we have all learned to manage discrediting information about ourselves' (1963b: 9). Some researchers studied stigma as a substantive area (for example in the context of the sociology of deviance, or medical sociology). Holland (2004) and Ucok (2002) applied Goffman's concept of spoiled identity to ground women's experiences of losing their hair on health grounds. Others focused on the discreditable aspects. Davies (2001) analysed a group of people for whom disguise is a way of life using Goffman's stigma management. He pointed out that the skills and stratagems of disguise employed by those with a discreditable stigma in order to avoid unembarrassed existence are transferable. He argued that this explains the high concentration of illegitimates and male homosexuals in the theatre, the entertainment industry and in espionage. Similarly, in her historical analysis of lesbian identity positions Beloff (2001) likened them to 'discreditable spoiled identities' which are negotiated within and outside straight gender stereotypes. This is managed through a set of subtle codes, from camouflage to understated elegant austerity which subverts the masculine look to create an alternative aesthetic. In Miller and Woodward's work on jeans (2012) – an ethnography of wearing blue jeans in North London – Goffman's work on stigma was used to explore how jeans were a means through which people who did not want to be marked as 'different' were able to pass as 'ordinary'. Wearing plain blue jeans was a means through which migrants managed to avoid a stigmatized identity.

All those examples refer to a discreditable identity as a potential negative attribute. In my own research I extended the discreditable stigma to include positive features. I argue that women's attractiveness (by whatever measure) can be seen as stigma due women's relentless cultural visibility and 'the fact that uncertainty is built into the construction of beauty as defining social and self-worth, followed by permanent insecurity of becoming ugly unless rigorous discipline is exercised' (Tseëlon, 1992c: 301). Thus 'women are stigmatised by the very expectation to be beautiful' (Tseëlon, 1995: 88). The knowledge that attractiveness must be publicly performed but can only ever be a temporary state, a fleeting moment bounded by insecurity, suggests that for women beauty is more appropriately considered a '*stigma symbol*' than a '*prestige symbol*'.

CONCLUSION

Goffman's method of meticulous observation of behaviour and cultural products, and of attending to deviant and extreme behaviours that challenge everyday order, established him as a forerunner of ideological critique. It is an intellectual tradition that seeks to unearth the implicit assumptions and explicit techniques that make possible social interaction on the mundane level of everyday behaviour. He established face-to-face interaction as an arena of study, which, however banal, is not trivial but central.

Goffman's approach provides the methodological and conceptual tools for combining micro (the wardrobe approach) and macro (the stereotype approach) analysis. By fusing together insights from a variety of sources – behaviours (observations, interviews or questionnaires), cultural practices (studying written rules and protocols, challenging rules, analysing ritualized behaviour), cultural products (media, fiction, popular culture) – the Goffmanesque approach facilitates the study of the social meanings of fashion as a process that is individual and collective.

REFERENCES

Beloff, H. (2001) 'Re-telling Lesbian Identities: Beauty and Other Negotiations' in E. Tseëlon (ed), *Masquerade and Identities*, London: Routledge.

Birnbaum, M.G. (2008) *Taking Goffman on a Tour of Facebook: College Students and the Presentation of Self in a Mediated Digital Environment* [PhD thesis], Tucson: University of Arizona.

Bolino, M.C., Kacmar, K.M., Turnley, W.H. and Gilstrap, J.B. (2008) 'A Multi-level Review of Impression Management Motives and Behaviors' in *Journal of Management*, 34 (6): 1080–109.

Cain, L.C. (2012) 'Integrating Dark Humor and Compassion: Identities and Presentations of Self in the Front and Back Regions of Hospice' in *Journal of Contemporary Ethnography*, 41 (6): 668–69.

Davies, C. (2001) 'Stigma, Uncertain Identity and Skill in Disguise' in E. Tseëlon (ed), *Masquerade and Identities*, London: Routledge.

Durr, M. and Harvey Wingfield, A.M. (2011) 'Keep Your "n" in Check: African American Women and the Interactive Effects of Etiquette and Emotional Labor' in *Critical Sociology*, 37 (5): 557–71.

Erlich, A. (1987) 'Time Allocation: Focus Personal Care'. Household Research Project, TIS No G87002, London: Unilever Research.

Fine, G.A. and Manning, P. (2003) 'Erving Goffman' in *The Blackwell Companion to Major Social Theorists*, Oxford: Blackwell.

Freud, S. (1955 [1919]) 'The "Uncanny"' in J. Strachey (ed), *The Standard Edition of the Complete Works of Sigmund Freud, Vol. 17 (1917–1919): The Infantile Neurosis and Other Works*, J. Strachey (trans), London: The Hogarth Press and the Institute of Psychoanalysis.

Frost, L. (2005) 'Theorising the Young Woman in the Body' in *Body & Society*, 11 (1): 63–85.

Geertz, C. (1980) 'Blurred Genres: The Refiguration of Social Thought' in *American Scholar*, 49 (2): 165–79.

Goffman, E. (1952) 'On Cooling the Mark Out: Some Aspects of Adaptation to Failure' in *Psychiatry*, 15: 451–63.

———(1953) *Communication Conduct in an Island Community* [PhD thesis], Chicago: University of Chicago.

———(1959) *The Presentation of Self in Everyday Life*, London: Penguin.

———(1961a) 'Role Distance' in *Encounters: Two Studies in the Sociology of Interaction*, Indianapolis, IN: Bobbs-Merrill.

———(1961b) *Asylums: Essays on the Social Situation of Mental Patients and Other Inmates*, Toronto: Anchor Books.

———(1963a) *Behavior in Public Places: Notes on the Social Organization of Gatherings*, New York: Free Press.

———(1963b) *Stigma: Notes on the Management of Spoiled Identity*, New York: Touchstone.

———(1967) 'Embarrassment and Social Organization' in *Interaction Ritual: Essays in Face to Face Behavior*, Chicago: Aldine.

———(1971) *Relations in Public*, New York: Doubleday.

———(1983) 'The Interaction Order' in *American Sociological Review*, 48: 1–17.

Holland, S. (2004) *Alternative Femininities: Body, Age and Identity*, Oxford: Berg.

Kumra, S., and Vinnicombe, S. (2010) 'Impressing for Success: A Gendered Analysis of a Key Social Capital Accumulation Strategy' in *Gender, Work and Organization*, 17 (5): 521–46.

Manning, P. (2008) 'Goffman on Organizations' in *Organization Studies*, 29 (5): 677–99.

Miller, D. and Woodward, S. (2012) *Blue Jeans: The Art of the Ordinary*, Oakland: University of California Press.

Nosko, A., Wood, E., and Molema, S. (2010) 'All About Me: Disclosure in Online Social Networking Profiles: The Case of FACEBOOK' in *Computers in Human Behavior*, 26: 406–18.

Phillips, H. (2014) *Do People Dress for Themselves?* [BA Hons dissertation], Leeds: University of Leeds.

Scheff, T. (2014) 'The Ubiquity of Hidden Shame in Modernity' in *Cultural Sociology*, 1–13, doi: 10.1177/1749975513507244.

Schlenker, B.R. (2003) 'Self-presentation' in M.R. Leary and J.P. Tangney (eds), *Handbook of Self and Identity*, New York: Guilford Press.

Tseëlon, E. (1989) *Communicating via Clothing* [PhD thesis], Oxford: University of Oxford.

———(1992a) 'Self-presentation through Appearance: A Manipulative vs. a Dramaturgical Approach' in *Symbolic Interaction*, 15 (4), 501–14.

———(1992b) 'Is the Presented Self Sincere? Goffman, Impression-management and the Postmodern Self' in *Theory, Culture & Society*, 9: 115–28.

———(1992c) 'What is Beautiful is Bad: Physical Attractiveness as Stigma' in *Journal for the Theory of Social Behaviour*, 22: 295–309.

———(1995) *The Masque of Femininity: The Presentation of Woman in Everyday Life*, London: Sage.

———(2001) 'Ontological, Epistemological and Methodological Clarifications in Fashion Research: From Critique to Empirical Suggestions' in A. Guy, E. Green and M. Banim (eds), *Through the Wardrobe: Women's Relationships with their Clothes*, Oxford: Berg.

————(2012). 'How Successful is Communication via Clothing? Thoughts and Evidence for an Unexamined Paradigm' in Ana Marta Gonzalez and Laura Bovone (eds), *Identities Through Fashion: A Multidisciplinary Approach*. Oxford: Berg.

Ucok, I.O. (2002) *Transformations of Self in Surviving Cancer: An Ethnographic Account of Bodily Appearance and Selfhood* [PHD thesis], Austin: The University of Texas at Austin.

Watt, G. (2013) *Dress, Law and Naked Truth: A Cultural History of Fashion and Form*, London: Bloomsbury.

Wong, W.K.W. (2012) 'Faces on Facebook: A Study of Self-presentation and Social Support on Facebook' in *Discovery–SS Student E-Journal*, 1: 184–214.

Woodward, S. (2007) *Why Women Wear What They Wear*, Oxford: Berg.

10

GILLES DELEUZE
Bodies-without-Organs in the Folds of Fashion

Anneke Smelik

'the self is only a threshold, a door, a becoming between two multiplicities'
(Deleuze and Guattari, 1987: 249)

INTRODUCTION

Imagine a philosopher who writes about the warp and woof of fabric; about
the entanglement of fibres in felt; the variables and constants of embroidery;
or the infinite, successive additions of fabric in patchwork. Gilles Deleuze
(1925–1995) was such a philosopher. His musings on textiles can be found
in the chapter 'The Smooth and the Striated' in the famous book *A Thousand
Plateaus* that he co-wrote with Félix Guattari (1987).

The example of the warp and woof of fabric shows both the richness
and the quirkiness of Deleuze's thought. In *A Thousand Plateaus*, fabric, but also
music or mathematics, serve as ways of thinking about something that at first
sight seems rather unrelated, in this case the organization of space. Deleuze
and Guattari take the warp and weft of woven fabric as a model of *striated*
(delineated) space, and the rolling or fulling of fibres in felt as a model for
smooth (affective) space (1987: 475–77). Knitting, crochet, embroidery and
patchwork are all interlacings between the striated and the smooth. From
fabrics and textiles, Deleuze and Guattari move via capitalism and art to
a revolutionary call for change, associatively throwing around ideas, in a
chapter without a clear beginning, middle or end, in a book with 'plateaus'
rather than a linear structure. Not only the structure of the book, but also the

language is feverish: 'streaming, spiralling, zigzagging, snaking' (499); or in a favourite word of Deleuze and Guattari, 'rhizomatic' – working through connections and networks instead of a hierarchical structure. No surprise, then, that their work often poses quite a challenge for a student.

Gilles Deleuze's work is exciting because the main aim of his philosophy is to come up with new concepts so as to rethink and revitalize life (Colebrook, 2002b: xliii). In that sense, he is quite a radical, post-structuralist thinker, challenging set ways of thinking. His innovation and creativity, introducing many original notions that at first may appear perplexing and even bizarre, make it both stimulating and arduous to enter Deleuze's thought. Many concepts are intertwined in such a way that it is not always easy to find a way to disentangle his rhizomatic network of concepts; here it is best to read introductory books or dictionaries (Colebrook, 2002a, 2002b, 2006; Parr, 2005; Stivale, 2005; Sutton and Martin-Jones, 2008). Although Deleuze's concepts have hardly been applied to fashion yet, in my view they can be highly illuminating for the study of fashion. In this chapter I hope to show how certain concepts – becoming, the body-without-organs and the fold – give new insights on contemporary fashion.

Like other philosophers discussed in this book, Gilles Deleuze's work is rich and prolific, but also dense and difficult. His thought can be situated within the post-structuralist endeavour of mostly French philosophers to recast Western metaphysics away from unitary identities and transcendental claims to truth. Contrary to a thinker like Derrida (see chapter 15) he abandons the linguistic frame of reference and critiques the concept of representation. Deleuze's many books can be divided thematically into three distinct but interwoven strands:[1] 1) a history of philosophy, in which he gives a counter-genealogy of classical philosophy by reinterpreting philosophers in the margins, for example Spinoza, Hume, Leibniz, Nietzsche and Bergson; 2) his psychoanalytically infused work, which is a sustained critique of psychoanalysis and semiotics. This is most visible in the co-authored books with psychoanalyst Félix Guattari, especially in the two volumes on 'capitalism and schizophrenia' (as the subtitle runs): *Anti-Oedipus* (1983) and *A Thousand Plateaus* (1987); and 3) books on literature (Proust and Kafka), art (Francis Bacon) and cinema.

For Deleuze, theory 'must be useful'; it must have a function and if it does not work, 'the theory is worthless or the moment is inappropriate', as he said in his conversation with historian Michel Foucault (1980 [1972]: 208). I therefore advocate a pragmatic approach, in that I am primarily interested in understanding fashion and not in philosophy or theory for its own sake. A student of fashion does not need to aim at full mastery of philosophical concepts, but can – at least initially – follow Deleuze's call to use theory 'like a box of tools' (1980 [1972]: 208). The first step is to get inspired by the creativity of Deleuze's thought. Using Deleuze's theories as a toolbox, this chapter discusses some of his most important concepts (some in co-authorship with Guattari) that are productive in relation to fashion: becoming, the body-without-organs and the fold. Of course, many other concepts are equally relevant or fruitful, but within the restricted space of an introductory chapter I have chosen these to illustrate how Deleuzean concepts can help grasp contemporary fashion.

BECOMING

Deleuze's thought is affirmative: he is fundamentally a creative and positive thinker who is interested in transformation and metamorphosis (Braidotti, 2002). It is not just a negative critique of what is wrong in the world, but rather a thinking-along with the world in order to change it. The main concept that runs throughout Deleuze's philosophy is 'becoming' (Colebrook, 2002a; Braidotti, 2006). Pitched against the static notion of 'being' that is so prevalent in the West (just think of Hamlet's famous words 'to be or not to be'), 'becoming' is a practice of change and of 'repetitions with a difference', to refer to the title of one of Deleuze's most important books (Deleuze, 1994 [1968]). With each repetition – of a gesture, a thought, a desire, a way of dressing – one can make little changes and hence differ from what one was before. The continuous process of creative transformations is what Deleuze and Guattari (1987) understand by 'becoming-other'. Becoming implies a different way of thinking about human identity: not rigid and fixed from cradle to grave, but fluid and flexible throughout life. Human identity is capable of morphing into new directions, participating in movement, crossing a threshold, finding a line of flight, or jumping to the next plateau.

Becoming is about creating alliances or encounters, not only with other living beings but also with art, fashion or popular culture (O'Sullivan, 2006). By focusing on the process of becoming, Deleuze is more interested in the affects, forces and intensities of life than in meanings and significations. For him, the central question of art, for example, is not what it means, but what it *does* (Colebrook, 2002b: xliv; O'Sullivan, 2006: 43). How does it affect you or me? What kind of encounter happens between the work of art and you or me? What possibilities does it open? Transposing it to fashion, the question then is not 'what does it mean?', but rather '*what does fashion do?*' Does dressing in a certain way enable you or me to develop new parts of identity? Or does it fix you or me in a role? A different line of enquiry would be what fashion does to consumer society, the environment or to workers in factories.

Fashion today, especially in more artistic representations like catwalk shows or fashion photography, is often about creative performances, affective experiences and flexible relations, defying any fixed meanings or stable identities. At the same time, the fashion system may fix identities, for example in specific class or gender roles. There is a certain paradox: on the one hand, fashion is, or rather pretends to be, forever changing and innovating. It sometimes shocks society, for instance by taking underwear as material for *haute couture* (Chanel's jerseys, Westwood's corsets), designing trousers for women (YSL's tuxedo), or skirts for men (Gaultier), turning clothes inside out, strewing them with holes, shredding sweaters and patchworking them together (Comme des Garçons), creating dresses upside down (Viktor & Rolf) or by making outrageous designs that no-one except a few pop icons could ever possibly wear in normal life. On the other hand, fashion follows change only with marginal differentiation (Lipovetsky, 2002), laying down rules as to what (not) to wear this season. As Georg Simmel already remarked at the beginning of last century, fashion is a social and cultural system that tells individuals and groups how to dress and behave, moulding people into static identities (Simmel, 1950; see chapter 4 in this book). While many people are convinced that the way they dress expresses their unique individuality, they are, in fact, highly conformist to the capitalist demands of a fashion system that sells and even brands authenticity (Smelik, 2011).

Becoming – a process of transformation and metamorphosis – implies what Deleuze and Guattari (1987) have called a process of territorialization, de-territorialization and re-territorialization. A certain territory – for example the field of fashion – is not necessarily a static notion, but rather an assemblage with 'a mobile and shifting centre' (Parr, 2005: 275). Such a territory can be de-territorialized by 'a line of flight', Deleuze and Guattari's term for an escape route out, stimulating a process of becoming (1987: 88). Given that change is inherent to any territory, it will also be re-territorialized in search of renewed stability and structure. Fashion design, catwalk shows and fashion photography thus sometimes de-territorialize ways of dressing, which means that they move beyond a representational meaning of garments, beyond the familiar contours of the human body, and hence beyond fixed forms of identity. Ready-to-wear fashion and the fashion system as a whole, however, often serve as a tool for territorialization. From production to consumption the fashion system appeals to guidelines on how to dress and shape identity in a mould (Brassett, 2005), and the media are an important part of this process; just think of make-over, make-under or how-to-dress-for-success programmes.

An analysis of fashion would on the one hand involve tracing processes of territorialization – how does a fashion design, show or photograph code meanings, organize bodies, segment groups, stratify production and consumption and striate space? On the other hand, one can look for the moments of de-territorialization, those instances where a fashion design, show or photograph opens up meanings, liberates bodies, escapes segmentation, creates lines of flight and produces rhizomes, assemblages and smooth space. In this chapter I mostly follow this latter line of enquiry. For Deleuze such a critical exploration is never a game of either/or, because flows of affect, forces and intensities rhizomically connect different nodes in multiple networks. On any plateau, any territory, there are moments in time or spots in space, where territorialization, de-territorialization and re-territorialization take place. A process of becoming thus implies continual moving, transforming and metamorphosing.

MULTIPLE BECOMINGS

'Becoming is a verb', write Deleuze and Guattari (1987: 239). But who or what does one become? To put it in a Nietzschean way, you become who you are.[2] However, in Deleuze and Guattari's view 'you' is an ego-centred, self-aggrandizing, narcissistic entity that is 'organized, signified, subjected' (1987: 161). This is the fixed and confined self that one should leave behind, if only temporarily, by experimenting and looking for new ways of becoming. In one of their most beautiful sentences, which also serves as the epigram for this chapter, they write: 'in fact, the self is only a threshold, a door, a becoming between two multiplicities' (Deleuze and Guattari, 1987: 249). The self is a node in a network of multiple relations, and to set its desires flowing, one has to create connections with others – animals, plants, machines, molecules. They want 'you' to stretch your boundaries and 'become-woman', 'become-animal', 'become-machine', 'become-molecular' and even 'become-imperceptible'.[3]

This may sound abstract, but when we turn to myth or art examples are easy to find: from Ovid's to Kafka's Metamorphosis people have turned into animals, trees or insects. Horror or fantasy movies are keen on such transformations, from a fly or rat to vampires and werewolves. Science fiction is a genre where many humans have changed into an alien, machine or cyborg. Fashion is a particularly interesting field, because it moves between the imaginary realm and the material object. While art and popular culture can still be dismissed as mere fantasy, fashion actually produces material objects to be worn on the body. Examples abound. Take the becoming-animal, and then not just the obvious use of fur, but rather the creeping, crawling and flying insects in the Lanvin collection of 2013. Or the use of fantastically coloured plumes and feathers in fashion, as in Alexander McQueen's spectacular 'bird' collection 'Voss' (2001), or Jean Paul Gaultier's equally flamboyant collection of 2011, and, in fact, in many of McQueen's or Gaultier's other collections as well.[4] Just as remarkable was Alexander McQueen's collection 'Plato's Atlantis' (2010) in which the models were dressed in reptile-patterned, digitally printed dresses. The alien look was enhanced by grotesque shoes and make-up, hairdo or accessories that made the models look like some fantastical breed of monster. Of course, the process of becoming does not literally mean that one transforms into an insect, bird or robot by donning 'animalistic' dresses, but rather that one forms alliances with different affects, forces and intensities of life. The models become-other in an assemblage of fur, feathers, bones and bodies.

Becoming-machine is also prominent in avant-garde fashion designs in what I call the field of 'cybercouture' (Smelik, 2016 forthcoming). Technology is one of the major factors in affecting our identity and changing the relation to our own body. The scientist who launched the term 'cyborg' in 1960, Manfred Clynes, said: '*Homo sapiens*, when he puts on a pair of glasses, *has* already changed' (cited in Gray, 1995: 49, original emphasis). If this is the case for normal glasses, just imagine how the human body and identity change with Google glasses; the new 'geek chic' (Quinn, 2002: 97) that Diane von Furstenberg brought to fashion in 2012.

Hussein Chalayan is one of those designers moving between fashion, art and technology. For his renowned 'Aeroplane Dress' from the collection 'Echoform' (1999) and the 'Remote Control Dress' from 'Before Minus Now' (2000) he worked with hi-tech materials that are also used in the construction of aeroplanes. The dresses were aerodynamic in form and equipped with a computer system that could move the different glass fibre panels of the dresses, revealing the skin of the model. In a short film that Chalayan made with Marcus Tomlinson in 1999, a female model wearing the 'Aeroplane Dress' revolves on a pedestal, while the panels of the dress move open at ever increasing speed, and then move down till they stand still again (Evans,

2003: 271). With the sound of a propeller, the film suggests that the model is like an aeroplane taking off and landing. The movements of the panels in the dresses reveal the vulnerable body under it. Rather than being wearable – the hard panels prevent sitting in them – the dresses reveal a reflection on the intimate relationship between the soft body and the hard technology (Evans, 2003: 274). Chalayan's designs explore and push the boundaries between body and technology, looking for new forms of embodiment and bodily experience. The becoming-machine suggests engaging affectively with the technology that surrounds us and vice versa.

The notion of 'becoming-machine' is particularly relevant in the field of 'wearable technology' (Quinn, 2002) or 'fashionable technology' (Seymour, 2009). Complex systems of microprocessors, motors, sensors, solar panels, LEDs or interactive interfaces are wired into the fabric, textile or clothing, turning them into smart garments that have a certain agency of their own. Some recent examples are wearable communication in the 'Twitdress' that singer Imogen Heap wore for the Grammy Awards in 2010; wearable robotics in the 'Robotic Spider Dress' by Anouk Wipprecht (2012), or wearable solar panels in the 'Solar Dress' by Pauline van Dongen (2013). Integrating technology into our clothes, for example as already actualized in sportswear, will have an impact on how we experience our bodies and our selves. By wearing them on our bodies, we relate intimately to technical objects and materials. Exploring the wearer's corporeal and sensorial boundaries, fashionable technologies enable the body to perform identity in and through the clothes. This extends the possibilities and functions of fashion as an embodied performance. Understanding identity as a bodily practice that is performed time and time again – that is, as a repetition-with-a-difference – fashionable technology offers alternative and new ways of transforming identities.

Becoming-animal and becoming-machine are examples of the transformative process of becoming through fashion designs. The de-territorialization of the human body through the extravagant designs of high fashion or the use of wearable technology invite a reflection on new forms of embodiment and even identity. By reshaping the human body beyond its finite contours, these designs offer an encounter with otherness, opening up to the alien world of insects, birds, or cyborgs and posthumans. Such encounters suggest 'that all bodies possess an inherent capacity for transformation', as Stephen Seely puts it (2013: 251). As such, fashion designs provoke a dynamic process of multiple becomings.

HOW DOES A BODY-WITHOUT-ORGANS DRESS?

Becoming, for Deleuze and Guattari, is a process of undoing the 'organized, signified, subjected' body. Becoming is therefore key to another of their innovative concepts: the 'Body-without-Organs'; often abbreviated as BwO (1987: 161). The idea of the body-without-organs is to undo the organization of the embodied 'self' as a fixed form of identity. This does not mean that the body should get rid of its organs – which would amount to suicide – but rather that one should re-organize the way in which the body is given meaning. Deleuze and Guattari claim that 'The enemy is the organism', that is, the way in which the organs are organized (1987: 158). As Seely argues, 'of all art forms, fashion is perhaps the one most bound to a normative image of the human body' (2013: 258). This is of course most true for idealized images of flawless femininity and perfect female bodies. The notion of the body-without-organs can therefore help to counter these normative images of what a body should look like. In undoing – tentatively and temporarily – the central organization of the body, identity can become more fluid and flexible. As fashion often probes the limits of what a body can do or what it can become, the notion of the body-without-organs helps to see how such designs set the body in motion, potentially freeing it from a territorialized understanding of its matter.

Let me expand on the de-territorializing designs of the Dutch fashion designer Iris van Herpen as examples of bodies-without-organs. In 'Biopiracy' (2014) the models were caught in something that looked like spider webs, and as in much of Van Herpen's work, the 3D printed designs seemed to be made out of wafts of smoke, falls of water, rings of twisted leaves or rhizomatic folds of bones. In a unique play of endless loops, folds, waves, bends, curls, wrinkles and circles, baroque shapes open and close. Forms undulate and fluctuate. Materials ripple, waver and swing. Van Herpen's sensitive visual language is not captured in traditional flowing fabrics like silk, satin, tulle or organza, but in hard materials such as leather, metal, plastic, synthetic polyesters and hi-tech fabrics. She succeeds in catching a wave of water in an intangible form, a becoming-water in 'Crystallization' (2011), or a becoming-smoke in a design from the collection 'Refinery Smoke' (2008). Through her designs the models cross the boundaries of what a body can look like and become in-between characters: between humans and animals in 'Fragile Futurity' (2008), between mummy and doll in 'Mummification' (2009), between skeleton and body in 'Capriole' (2011), between man and cyborg in 'Chemical Crow' (2008), between the virtual and material in 'Escapism' (2011) and between organic

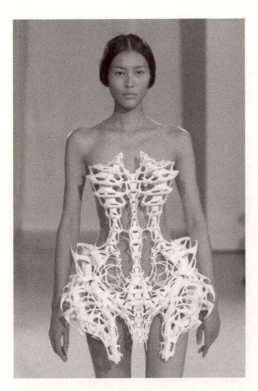

10.1 Capriole, F/W 2011, by Iris van Herpen, photograph by Peter Stigter.

and artificial in 'Hybrid Holism' (2012) or 'Wilderness Embodied' (2013). The multiple becomings are then effectuated by bodies-without-organs, challenging a stratification of self and identity.

As Deleuze and Guattari claim, 'we are continually stratified' (1987: 159); and this is often the case for the field of ready-to-wear. Van Herpen's futuristic designs, however, point to ways of de-organizing, de-stratifying and de-territorializing the human body. In her experiment with form and matter she calls for a different relation to the, mostly female, body. The designs come across as futuristic, morphing new silhouettes, inviting the wearer to inhabit the freedom of co-creating the body into new shapes. It is in that sense that she produces bodies-without-organs. Looking at any of her innovative designs one can see how the body-without-organs is dynamic, opening up to a multiplicity of lines, notches, gaps, holes and fissures. Considering the territorializing function of much of the fashion system, Van Herpen's bodies-without-organs are highly revolutionary and politically relevant. There are, of course, darker examples of bodies-without-organs in the world of fashion, for example the anorexic body of models or the heroin

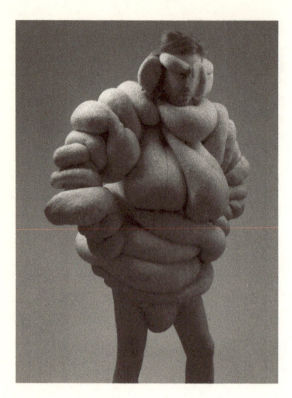

10.2 LucyandBart,
Germination Day
One, 2008.

chic aesthetic of fashion photography of the 1990s, portraying bodies that
'are moving fast toward their limit-points: toward schizophrenia, overdose,
unconsciousness, death' (Malins, 2010: 175).

Not only images in fashion media, but perhaps many high fashion
designs are slightly frightening for people precisely because they push the
boundaries of what a body could do, unleashing normative ideas of what a
body should look like. A most fascinating example is provided by the Dutch
artist Bart Hess, who has produced many body-without-organs by dressing
the naked, often male, body in a range of materials like toothpicks, shaving
foam, grass, pins and needles, earth, shards of plastic and even dripping
slime. Bart Hess alters the appearance of the human body or the human face
into fascinating forms beyond recognition. The pictures here show the project 'Germination' that Hess developed together with artist Lucy McRae as the
duo LucyandBart. A male body is dressed in a padded suit that was created by
stuffing tights with sawdust. This image is reminiscent both of the 'Lumps
and Bumps' collection by Rei Kawakubo from 1997 and the Michelin logo
of the little man made of tyres. The image changes, however, because the

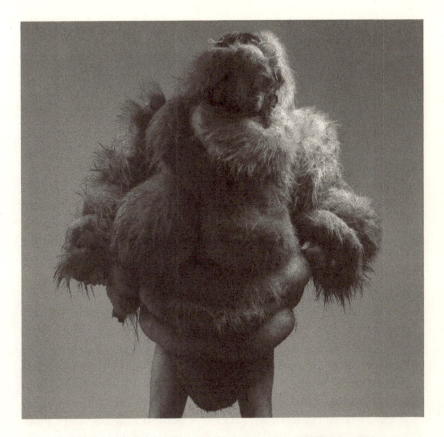

10.3 LucyandBart,
Germination Day Eight, 2008.

material was covered in grass seed and left in a wading pool for over a week, after which it had grown into real grass. Here we find images that express perfectly, if not literally, the becoming of a Deleuzean body-without-organs.

This is a body-without-organs at its most extreme; it is a dis-organized and de-territorialized body without a pre-ordained meaning or function. By growing the grass slowly, LucyandBart almost literally show the temporal process of becoming; it takes time to become-other. In 'Germination' they have produced a body-without-organs through a process of 'becoming-grass'. High fashion, like art, can thus liberate the materiality of the body into 'flows of intensity, their fluids, their fibers, their continuums and conjunctions of affects' (Deleuze and Guattari, 1987: 162). Weird perhaps, but in the very lumps and bumps covered by grass, LucyandBart radically undercut any notion of an idealized, stratified, body. As the grass grows, the human body reveals the constant flux of becoming.

FOLDS OF FASHION

Another way of approaching the transformative process of becoming is through Deleuze's notion of 'the fold', which he develops in his book on the philosopher Leibniz and the Baroque (Deleuze, 1993).[5] For Deleuze, the Baroque is a world where 'everything folds, unfolds, refolds' (Conley, 2005: 170). While Deleuze – rather abstractly – argues that the fold is a dynamic and creative force equivalent to a process of infinite becoming, he takes the fold quite literally in his discussion of the typical mannerism of the Baroque period. This is expressed not only in painting or sculpture, but also in the Baroque style of dress:

> The fold can be recognized first of all in the textile model of the kind implied by garments: fabric or clothing has to free its own folds from its usual subordination to the finite body it covers. If there is an inherently Baroque costume, it is broad, in descending waves, billowing and flaring, surrounding the body with its independent folds, ever-multiplying, never betraying those of the body beneath: a system like rhingrave-canons – ample breeches bedecked with ribbons – but also vested doublets, flowing cloaks, enormous flaps, overflowing shirts, everything that forms the great Baroque contribution to clothing of the seventeenth century.
>
> (Deleuze, 1993: 121)

We don't have to go back to the period of the Baroque to find pleats, creases, draperies, furrows, bows and ribbons; contemporary fashion overflows with them. The fold can be taken literally in garments, but also metaphorically as a concept to understand the process of becoming. In both cases it functions as an interface between the inside and the outside, depth and surface, being and appearing, and as such demolishes binary oppositions.

Deleuze suggests that clothing surrounds the body and that consequently the fold is autonomous and no longer submitted to the human body that it covers (1993: 122). In the extravagance of Baroque clothing – but one can equally think of designs by John Galliano or Alexander McQueen, the deconstructionist fashion of Japanese designers[6] or even of the pleats and bows in ready-to-wear – the fold is no longer tied to the body, but takes on a life of its own. It is this gap that allows the person who wears the clothes to commence a process of becoming.

The key point here is that Deleuze's notion of the fold undoes a binary opposition between inside and outside, between appearance and essence: 'for the fold announces that the inside is nothing more than a fold of the outside' (O'Sullivan, 2005: 103). Identity is made up of a variety of foldings, from the material body and its dressings to the immaterial time of memory or desire. This insight involves a fundamental critique of the idea that fashion is a superficial game of exteriority covering over a 'deep' self hidden in the interior folds of the soul. Such a simple opposition does not hold. Rather, the self is a set of folds – folding-in and folding-out – not unlike the folds of the garments we wear in daily life. As fashion often probes the limits of signification or of what a body can do, the notion of the fold helps to see how designs set the body in motion, liberating it from the dominant modes of identity in the consumerist world of fast fashion. In the following paragraph I further explore the fold, or the process of folding, as a practice of becoming (Deleuze, 1993: 37; see also O'Sullivan, 2005: 102–4), through the fashion designs of yet another Dutch example, the duo Viktor & Rolf.

VIKTOR & ROLF: SPIRALLING UP WITH BOWS AND RIBBONS

Known for 'their exaggerated silhouettes and noteworthy runway performances' (Chang, 2010: 710), Viktor & Rolf's haute couture designs often centre on provocation and the baroque. Take for instance the potentially de-territorializing function of the collection 'Atomic Bomb' (1998–99). Viktor & Rolf stuffed the garments with large balloons or padding, resembling the mushroom cloud shape of a nuclear bomb. They showed the colourful clothes twice, once with the balloons or paddings, and once without them. The 'anticlimax', as they dubbed the unstuffed designs, hung in loose large folds around the body, festively enhanced with garlands. The designs thus integrated the elements of festivity and war, indicating the confusion whether people would 'either be partying or become victims of weapons of mass destruction' in the approaching millennium (Spindler and Siersema, 2000: 26).

The collection is an exploration of the potential function of clothes to de-territorialize the familiar form of the body, and especially of the idealized body shape circulating in contemporary consumer culture. Deforming the body through padding is a recurrent element in Viktor & Rolf designs, which is important in understanding how 'the process [of becoming] also has the power to deterritorialize bodies from certain dominant modes of stratification' (Seely, 2013: 263). This kind of fashion pushes the limits of what a body can become. De-territorialization is a logistical precondition for a process of becoming, which unsettles the familiar territory of the striated world of fashion. The fold can be understood as such a movement of de-territorialization by which one leaves the familiar terrain of idealized body shapes, unified wholes or striated structures.

Viktor & Rolf's 'Flowerbomb' collection (2005) showed the same principle of reversal. In the extravagant show of the 'Flowerbomb' collection, the models first donned black motor helmets and black clothes. After the spectacular launch of Viktor & Rolf's first perfume, called Flowerbomb, the models returned with their faces made up in pink and dressed in the same designs but now in exuberant colours. The dresses were constructed out of giant bows and ribbons, which have since become a trademark of Viktor & Rolf; their latest perfume launched in 2014, 'Bonbon' also takes the bow as its main aesthetic form. Bows, knots, ribbons, frills, ruffles and all such trimmings can be taken as variations on the fold. Watching the models walk down the catwalk one sees the bows and ribbons bob up and down, flowing and billowing around the body.

The motion of the clothes gives an idea of the body as in-corporeal, a body of passions, affect and intensity. Giuliana Bruno has pointed to the quality of motion as emotion in clothes: 'Home of the fold, fashion resides with the reversible continuity that, rather than separating, provides a breathing membrane – a skin – to the world. Sensorially speaking, clothes come alive in (e)motion' (Bruno, 2010: 225). Take for example Viktor & Rolf's collection 'Bedtime Story' (2006/7), where the garments were enwrapped in or as duvets and cushions: satin pillows with *broderie anglaise* became gargantuan collars; bed sheets became sumptuous gowns; duvets became quilted coats and ruffled sheets became cascading gowns of folds (Evans and Frankel, 2008: 164). The bedroom theme created warmth and intimacy, where the many folds of the sculptural clothes presented opportunities to relate differently to the surrounding world. This kind of 'affective fashion', as Seely (2013) calls it, reveals the transformative power of avant-garde fashion; in their exaggeration and excess Viktor & Rolf's designs defy the commodification of the female body.

The fold is a concept that helps us to think of identity as a process of becoming, functioning as an interface between the inside and the outside, depth and surface, being and appearing. In that context, we can understand

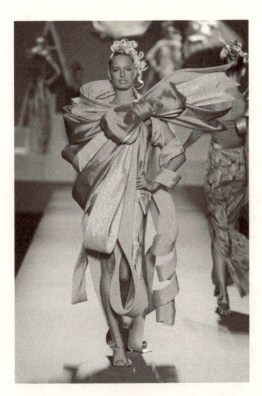

10.4 Flowerbomb, S/S 2005, by Viktor & Rolf, photograph by Peter Stigter.

Viktor & Rolf's experimental designs as an invitation to engage the wearer in the creative process of becoming, by transforming the body, and perhaps reinventing the self. In creating fold after fold, crease after wrinkle, bow after ribbon, Viktor & Rolf's designs create an infinite play of becoming.

In the examples that I discussed I primarily looked at avant-garde fashion designs worn by models on the catwalk or in artistic photo shoots. The question is whether the creative process of becoming can be attributed to this kind of fashion that is closer to art than to commercial commodity. I want to suggest that the process of becoming can move beyond the model on the catwalk or in the picture, onto the viewer or consumer, in that she or he desires or imagines wearing the designs. Fashion functions in-between, because the potential consumer moves in-between looking at a design and desiring to or imagining wearing it. Through that moment of desire and identification the viewer becomes the model who is wearing the avant-garde design. While consumers may never wear actual designs with lumps on the back, a pillow on the head, bows billowing in the air, they are familiar with the feel of folds, ruffles and pleats surrounding the body. They can imagine the endless potentialities of the fold and of the body-without-organs that it produces. They may see how such dress design frees the body from the territorialized understanding of its matter; liberating the materiality of the body into something continuously changing, mobile and fluid. Or, to put it differently, fashion designers create conditions to actualize multiple becomings.

CONCLUSION

In this chapter I have arranged an encounter between the different fields of Deleuze's thought and contemporary fashion. I have shown how the concepts of becoming, body-without-organs and the fold can illuminate certain aspects of fashion, and vice versa, how fashion can in turn re-animate those concepts. This chapter can only suggest a few ways in which Deleuze's work can be applied to fashion; it is up to students and scholars of fashion to open up the toolbox and focus on the many creative, intensive and affective aspects of dress and adornment. There is certainly a high potential for understanding contemporary fashion through Deleuzean concepts like 'rhizome', 'faciality', 'assemblage' or 'difference'. For example, one can think of the rhizomatics of trends in fashion, or analyse the faces of top models as the empty containers of normative perfection. Another compelling path could be to pursue Deleuze's claim that we have moved from a disciplinary society to a society of control (Deleuze, 1992); what are the implications for fashion? A possible take is a political critique of fashion, by focusing on the schizophrenic aspects of capitalism, as demonstrated by consumers' callous denial of the rude exploitation of people and resources in the fashion industry. But capitalism today is also about the insidious commodification of emotion or the ruthless capitalization of the self, new systems of affect in which fashion is a prominent and complicit actor. Yet another possibility is to develop an ecological perspective on sustainability through the idea of a 'becoming-world' (Deleuze and Guattari, 1994).

The main point of Deleuze's thought is to understand the prevailing regime of affect today, and fashion may be one of the best entries to take the temperature of the present. The next step is to search for possible pockets of resistance; how and where does fashion resist the present? For Deleuze resistance can be achieved by creativity. The question then becomes where and how fashion designers or the fashion system co-opt, solidify and territorialize, and where and how they create a critical engagement with our times or a new orientation towards the future. The act of thinking is for Gilles Deleuze an encounter with what you do not know (yet). It is therefore always a creative act: 'rather, it is a question [...] of inventing vibrations, rotations, whirlings, gravitations, dances or leaps which directly touch the mind' (Deleuze, 1994: 8). Deleuze's work is thus a call to 'think through fashion' differently; that is, to invent, rotate, whirl, gravitate, dance or leap through the field of fashion.

ACKNOWLEDGEMENTS

I thank Daniëlle Bruggeman, Roos Leeflang, Lianne Toussaint, and co-editor Agnès Rocamora for their constructive feedback on earlier versions of this chapter.

NOTES

1   I take this characterization of Deleuze's work from a research seminar that Rosi Braidotti and I have taught for the Dutch Research School of Literary Studies in The Netherlands, from 2006 to 2012.
2   'Become who you are' is a famous idea from Friedrich Nietzsche's philosophical novel *Thus Spoke Zarathustra* (1883–1885).
3   Deleuze and Guattari claim in *A Thousand Plateaus* that each series of becomings starts with the 'becoming-woman', because in patriarchy woman is always the 'other' of man, as the classical feminist analysis of Simone de Beauvoir argued. The 'becoming-woman' has been criticized by Deleuzean feminists, for example Braidotti (2002, 2006) and Buchanan and Colebrook (2000) and for fashion by Thanem and Wallenberg (2010: 7). A gender-sensitive analysis of 'becoming-woman' would be highly welcome in the field of fashion, considering the demands on the 'body beautiful' for both genders.
4   The Fashion Museum of Antwerp dedicated an exhibition and symposium to the use of plumes and feathers in fashion, entitled 'Birds of Paradise' (2014).
5   This part of the chapter is based on an article in which I have explored more extensively the notion of Deleuze's 'Fold' for fashion (Smelik, 2014).
6   The folding, wrapping and tying of cloth in non-Western styles of dress and fashion achieve similar modes of becoming; see Smelik (2014) for a first exploration of Japanese designers in this respect.

REFERENCES

Braidotti, R. (2002) *Metamorphoses: Towards a Materialist Theory of Becoming*, Cambridge: Polity.
———(2006) *Transpositions: On Nomadic Ethics*, Cambridge: Polity.

Brassett, J. (2005) 'Entropy (Fashion) and Emergence (Fashioning)' in C. Breward and C. Evans (eds), *Fashion and Modernity*, Oxford: Berg.

Bruno, G. (2010) 'Pleats of Matter, Folds of the Soul' in D. Rodowick (ed), *Afterimages of Gilles Deleuze's Film Philosophy*, Minneapolis: University of Minnesota Press.

Buchanan, I. and Colebrook, C. (eds) (2000) *Deleuze and Feminist Theory*, Edinburgh: Edinburgh University Press.

Chang, A. (2010) entry on 'Viktor & Rolf' in V. Steele (ed), *The Berg Companion to Fashion*, Oxford: Berg.

Clynes, M., interview in C. Hables (ed) (1995), *The Cyborg Handbook*, London: Routledge.

Colebrook, C. (2002a) *Gilles Deleuze*, London: Routledge.

————(2002b) *Understanding Deleuze*, Crows Nest: Allen & Unwin.

————(2006) *Deleuze: A Guide for the Perplexed*, London: Continuum.

Conley, T. (2005) 'Folds and Folding' in C. Stivale (ed), *Gilles Deleuze: Key Concepts*, London: Acumen.

Deleuze, G. (1980 [1972]) 'Intellectuals and Power: A Conversation between Michel Foucault and Gilles Deleuze' in D.F. Bouchard (ed), *Language, Counter-Memory, Practice: Selected Essays and Interviews by Michel Foucault*, Ithaca, NY: Cornell University Press.

————(1992) 'Postscripts on the Societies of Control' in *October*, 59: 3–7.

————(1993 [1988]) *The Fold: Leibniz and the Baroque*, T. Conley (trans), Minneapolis: University of Minnesota Press.

————(1994 [1968]) *Difference and Repetition*, P. Patton (trans), New York: Columbia University Press.

Deleuze, G. and Guattari, F. (1983 [1972]) *Anti-Oedipus: Capitalism and Schizophrenia*, R. Hurley, M. Seem and H.R. Lane (trans), Minneapolis: University of Minnesota Press.

————(1987 [1980]) *A Thousand Plateaus: Capitalism and Schizophrenia*, B. Massumi (trans), Minneapolis: University of Minnesota Press.

————(1994 [1991]) *What Is Philosophy?*, H. Tomlinson and G. Burchell (trans), New York: Columbia University Press.

Evans, C. (2003) *Fashion at the Edge: Spectacle, Modernity and Deathliness*, New Haven, CT: Yale University Press.

———— and Frankel, S. (2008) *The House of Viktor & Rolf*, London, New York: Merrell.

Gray, C.H. (ed) (1995) *The Cyborg Handbook*, London: Routledge.

Lipovetsky, G. (2002 [1987]) *The Empire of Fashion: Dressing Modern Democracy*, C. Porter (trans), Princeton, NJ: Princeton University Press.

Malins, P. (2010) 'An Ethico-Aesthetics of Heroin Chic' in I. Buchanan and J. Hughes (eds), *Deleuze and the Body*, Edinburgh: Edinburgh University Press.

O'Sullivan, S. (2005) entry on 'Fold' in A. Parr (ed), *The Deleuze Dictionary*, Edinburgh: Edinburgh University Press.

————(2006), *Art Encounters Deleuze and Guattari: Thought beyond Representation*, Basingstoke: Palgrave/Macmillan.

Parr, A. (ed) (2005) *The Deleuze Dictionary*, Edinburgh: Edinburgh University Press.

Quinn, B. (2002) *Techno Fashion*, Oxford: Berg.

Seely, S.D. (2013) 'How Do You Dress a Body without Organs? Affective Fashion and Nonhuman Becoming' in *Women's Studies Quarterly*, 41: 247–65.

Seymour, S. (2009) *Fashionable Technology: The Intersection of Design, Fashion, Science and Technology*, Vienna: Springer.

Simmel, G. (1950 [1905]) 'The Philosophy of Fashion and Adornment', K.H. Wolff (trans), *The Sociology of Georg Simmel*, New York: The Free Press.

Smelik, A. (2011) 'The Performance of Authenticity' in *Address: Journal for Fashion Writing and Criticism*, 1(1): 76–82.

———(2014) 'Fashioning the Fold: Multiple Becomings' in R. Braidotti and R. Dolphijn (eds), *The Deleuzian Century: Art, Activism, Society*, Amsterdam: Rodopi.

———(2016, forthcoming) 'Cybercouture: The Fashionable Technology of Pauline Van Dongen, Iris Van Herpen and Bart Hess', in *From Delft Blue to Denim Blue: Contemporary Dutch Fashion*, London: I.B. Tauris.

Spindler, A. and Siersema, D.J. (2000) *Viktor & Rolf Haute Couture Book*, Groningen: Groninger Museum.

Stivale, C.J. (ed) (2005) *Gilles Deleuze: Key Concepts*, London: Acumen.

Sutton, D. and Martin-Jones, D. (2008) *Deleuze Reframed: Interpreting Key Thinkers for the Arts*, London: I.B. Tauris.

Thanem, T. and Wallenberg, L. (2010) 'Buggering Freud and Deleuze: Toward a Queer Theory of Masochism' in *Journal of Aesthetics & Culture*, 2: 1–10.

11

MICHEL FOUCAULT
Fashioning the Body Politic

Jane Tynan

INTRODUCTION

The French historian and philosopher Michel Foucault (1926–1984) has profoundly impacted disciplines in the social sciences and humanities. For Foucault, power lies not in political leadership, but in the productive forces of everyday life, which is why he has become, as it were, fashionable again. Foucault's ideas have been used to describe the control modern institutions have over us, but in the aftermath of the global financial crisis, we are also witnessing remarkable displays of power from below.

In this chapter, I consider how Foucault's work might frame the social, political and economic meanings arising from fashion as a cultural system, a discourse, a practice and an industry. More interested in the political significance of material reality than in who appears to be in charge, Foucault set out the various techniques of social control that characterize modern life. Its disciplines and practices were for him critical to the judgements we make about ourselves and each other. The medical procedures available to us, our systems of learning and justice, how we are housed, the treatment of prisoners, all contribute to our sense of what is wrong, of who is rightfully in charge and what kind of speech is permitted. Are these modern systems and technologies that promote surveillance far removed from the glamour of fashion? Possibly, but they are also clearly relevant to mass fashion. Foucault's perspective on social structures directs our attention away from the spectacle of fashion to perhaps consider how it is constructed, to discover who is involved, to reflect on how fashion is articulated, who it benefits and whose concern it is thought to be. In other words, Foucault might ask what constitutes fashion as a social, cultural and economic practice. One thing is clear: most studies of fashion nod in Foucault's direction, which suggests that writers on fashion, identity and the body recognize his influence and many feel compelled to at least mention him in passing (Craik, 1993: 125; Benstock and Ferriss, 1994: 8; Svendsen, 2006: 143; Finkelstein, 2007: 211; Kaiser, 2012: 20).

Would the field of fashion studies be so rich and varied were it were not for Foucault? It is doubtful. Perhaps unwittingly, he demonstrated that the body is 'fashioned' by various institutions and practices. He politicized the transformation of the body, which subsequent theorists found in the various practices linked to fashion, beauty, style and regulation clothing. If garments shape body gestures and actions, they can also limit human experiences and, as I will show, various authors find in Foucault's work a critical framework to analyse clothing and the fashion system. However, despite the compulsion to name check Foucault in fashion studies, there continues to be a reluctance to build sustained analyses drawing on his theories. A notable exception is Joanne Entwistle, whose work has shown how discursive practices of dress make the body meaningful in a range of social and institutional contexts (Entwistle, 1997, 2000, 2001, 2009). Fashion clearly lends itself to a Foucauldian analysis. What we wear is significant to how we experience the world, but Foucault's most important contribution to fashion studies is a perspective on clothing that is embodied and socially meaningful. Most of all, his work suggests that we should treat clothing as an object that is worn rather than an image to be observed.

FOUCAULT'S CONCEPTUAL FRAMEWORK

One of the most basic facts about fashion is its ubiquity. Spectacular examples of fashion may be for the wealthy, but most ordinary, everyday dressing incorporates some form of fashion. As Joanne Finkelstein observes, fashion is a disciplinary power that coerces us to shape and transform our bodies: 'Fashion is collective, systematized and prescriptive' (Finkelstein, 2007: 211). Such perspectives are Foucauldian; they ask us to consider the demands fashion makes on our bodies. There are many aspects to fashionable dressing, from avant-garde catwalk shows to the most mundane wardrobe choices people make on a daily basis. However, key critical concepts in Foucault's body of philosophical thought have the potential to develop a neglected area in fashion studies: clothing for everyday life. Foucault was interested in how power is enacted through bodies; thus his theories are particularly useful to the analysis of the practices and rituals around regulation clothing and everyday dress. Whatever private meanings clothes hold, they also have a profoundly social role. Without mentioning fashion or dress, Foucault has provided us with a conceptual toolkit to consider how clothing is implicated in power structures.

This chapter surveys both the work of Michel Foucault and those who have employed his ideas to suggest how we might apply his concepts to the study of fashion. For Foucault, the body is critical to how power works: its visible construction shapes social and political discourses. One of the most compelling concepts that Foucault developed was discourse, which describes how knowledge is created and organized. Agnès Rocamora draws on both Bourdieu (see chapter 14) and Foucault to develop the notion of a 'fashion discourse': she explores the complex formation of texts, statements and ideas on Paris articulated in the French fashion media to demonstrate how and where fashion discourses proliferate and the social and material practices that give them life and meaning (Rocamora, 2009). It is clear that fashion discourse is critical to the maintenance of the fashion system, but fashion also constructs dominant narratives about health, gender, sexuality, class and race. Or at least fashion colludes with dominant narratives in any given social framework.

Discourse became a particularly influential concept for post-structuralists who sought to question positivist views of history. Discourse, developed in Foucault's books *The Archaeology of Knowledge* and *History of Sexuality, Vol. 1*, referred to the creation and organization of knowledge, which determines how and what we know, as individuals and as a society (Foucault, 2004, 1990). For Foucault, modern systems for knowledge classification represented a break from the system of classical thought. The role of history is critical to constructing discursive formations, what he called a 'history of the present', which made Foucault's work particularly influential in gender studies, queer theory, education theory, cultural studies, sports and criminology. Foucault was an anti-essentialist for whom everything was historically constructed, according to systems of knowledge that served specific power interests. Historically situated fields of knowledge have the power to make subjects and objects come into existence only through the discursive formations that make speech possible (Rouse, 1994: 93). If material things become articulate only within a field of knowledge, then discourse can demonstrate how these objects become carriers of social and cultural meaning. In many ways, Foucault materializes social theory, a useful perspective for scholars of design history and material culture.

Finding parallels across 'discursive fields' prompted Foucault to consider social life in terms of systems of representation and their reproduction through the operation of institutional structures (Rouse, 1994: 94). This is why Foucault viewed sexual identities as dangerous, turning on its head the notion that identity politics is empowering. He argued that the impulse to categorize human behaviour is a sinister feature of modernity, whereby the classification of human life reflects new forms of social control. He sought to uncover how social categories made bodies politically and economically useful. For instance, verbalizing sexual matters became a means to disperse the policing of sex in the nineteenth century. These discourses may have been negative and repressive, but Foucault was attentive to their tendency to 'demand truth' about sexual matters. The desire to categorize sexual desires stabilizes them, forming stereotypes to which we are all held and judged. Foucault saw the drive to categorize and objectify people as reactionary, a system primarily concerned with re-creating the body as an object of knowledge and target of power.

A frequent criticism of Foucault is that he attributes more power to institutions than to people. Jurgen Habermas criticized the limitations of his totalizing notion of power (Habermas, 1990), while Pierre Bourdieu, at various times, took issue with his methodological approach (Callewaert, 2006). Charles Taylor saw flaws in Foucault's model of domination and subjugation (Taylor, 1984) and Nancy Fraser questioned whether his anti-humanism made him a philosophical rejectionist or a nihilist (Fraser, 1985). Undoubtedly, Foucault was convinced of the power of modern institutions and the strategies they use to dominate people. He argued that despite nurturing an image of care and rehabilitation, prisons, hospitals and schools are designed to reform people, a set of power relations he described as 'biopolitics'. His contribution to thinking on the body in culture is clear, but it has fallen to subsequent thinkers to explore exactly how specific body practices reflect the workings of power. Discourse and biopolitics became part of what became known as Foucault's governmentality thesis, which was formulated in the 1970s.

Governmentality offers a conceptual framework with which to explore the shape and texture of the minutiae of everyday life to discover how they are harnessed for social control. This clearly has scope for interrogating the politics of fashionable consumption. As John Rajchman argues, he offers not a history of things 'but of the terms, categories, and techniques through which certain things become at certain times the focus of a whole configuration of discussion and procedure' (Rajchman, 1983–1984: 8). Foucault's work is concerned with exposing illusions, particularly conventional histories of 'development' and 'continuity' (Foucault, 1994: 419). He was interested in how things are 'constituted' and discourse became a key concept to describe conscious knowledge about a given subject, such as madness, health, sexuality, class or race, but also involved an unconscious substructure of beliefs, myths and ideologies.

'Biopolitics' offers a compelling conceptual framework to explore the social behaviour that specific body practices promote. His work on the body is critical to a Foucauldian analysis of fashion, particularly his book on the prison. Foucault's work extensively explores the key role of the body in modern institutions (Foucault, 2001, 1991). He carefully outlines how bodies are rearranged, improved and transformed within various institutional structures. In *Discipline and Punish* he explores how institutions have created knowledge by acting directly on the body (Foucault, 1991), which has implications for any study of social or spatial formations, but its real novelty lies in its conflation of both. Foucault argues that discipline creates certain kinds of individuals, employing Jeremy Bentham's Panopticon as a metaphor for the functioning of a disciplinary society (Foucault, 1991).[1] New discourses on criminality gave rise to new forms of prison punishment, which from the late eighteenth century were likely to include efforts to 'reform' prisoners. Physical punishment was replaced by surveillance installed to observe prisoners, a new strategy of domination intended to make them acutely aware of their bodies and to alter their conduct.

The Panopticon is the 'perfect' prison where inmates exist in a state of permanent, total visibility. The architecture is itself a technology of surveillance. A device whereby self-discipline can be induced by the threat of surveillance, the Panopticon imposes the pervasive normalizing gaze, which takes the place of physical force; order is achieved through the 'trap' of visibility (Foucault, 1997: 361). This has resonance with contemporary forms of surveillance, such as the routine use of CCTV cameras. Of course, Foucault uses Bentham's Panopticon purely as a metaphor for a society built on surveillance. For Foucault subjectivity is not just ideologically constructed, but the discursive leaves its imprints on the body. In *Discipline and Punish* Foucault outlines the emergence of a specifically modern form of disciplinary power, a set of relations involving techniques of control and regulation. He identifies the techniques of the disciplinary society as hierarchical observation and examination, procedures designed to make normalizing judgements. Do the principles of hierarchical observation and its goal to separate the normal from the abnormal resonate with the fashion system? A Foucauldian analysis offers scope for an exploration of the techniques of control and regulation in fashion. Indeed, control and subjection are the focus of a study by Alexandra Warwick and Dani Cavallaro, who use Foucault's work to frame a discussion of both discipline and transgression in relation to the dressed body (Warwick and Cavallaro, 1998).

USING FOUCAULT'S METHOD TO STUDY FASHION

Foucault's disciplinary power constitutes subjectivity, but his work suggests that these normalizing judgements are often made through visual means. He deploys the image of the Panopticon to describe the circulation of power, an architectural metaphor that is all about gazing. One of his key insights is that disciplinary power captures the body, manages its movements and shapes its behaviour, a far more effective tool of social control than, say, physical coercion. Punishment is not a penalty but a corrective; it trains the body to behave in certain ways. Once the prison becomes a metaphor for how people are organized throughout modern society, we can see how Foucault saw social life as embodied subjectivity. The anxiety we feel about our bodies – particularly concerns about appearance – result from this scopic regime of modernity.

However, it would be a mistake to confine Foucault's conception of a surveillance culture to the realm of the visual. As Cressida Heyes argues, Foucault draws our attention to normalizing technologies that encroach upon the micro-territory of the body, helpfully presented as 'solutions' such as diet regimes and cosmetic surgery (Heyes, 2007). It is not just idealized images of perfect bodies that serve as a reminder of the prevailing norms of beauty. The normalizing gaze is far more searching and intrusive; its reach onto every surface of our bodies serves as a painful reminder of just how badly our bodies are 'failing' to live up to socially constructed ideals. The point is that we do not require the judgement of an authority. We continually search for deviance, excess or fault in ourselves. Panopticism is a metaphor for the generalized anxiety that accompanies modern life, in particular the compulsion to maintain a critical view of our bodies. Fashion is the practice of self-presentation that fits with Foucault's concerns about the power that lies in the governance of everyday life. Foucault's contribution is valued precisely because his approach transcends politics; he sees power as everyday, socialized and embodied.

Foucault may not have said anything about fashion, but in *Discipline and Punish* he does discuss the appearance of the modern soldier in terms of the colour and shape of his uniform, which he cites as evidence of the emergence of a disciplinary regime (Foucault, 1991: 135–36). Foucault continually described how human beings become social, how they are transformed into certain types of subject, through various modes of knowing the world (discourses). How identities are made or constructed is of interest to anybody concerned with the regime of appearances that constitute social reality, particularly feminists, many of whom have taken up Foucault's work with enthusiasm (Sawicki, 1991; Bartsky, 1998; Bordo, 1998; McLaren, 2002), but there have also been some skirmishes. Admittedly, Foucault's analysis of power was not gendered. However, the disciplinary practices he describes have resonance with the feminist project to expose the cultural construction of femininity and the self-discipline it demands of women. For feminists, Foucault's work illuminates the discourses that form patriarchial power.

Sandra Lee Bartsky argues that his concept of 'docile bodies' perfectly describes the embodiment of the feminine, an obedience to patriarchy, which accounts for the insidious forms it takes in modern society (Bartsky, 1988: 93–111). As Efrat Tseëlon observes, the visibility of women traps them in the disciplinary gaze – and constantly maintains this – through the demand that they make themselves objects for men (Tseëlon, 1995: 69). Foucault's conception of power as socialized and embodied gave feminist scholars the scope to extend and problematize debates on spectatorship. Bodies subject to social scrutiny are not, however, exclusively female. Men's bodies are also subject to various normalizing judgements. Indeed, the range of practices that make the body available to an inspecting gaze goes beyond fashion to include beauty, dieting, fitness and cosmetic surgery.

Foucault's governmentality thesis offers ways of thinking about fashion on the micro and macro levels. Ingrid Jeacle argues that calculative technologies follow a normalizing process, to increase control in the production of fashion goods, separating the fashionable from the unfashionable (Jeacle, 2012: 82–98). Thus, in her analysis of fast fashion techniques, she points to a major theme in Foucault's work: the concern with accountability. In the case of fast fashion, the minute means of record-keeping is for her 'a surveillance system, which shapes the form of fashion, and ultimately the dress of the masses' (Jeacle, 2012: 95). But this flexible approach to manufacturing also bears down on the bodies of garment workers, whose employment conditions are often made hazardous and precarious by a globalized fashion industry. Jeacle draws attention to how these new technologies intensify the

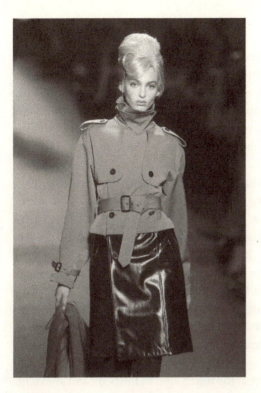

11.1 A model walks the runway at the Jean Paul Gaultier fashion show during Paris Fashion Week on 5 March 2011 in Paris, France. Photograph by: Anton Oparin.

power/knowledge formation by building calculative knowledge of bodies and spaces far removed from the centre of the industry. Whether we are examining the experience of retail workers, shoppers or garment workers, it is clear that industry micro-practices are giving rise to new and pernicious formations of power/knowledge. Studies such as these might divert scholars from the more seductive aspects of fashion – the episodic shows of novelty – to consider instead, as Foucault might, how power is dispersed throughout a complex system, and the impact this has on the lived reality of vast numbers of people.

The experience of the fashion model has also been explored from the perspective of Foucault's 'docile bodies'. In her ethnographic study, Ashley Mears argues that the work of fashion modelling is a disciplining process. It transforms women's bodies into commodities, particularly stringent due to 'floating norms' that characterize the uncertainties of both gender and markets that intertwine to produce fashion models (Mears, 2008: 429–56). Modelling professionalizes gender performance, where discipline and surveillance are enlisted to achieve high standards in an uncertain business. Mears draws attention to modelling as a physical, laborious, painful process characterized by a punishing regime of surveillance. Foucault's method highlights the processes that underpin the making of a fashion system. He emphasizes the visual, but is less concerned with aesthetics and more with *what images do*. In this way, panopticism offers a useful model to understand the mechanisms whereby idealized images of women in magazines and on the catwalk might result in unhealthy levels of self-monitoring by fashion consumers.

If the panoptic gaze works through public discourses such as health, dieting, fitness, exercise and beauty, does it operate to induce shame and subsequent adoption of a new regime? In one particular article, the metaphor of the Panopticon is utilized to trace the actual steps of self-monitoring that, in this case, a fitness magazine might induce in women readers (Carlisle Duncan, 1994: 48–65). Theories of spectatorship which gave rise to the influential theory of the 'male gaze' in the 1970s (Berger, 1972; Mulvey, 1975; Kaplan, 1983; Nochlin, 1994) anticipated some of Foucault's ideas, despite their use of psychoanalysis. What Foucault offers is a deeper sense of the effects of dominant patriarchal discourses, not just their ideological effects, but also the real ways in which they shape women's bodies. Discourses, or regimes of knowledge, are put into practice at the micro level of the body, and as Joanne Entwistle argues, are no less oppressive today than they were when women wore corsets in the nineteenth century (Entwistle, 2000: 20–21). Foucault's impact on fashion studies might bring to mind more extreme examples such as the corset, which Valerie Steele saw as a project to discipline the body (Steele, 2001: 155–65). But the important point that Entwistle makes is that body disciplines are at work in a range of fashioning practices: when men aim for muscularity, when women use dieting to achieve thinness, and when people elect for cosmetic surgery to improve their appearance. The demands made on women's bodies in the past, for instance, were not greater, but as both Entwistle and Steele argue, the type of clothing might change but the emphasis on body discipline remains the same.

Foucault's thinking on discourse and the body has also enhanced research into the various 'uniforms' that people wear, from civilian and military organizations to subcultural styles. Various thinkers concerned with social appearance have adopted Foucault's model of power/knowledge, but some use uniform clothing to describe how body cultures enhance citizenship and embody collective disciplines. The anthropologist Brian McVeigh draws on Foucault's governmentality thesis to consider how the Japanese high school uniform reflects state power, causing students to internalize the 'normalising gaze' as part of strategic schooling in Japan (McVeigh, 1997: 195). Thus, the collective discipline of the uniform – particularly the daily habit of putting on the uniform – offers new ways of understanding how clothing is critical to political projects. Foucault's concepts illuminate the role of the uniform to inscribe bodies, to construct specific forms of citizenship.

Those concerned with the cultural politics of education have also utilized Foucault's work to consider how the uniform acts as a form of power over the bodies of students. Daphne Meadmore and Colin Symes see uniform appearance as a potent symbol of school discipline, but also a significant technique of governmentality in Australian schools (Meadmore and Symes, 1996: 209–25). A 'dividing practice', the uniform validates certain subjectivities and excludes others, atomizing individual bodies to enforce discipline (Foucault, 1982). Uniforms are as much about promoting correct appearance as they are about locating deviation and fault. How the uniform looks, the various ways it is worn, and the acts of resistance it inspires are usefully analysed through Foucault's concepts. Studying the rituals and practices of the uniform is critical to understanding how a technology of the body achieves social and political goals. Inés Dussell argues that uniforms are part of long-standing technologies of the body that combine 'aesthetic, scientific, political, and moral discourses' (Dussell, 2004: 86). She uses Foucault's work on bodies and power to argue that subjectification takes place primarily through the body, revealing clothing as a powerful tool of social regulation.

She concludes that uniforms embody resistance as well as power. Despite perceptions of the monolithic nature of uniform wearing, her analysis instead reveals the plural and contradictory features of regulation clothing. Just because systems are created to govern bodies does not mean that they always succeed. Shauna Pomerantz, in her a study of dress code policy for girls in North American schools, finds discourses positioning girls as irresponsible and deviant by normalizing power and control over their bodies (Pomerantz, 2007: 373–86). Dress codes promote students' consciousness of their bodies, and train students to regulate themselves in school and in society, but as these studies demonstrate, there is also the potential to explore creative resistance. Reluctant to characterize school uniform as a rigid system, these scholars use a Foucauldian analysis to reveal the versatility and changing nature of these disciplinary projects.

Foucault has also been used to better understand the social role of the military uniform. Daniel Purdy contrasts two modes of visibility, the tactical

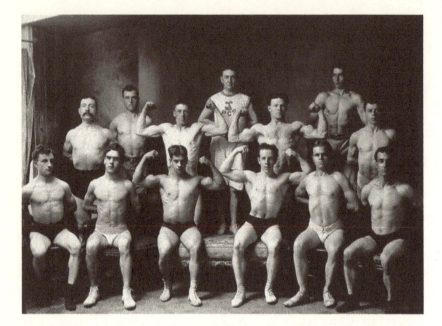

11.2 Male body-builders or wrestlers of the Physical Culture Society of Montreal, Canada, posing with their trainer in a photographic studio, Photograph by: Gordon 1905.

and the fashionable, in his article on the uniform of the Prussian army in the eighteenth century, to consider how the dress of this soldier served the interests of power (Purdy, 2003: 23–45). Purdy suggests that the simplicity of the clothes of the Prussian soldier reflected a disciplinary field of vision: 'The clothes cover the body with such intensity that they become almost a second skin, a natural part of the body, and thereby are almost no covering at all […]. The uniform was both invisible and visible' (Purdy, 2003: 45). For Foucault, disciplines are the various techniques that form a sustainable strategy for sorting people into disciplined groups, but the aesthetic employed in the design of modern uniforms reflects his 'dividing practices', the drive to individualize people within groups. In this sense, the utility aesthetic of modern uniform design is linked to strategic projects of institutional control.

And yet, McVeigh insists that however powerful the repetitive act of don-ning uniform, norms are often 'imperfectly reproduced' (McVeigh, 1997: 208). Wherever control is imposed there is also excess and resistance. In my work on the military uniform I explore personal accounts from con-scientious objectors who experienced brutal treatment when they refused to wear khaki, extreme actions that exposed the official drive to police mas-culine appearance in Britain during World War I (Tynan, 2012: 86–102). Army authorities responded to their protest with excessive force, a measure of the strategic role clothing had in this military project. Also, in my study on uniforms worn by British combatants in World War I, I use a Foucauldian critical framework to argue that a range of images of soldiers and texts on soldiering formed a powerful discourse about what constituted military masculinity during wartime (Tynan, 2013). Despite the force of discursive formations, the judgements that arose and the consequences of dissent tell a story of negotiation, resistance and improvisation, whereby collective dis-ciplines and subcultures of creative activity became equally critical to the war effort. Thus, the beauty of Foucault's vision of a disciplinary society is that it contains the potential for resistance and negotiation.

Modern uniforms offer a system to mark – and make visible – bodies for classification and discipline, which illustrates why Foucault described mod-ern society as the move from spectacle to surveillance (Shapiro, 2003: 302). For Foucault knowledge and power are inseparable, directing our attention to how things are constituted. Ku Hok Bun argues that 'the purpose of div-ision and scientific classification is for rejection' (Hok Bun, 2006: 290). By describing the techniques of racism and exclusion against Pakistani women in Hong Kong, Hok Bun explores dress as a critical object to constitute normality in terms of bodily appearance and social interaction. The bodies of Pakistani women become a battlefield between two sets of knowledge systems: the strict religious Islamic value system and the local Hong Kong system. Foucault's work offers opportunities to expose the techniques and objects enlisted to enact social exclusion and to express racism. 'The severity of restrictions placed on dress and body, and by extension on our lives (such as work and education), is directly proportional to the degree to which we exceed our culture's norm' (Hok Bun, 2006: 300). Restrictions placed on Pakistani women's dress reflect the degree of stigma attached to their bodies – how uncivilized they are thought to be.

Research on veiling also looks to Foucault to explore how identities are constituted within discursive regimes, whereby dress maintains col-lective identities, but also makes visible the dynamics of identity conflicts

(Humphreys and Brown, 2002, 927–52). In a study of the veil in urban space in Istanbul, Anna Secor uses Foucault's ideas to establish how the body is inscribed with power and knowledge (Secor, 2002: 5–22). Veiling is revealed as more than a symbol, and through Foucault's ideas, becomes a spatial practice that both constrains and enables mobility in urban space. The complexity of the outcomes of all of these studies demonstrates that Foucault's concepts are not as over determined as many have suggested. Foucault was reluctant to 'race' or 'gender' his subjects, but he offered a conceptual toolkit that has given rise to invaluable insights throughout the humanities and social sciences. For the arts, Foucault has particular resonance. He is concerned with modes of visibility but questions their instrumental uses. He reminds us that we should question how images are put to work within the wider political field. This fits with a general scepticism about aesthetics and the embrace of cultural studies methods in art and design history since the 1980s, a shift that has illuminated how images and appearances maintain power structures. Foucault's concern with the body as the target of power gives scholars and students of fashion studies much scope to consider how dress unites communities but also potentially how it can divide them.

CONCLUSION

Foucault saw discourse as a site of power but also resistance. He expanded his model of human society to consider how people challenge and subvert the dominant order. This is why Foucault has gained increased relevance in the context of recent outbursts of civil disobedience globally. Arguably, the politics of everyday clothing, such as the adoption of 'hoodies' to evade police cameras in street protests and the use of civilian uniforms by new anarchists *Black Bloc* all suggest that people are conscious of the potential for clothing to mark them out and re-create them as docile bodies. The pattern to resist the expected norms of everyday appearance is propaganda feedback, a technique used particularly by young people. Having lived under a regime of surveillance all of their lives they are only too aware of the consequences of its judgements.

There are so many potential projects in this area, for instance, how dissenters improvise uniform, to see whether the panoptic gaze is always available to test and neutralize new modern social formations. To explore examples where clothing marks people out could test levels of tolerance in our society for people whose bodies 'exceed our culture's norm'. There is also enormous potential for work on how fashionable dressing reflects the actual disciplines and procedures of production and marketing. More work could be done on subversive fashion from a Foucauldian perspective. Recent groups such as Femen and Slutwalk adopt styles of public protest that echo 1970s feminist activism, in an effort to draw attention to the various ways in which the female body is treated as a battleground in modern society. The public 'pyjama wearing' of young urban working class women, in Dublin and Liverpool in particular over the past few years, is also an intriguing practice whereby women are resisting the dominant code of feminine propriety. Certainly, the response to ban these young women from shops confirmed that this fashion practice was considered deviant. Most of all, it exposed the means of feminine production, representing a bold refusal to fear the censure of a society that demands the concealment of an unfinished and chaotic femininity. Subversive fashion practices challenge the forces that seek to normalize power over bodies. To what extent will body excess be tolerated? And who decides where the lines are to be drawn? Foucault offers us a sense of the all-pervading judgemental gaze, but he also reminds us that the body is the ultimate site of resistance in everyday struggles for power.

NOTES

1   Jeremy Bentham (1748–1832): English philosopher, jurist and social reformer, who planned a school and a prison, and founded University College London.

REFERENCES

Bartsky, S. (1998) 'Foucault, Femininity and the Modernization of Patriarchal Power' in L. Diamond and L. Quinby (eds), Feminism and Foucault: Reflections on Resistance, Boston, MA: Northeastern University Press.

Benstock, S. and Ferriss, S. (eds) (1994) On Fashion, New Brunswick, NJ: Rutgers University Press.

Berger, J. (1972) Ways of Seeing, London: Penguin.

Bordo, S. (1998) 'Anorexia Nervosa: Psychopathology as the Crystallization of Culture' in L. Diamond and L. Quinby (eds), Feminism and Foucault: Reflections on Resistance, Boston, MA: Northeastern University Press.

Callewaert, S. (2006) 'Bourdieu, Critic of Foucault: The Case of Empirical Social Science against Double-Game-Philosophy' in Theory, Culture & Society, 23 (6): 73–98.

Carlisle Duncan, M. (1994) 'The Politics of Women's Body Images and Practices: Foucault, the Panopticon and *Shape Magazine*' in *Journal of Sport and Social Issues*, 18 (1): 48–65.

Craik, J. (1993) *The Face of Fashion: Critical Studies in Fashion*, London: Routledge.

Dussell, I. (2004) 'Fashioning the Schooled Self' in B.M. Baker and K.E. Heyning (eds), *Dangerous Coagulations: The Uses of Foucault in the Study of Education*, New York: Peter Lang.

Entwistle, J. (1997) ' "Power Dressing" and the Construction of the Career Woman' in M. Nava et al. (eds), *Buy This Book: Studies in Advertising and Consumption*, London: Routledge.

———(2000) *The Fashioned Body: Fashion, Dress and Modern Social Theory*, Cambridge: Polity.

———(2001) 'The Dressed Body' in J. Entwistle and E. Wilson (eds), *Body Dressing*, Oxford: Berg.

———(2009) *The Aesthetic Economy of Fashion: Markets and Values in Clothing and Modelling*, Oxford: Berg.

Finkelstein, J. (2007) *The Art of Self-Invention: Image and Identity in Popular Visual Culture*, London: I.B. Tauris.

Foucault, M. (1982) 'The Subject and Power' in H.L. Dreyfus and P. Rabinow (eds), *Michel Foucault: Beyond Structuralism and Hermeneutics*, New York: Harvester-Whatsheaf.

———(1990 [1976]) *The History of Sexuality, Vol. 1*, R. Hurley (trans), London: Penguin.

———(1991 [1977]) *Discipline and Punish: The Birth of the Prison*, A. Sheridan (trans), London: Penguin.

———(1994) 'Return to History' in J.D. Faubion (ed), *Aesthetics, Method and Epistemology*, London: Allen Lane.

———(1997) 'Panopticism' in N. Leach (ed), *Rethinking Architecture*, London: Routledge.

———(2001 [1967]) *Madness and Civilization: A History of Insanity in the Age of Reason*, R. Howard (trans), London: Routlege.

———(2004 [1969]) *The Archaeology of Knowledge*, London: Routledge.

Fraser, N. (1985) 'Michel Foucault: A "Young Conservative"?' in *Ethics*, 96 (1): 165–84.

Habermas, J. (1990) *The Philosophical Discourse of Modernity*, Lawrence, MA: The MIT Press.

Heyes, C. (2007) *Self-Transformations: Foucault, Ethics, and Normalized Bodies*, Oxford: Oxford University Press.

Hok Bun, K. (2006) 'Body, Dress and Cultural Exclusion: Experiences of Pakistani Women in "Global" Hong Kong' in *Asian Ethnicity*, 7 (3): 285–302.

Humphreys, M. and Brown, A. (2002) 'Dress and Identity: A Turkish Case Study' in *Journal of Management Studies*, 39 (7): 927–52.

Jeacle, I. (2012) 'Governing and Calculating Everyday Dress' in *Foucault Studies*, (13): 82–98.

Kaiser, S.B. (2012) *Fashion and Cultural Studies*, London: Berg.

Kaplan, A. (1983) *Women and Film: Both Sides of the Camera*, London: Methuen.

McLaren, M.A. (2002) *Feminism, Foucault and Embodied Subjectivity*, New York: SUNY Press.

McVeigh, B. (1997) 'Wearing Ideology: How Uniforms Discipline Minds and Bodies in Japan' in *Fashion Theory*, 1 (2): 189–214.

Meadmore, D. and Symes, C. (1996) 'Of Uniform Appearance: A Symbol of School Discipline and Governmentality' in *Discourse: Studies in the Cultural Politics of Education*, 17 (2): 209–26.

Mears, A. (2008) 'Discipline of the Catwalk: Gender, Power and Uncertainty in Fashion Modeling' in *Ethnography*, 9 (4): 429–56.

Mulvey, L. (1975) 'Visual Pleasure and Narrative Cinema' in *Screen*, 16 (3): 6–18.

Nochlin, L. (1994) *Women, Art and Power and Other Essays*, London: Thames and Hudson.

Pomerantz, S. (2007) 'Cleavage in a Tank Top: Bodily Prohibition and the Discourses of School Dress Codes' in *The Alberta Journal of Educational Research*, 53 (4): 373–86.

Purdy, D. (2003) 'Sculptured Soldiers and the Beauty of Discipline: Herder, Foucault and Masculinity' in M. Henn and H.A. Pausch (eds), Body Dialectics in the Age of Goethe, Amsterdamer Beiträge zur neuren Germanistik, Vol. 55, Leiden: Rodopi.

Rajchman, J. (1983–84) 'The Story of Foucault's History' in Social Text, 8: 3–24.

Rocamora, A. (2009) Fashioning the City: Paris, Fashion and the Media, London: I.B. Tauris.

Rouse, J. (1994) 'Power/Knowledge' in G. Cutting (ed), Cambridge Companion to Foucault, Cambridge: Cambridge University Press.

Sawicki, J. (1991) Disciplining Foucault: Feminism, Power, and the Body, Hove: Psychology Press.

Secor, A. (2002) 'The Veil and Urban Space in Istanbul: Women's Dress, Mobility and Islamic Knowledge' in Gender, Place and Culture, 9 (1): 5–22.

Shapiro, G. (2003) Archaeologies of Vision: Foucault and Nietzsche on Seeing and Saying, London: University of Chicago Press.

Steele, V. (2001) The Corset: A Cultural History, New Haven, CT: Yale University Press.

Svendsen, L. (2006) Fashion: A Philosophy, London: Reaktion Books.

Taylor, C. (1984) 'Foucault on Freedom and Truth' in Political Theory, 12 (2): 164–65.

Tseëlon, E. (1995) The Masque of Femininity: The Presentation of Woman in Everyday Life, London: Sage.

Tynan, J. (2012) ' "Quakers in Khaki": Conscientious Objectors' Resistance to Uniform Clothing in World War I' in S. Gibson and S. Mollan (eds), Representations of Peace and Conflict, Basingstoke: Palgrave Macmillan.

———(2013) British Army Uniform and the First World War: Men in Khaki, Basingstoke: Palgrave MacMillan.

Warwick, A. and Cavallaro, D. (1998) Fashioning the Frame: Boundaries, Dress and the Body, Oxford and New York: Berg.

12

NIKLAS LUHMANN
Fashion between the Fashionable and Old-fashioned

Aurélie Van de Peer

INTRODUCTION

Prior to the January 2013 collections, Andrew Tuck, editor of lifestyle magazine *Monocle*, worried on the periodical's internet blog that for today's fashion aficionados 'fashion is no longer fashionable', and you better not 'say you like fashion, you'll get yourself a terrible reputation' (Tuck, 2013). It seems that in today's fashion world, wanting to be in fashion is considered old-fashioned. This observation is a fashion insider form of distinction, but might also be suggestive of hostility towards fashion. Despite contemporary fashion theorists' continuous efforts to prove the critics wrong, fashion has been condemned time and again for its frivolous and ephemeral features. For instance, by comparing fashion to more timeless cultural formations that allegedly express deeper, hidden meanings, such as the fine arts, critics continue to allocate fashion with its purported lack of depth and rationality to the lower steps of the ladder of cultural worth. By taking up the grand theoretical framework of the German sociologist Niklas Luhmann (1927–1998), this chapter considers whether there is logic to the operations of fashion and whether Luhmannian theory may aid fashion scholars in addressing the repudiation of their object of inquiry.

ALL THINGS SOCIAL

In his 30 year career the German sociologist Niklas Luhmann touched upon a wide range of topics, from mass media to time and from education to the arts. Authoring over 50 books and 400 articles, of which so far only a few have been translated into English, his work has had a major influence on several disciplines. Suffice it to say that this chapter will be an introduction to his comprehensive theoretical framework.

In the above section I describe Luhmann's theoretical framework as 'grand'. This is exactly what he intended his work to be. Reasoning in a highly abstract manner, Luhmann was often critiqued for his nearly indigestible prose. After introducing Luhmann's key concepts, this chapter seeks to transform a possible conceptual intimidation into an understanding that his 'supertheory' (Luhmann, 1995a: 4) of all things social contributes some important theoretical tools for fashion scholars. Thinking of fashion through the work of Niklas Luhmann offers a pathway to strengthen the position of those who wish to theorize further how it can be that the power of fashion remains so hard to overcome, despite all the criticism addressed to it.

The next section highlights Luhmann's major concepts following Borch's (2011) three phases in the sociologist's oeuvre: his focus on the relation between system and environment of the 1970s, the autopoietic turn of the 1980s and the paradoxical turn of the 1990s. The section likewise outlines Luhmann's view of modern society. The subsequent part of the chapter discusses his scarce writing on fashion and explores the existing Luhmannian theoretical analyses of fashion (Esposito, 2004, 2011; Loschek, 2009; Schiermer, 2010). I conclude by pointing to the insights a Luhmannian perspective might spark in fashion studies.

LUHMANN IN CONTEXT

Niklas Luhmann's interest in sociology was sharpened by a stay at Harvard University in 1960–1961 under the supervision of Talcott Parsons, the renowned American proponent of functional systems theory (see Parsons, 1951). Luhmann quickly realized how Parsonian systems theory was incompatible with his own view of *systems*. A system in general refers to a unified entity that can operate on its own separate from the environment (Luhmann, 1995a). The difference between Parsons' and Luhmann's interpretation of a system is that Parsons considers the actions of people taking up important positions structured by role expectations to be the building blocks of a system, where Luhmann sees communications (infra) as the constituents of a system.

Luhmann was primarily interested in social systems and wanted to draw attention to the question of how social systems 'make sense' of their environment. In analysing systems, Luhmann emphasizes the *boundaries* between systems and their environment. Diverse types of system appear only because they differentiate themselves vis-à-vis what they are not, meaning whatever lies outside the boundaries of the system.

Being interested in social systems, Luhmann's analysis of the social realm begins with the broad claim that *distinction* determines the social sphere. In developing his understanding of the concept of distinction, Luhmann (1993) aligned his systems theory with the post-modern French thinking on difference, which found its most known arbiter in Jacques Derrida (1974, 1978; see chapter 15 on Derrida) and his theory of deconstruction. Both theorists share the idea that self-reflection, or what Luhmann calls *observations of the second-order*, that observe how others and you as the 'Other' observe, are predicated on 'differences, to look at distinctions without the hope of regaining unity at a higher (or later) level' (Luhmann, 1993: 766). Consequently, systems cannot be understood as unities; rather it is *difference* that characterizes them most. Luhmann likewise employs his understanding of distinction to distance himself from contemporary sociologists, such as Pierre Bourdieu (see chapter 14), who hold the common sense view of distinction as individuals and groups seeking to set themselves apart from others through identifying with aesthetic or social values and practices associated with specific social groupings such as, in the case of Bourdieu, classes.

THREE PHASES

Draw a Distinction

Luhmann's concept of *distinction* marks the first phase in his oeuvre. As stated, this does not entail the dynamic between belonging and setting oneself apart. Rather he draws on the notion of *observation* in the philosophical logics of George Spencer-Brown's 'Laws of Form' (1969) to understand distinction. Luhmann sees it, simply put, as a concept of demarcation (Luhmann, 1998). When systems observe, they distinguish between two elements, while relying on only one side of the distinction. The totality of the observation thus remains out of sight. Systems construe an understanding of reality in a *first-order observation* that produces its own blind spot: the two poles of the distinction. Following Spencer-Brown, Luhmann labels such an observation as a form or, in German, a *Leitdifferenz*. Systems employ these operations of distinction to perform their main goal: *the reduction of complexity*. Let me give an example related to fashion.

Imagine you need to decide what to wear to work in the morning. You open up the wardrobe that you share with your spouse and are overwhelmed by the complex tangle of garments you see. First you distinguish based on the observation 'my stuff/partner's clothes'. Next you distinguish between the various categories of garments, demarcating between skirts and trousers (lower body garments), tops and blouses (upper body garments). In each of those established categories, you then select one option, because in reality you cannot wear two pairs of trousers at once. In the end, you choose your red pair of jeans. Two elements here are essential to grasping Luhmann's notion of distinction. First, your series of observations are not necessarily conscious or deliberate. Second, when focusing on your clothes only, you forget the first step you took to simplify the complex decision of what to wear based on the two poles of the observation. The distinction 'my stuff/spouse's clothes', thus becomes the blind spot of your first observation.

Hence distinction is the most basic operation through which something meaningful is constructed. Meaning is a notion Luhmann (1995a: 60) understands, however, in the Husserlian sense of *Sinn*, which finds a better translation in the English word *sense*, as employed in 'making-sense' through selection within the horizon of whatever is possible. The red jeans you wear are meaningful because you selected one possibility from the mass of garments you own, not because the trousers 'mean' something in the sense of 'representation'. Moreover, your choice excluded all other skirts and trousers. Yet these selections remain open, since the other possibilities in your wardrobe are only temporarily closed off. You may wear those options at some other time. In addition, you could have chosen other trousers. Therefore selections are *contingent* or, as Luhmann (1998: 45) likes to put it, 'neither necessary nor impossible'.

Perhaps the discussion on what to wear to work gave you the impression that in Luhmann's work the subject is central to sense-making. Of course people, who Luhmann terms *psychic systems*, make sense of the world through mental acts of distinguishing between the various options available. Yet contrary to phenomenology, which sees meaning as attributed by the individual's 'experience', Luhmann does not privilege the subject as observer (Luhmann, 1990a: 23). He argues that all types of systems, thus also *social systems*, make sense of themselves and their environment through observation. In keeping with the de-subjectified nature of his conceptual frame, Luhmann finds that there are two kinds of observers: *psychic systems* (persons) that observe via consciousness and *social systems* that observe via communication. When we turn to the question of how systems create and maintain their boundaries, we enter a new phase in Luhmann's thinking, regarding the autopoietic.

Functional Differentiation and Autopoiesis

During the 1980s the notion of *autopoiesis*, from the Greek words 'auto' (self) and 'poiesis' (production), received most of Luhmann's (1995a) attention. Central to the concept is that all systems maintain their boundaries by self-producing their own meaning-constructions: people self-produce cognition and the different social systems self-produce communications. These systems thus follow an *operative closure*, although they are not disembedded from their environment. Remember that systems come into being through construing a difference with their environment. Yet because of this difference the system and its environment remain co-dependent. This mutual dependence Luhmann terms *structural couplings*. As a consequence, systems co-evolve in the sense that a change in one system, constituting the environment of other systems, will give an impetus for change in another system.

For instance, the operative logic of fashion may influence the sciences: think of the recent linguistic, performative and material turns in the humanities and social sciences which seem to express the desire of scholars to engage with the temporal logic of fashion in adopting a fashionable or 'of the moment' theoretical perspective. This interference of fashion within the science system, however, does not occur in a simplistic pattern of cause and effect. Systems cannot straightforwardly influence the operations of other systems. When a new academic book frames its narrative within a popular conceptualization, the scholarly public may recognize that the fashionable element is part of the book's appeal. Yet scholars would never approve of such research solely because it adheres to the latest academic fad. Instead, they privilege studies that represent and explicate the research questions in a highly plausible manner. Fashion merely *irritates* science, so to speak. It produces a perturbation in the science system, which science then deals with in its own communications.

Luhmann sees modern society as made up of various *functionally differentiated social subsystems*. Yet theorizing modern society in this light is not new. Various theorists in the sociological tradition embraced the concept of a differentiated society, from Karl Marx to Georg Simmel. Niklas Luhmann added his idea of autopoiesis to the differentiation thesis. In modern society we find various self-producing subsystems that offer society something only they can deliver. Luhmann explored science (1990a), economics (1999), education (2002a), politics (2000) and art (2000) as such functional subsystems, which are entirely self-producing or autopoietic. Indeed in Luhmann's strict vision (2002b: 116–17), if systems do not produce their own operations through system-specific communications, they are not systems.

With functional differentiation, initiated between the sixteenth and eighteenth centuries, modern society grew radically different from earlier societal formations (Luhmann, 2012). Archaic societies are defined by *segmentary differentiation*, for instance, with kinship as a principal organizational form. *Stratification differentiation* characterizes high-culture societies divided by hierarchical social strata, classes or castes. Luhmann argues that modern society is the most complex societal formation because it has incorporated the two other forms of societal organization. Think of how, in the fashion world of the early twentieth century, Parisian houses such as Lanvin and Worth mostly kept business succession within the family (segmentary) or how most fashion companies today still rely on the unpaid labour of interns who are lowest in rank (stratification). Moreover, in our modern differentiation, societal forms occur that have not yet reached functional differentiation; for example, the caste system in India is still present today.

How does a functional subsystem come into being and how does it operate? *Success media* trigger the differentiation of function systems through providing a binary code structure around which the communications in the subsystem can revolve (Luhmann, 2012: 358–59). These media are not the mass media, however, but instances that increase the probability of the success of communications, such as money (Luhmann, 1990b). In the economic system money allows you to buy that pair of red jeans. Yet you cannot rely on it to bring successful outcomes for any operation outside the economic system, if a scientist uses money to convince a publisher to disseminate his or her work, that would be regarded as a bribe. The *binary codes* these success media spark likewise pertain only to one functional subsystem. Furthermore, the codes are strictly binary. The economy oscillates between payment and non-payment, for instance, and the sciences between true and false. In other words, you cannot 'more or less' pay someone, just like a specific scientific assertion cannot be 'a bit' true. This implies that, like all other social systems, functional subsystems are operationally closed, meaning that they are not at all interested in the workings, communications and perspectives of other subsystems. Every subsystem, therefore, produces its own reality and may operate along its self-produced operative logic (Luhmann, 1990c: 693). Operative logic will differ in a legal perspective from that in an art perspective, for example. In Luhmann's theory, binary codes remain closed off to change. Nonetheless, subsystems themselves are highly flexible and open. A subsystem's binary code does not decide itself how and when it should be applied. Instead, *programmes* are the criteria for the application of the code. They control how to attribute the code correctly. Programs may undergo considerable change and may even be replaced by new programmes (Luhmann, 1995a: 317). Think of a paradigm shift in the sciences which incites the need for new theories and methodologies without touching its basic operative code. Luhmann's understanding of the functional differentiation of modern society has several important consequences. First, because every functional subsystem may produce its own operative logic, a societal problem will be regarded and acted upon differently by every subsystem (Luhmann, 1995b). This has both discursive and temporal implications. Every subsystem speaks its own language. For instance, fashion aficionados have adopted a specific fashion discourse, or in Luhmann's words *semantics*, which is often foreign to the non-interested. Likewise systems operate in different temporal horizons. The timeframe for legal jurisdiction is different from the timeframe of fashion, known for its short-lived temporality. Second, Luhmann imagines society as flat: no subsystem has the power to intervene in another. Unlike scholars working in the Marxist tradition, who Luhmann believes overestimate the importance of the economic system, Luhmann privileges no subsystem. There is no vantage point from which we can observe all of society, which implies that every perspective we take inevitably has a blind spot. Furthermore, because of the absence of an overarching perspective, every social system continuously produces its own 'ways of not seeing'. This brings us to *paradox*: the notion Niklas Luhmann meticulously developed in the 1990s.

Paradox

Every system produces its own blind spot, which ultimately leads to a paradox. When we return to the principal elements of sense-making, that is, observation and distinction, we will comprehend paradox better. Recall that you decided to wear the red jeans. Now assume your friend asks you why you chose to wear the garment. You maintain you selected the trousers because 'these are in fashion nowadays'. Luhmann calls such statement a *first-order observation* in which you claim something to be the case. Imagine that your friend replies with the following *observation of the second-order*: 'It's so interesting you say that. I just read this article that asked whether wanting to be in fashion is actually still fashionable.' Citing the *Monocle* journalist, your friend here observes your initial justification that the jeans were fashionable through applying that very same distinction. At this moment a paradox appears that blocks further observations, because how can one reply to the statement questioning whether wanting to be in fashion is still fashionable? Unlike traditional epistemologies that view paradoxes as indicators of conceptual flaws, they do not worry Niklas Luhmann at all. In his later work he proposed that the recognition of paradoxes may actually reveal that which remains beyond reach: the strategies systems employ in practice to function despite paradoxes (Luhmann, 1995b: 52). This is why Luhmann's later project paid so much attention to second-order observations, because this type of observation allows you to observe the blind spot of your own and other systems' observations. He finds that modern society consists of a plethora of paradoxes (Luhmann, 1995b). Fashion too, as I explain below, is predicated on myriad paradoxes (Esposito, 2004, 2011). One trajectory fashion scholars can take to conceptualize further the power of fashion is to probe the paradoxes at its heart.

THE PARADOXES OF FASHION

Luhmann's writings on fashion are scarce. The only text in which he addresses the question of fashion directly is a book review (Luhmann, 1984) of Udo Schwarz's monograph (1982) *Das Modische*. There Luhmann proposes that fashion enables systems to deal with a great amount of contingency or uncertainty because it finds its own rationality or operative logic in the reliability of the changeable. Recently Elena Esposito (2004, 2011) developed this line of thought further in arguing that the nature of fashion is inherently paradoxical. Such paradoxes find a clear articulation in both the temporal and social dimensions of fashion.

First, fashion developed its own operative logic from the continuity of its changeable character. In other words, fashion proffered 'the stability of the transitional' (Esposito, 2011: 607). Where in early modernity this proposal was still met with distrust, soon it acquired a sense of factuality and, I would add, normativity, in the sense that the modern individual only finds the changeable to be likeable, approvable and to be the object of reference for all items of fashion deemed to be 'good'. In fashionable dress, it seems that only a 'scheduled transitoriness' (Luhmann, 1989: 256 cited in Esposito, 2011: 608) grants us firm ground, to the extent that we now constantly expect things to differ from whatever dress style came before. Second, modernity became obsessed with individuality and originality because its subject paradigm made it the ultimate carrier of agency and change. Whether trickle-down or bubble-up, particular fashion-forward individuals or groups (in the sense of a community of early adopters) set the example for all others to follow. Yet it is paradoxical that an individual should do what others do in order to be an individual (Esposito, 2004).

Furthermore, this mimetic side of fashion holds such penetrating power into both fashionable dress and other cultural formations because it looks so harmless (Esposito, 2011). The power of fashion lies exactly in its frivolous and transient character. Fashion can acquire a mask of harmless ephemerality because it knows how to neutralize its paradoxes. For instance, we constantly expect to be surprised by the newness and difference of the latest fashions. Yet this temporal expectation is paradoxical in the normality it has acquired. Through attributing these expectations of surprise to the originality of individuals, however, the social paradox compensates for the temporal one. For instance, through picturing fashion designers as creative autonomous artists or particular celebrity fashion icons as the arbiters of the new, we neutralize the temporal paradox that lays bare how fashion in its changeability is compared to the continuous.

Engaging with the question of whether fashion is a functional subsystem of modern society further offers a Luhmannian route to tackling the lower cultural status of fashion. Remember that Luhmann privileges no societal subsystem. The next section proposes that if fashion is such a functional subsystem, there is conceptual space to rebuff the ladder of cultural valorization which tends to allocate fashion to its lower steps.

IS FASHION A FUNCTIONAL SUBSYSTEM OF MODERN SOCIETY?

The answer to the above question seems a straightforward, affirmative one. Just a quick glance at the contemporary fields of luxury, mass fashion production and consumption seems to yield the insight that other societal subsystems have no say in determining the next fashion. Yet the few fashion scholars who have turned to Niklas Luhmann for theoretical guidance have not yet settled the debate. Where Doris Schmidt (2007) and Ingrid Loschek (2009) see fashionable dress as a functional subsystem, Elena Esposito (2004, 2011), Bjorn Schiermer (2010) and Udo Schwarz (1982) have their doubts. Let us first turn to the work of those scholars who theorize that fashionable dress is a subsystem that operates by following self-produced communications.

Both Schmidt (2007) and Loschek (2009: 21–28) picture fashionable dress as a subsystem in which all communications ultimately revolve around the binary code of In and Out. Fashion media that structure their reports on fashion items in 'In and Out' columns, for example, clearly evidence this binary code. Loschek and Schmidt differ, however, on the subject of material fashion objects. For Schmidt (2007: 46) the cut, fabrics, patterns and textures are the very communications of fashion. Loschek (2009: 133–36) instead perceives such features as parts of the programs of the system, in which the changeable nature of fashion manifests itself most clearly. Because the binary code of In and Out implies the additional code of Fashionable and Old-fashioned, Loschek maintains that the system-specific communications of fashion are centred around social validity. She writes: 'the question of which clothing is fashion is an exclusively social, communicatively negotiated definition' (Loschek, 2009: 25).

Yet this idea seems foreign to a traditional Luhmannian perspective. In his work on the art system, for instance, Luhmann (2000) claims that works of art put themselves forward as 'art' by means of 'communications through art' (Schinkel, 2010). I would argue that we can extrapolate Luhmann's assumption to other cultural products, and that he views the material fashion objects as communicating 'I am fashion'; much like Doris Schmidt described the communications of the fashion system occurring through the stuff of fashion. This is to say that Luhmann refers communications *about* art or *about* fashion (museums, buyers, journalism), in deciding which objects count as art or fashion, to the environment of the systems of art and fashion. Nonetheless, Loschek writes that 'any garment other than what has been agreed upon as fashion is simply clothing' (Loschek, 2009: 136). This begs the question as to who communicates fashion-status *about* clothing and how they legitimately do so. Luhmann (2000) tends to assume an object or practice to be art a priori; however, the question above points us to the work of the 'cultural intermediaries' (Bourdieu, 1996) of fashion, such as journalists, buyers, photographers and stylists. They not only disseminate the latest trends but negotiate decisions on fashion status. Consequently, I contend that scholars who seek to theorize fashion as a self-producing system should include the communications *about* fashion, because in reality these ground, judge and stabilize communications *through* fashion.

For example, in 1982 Rei Kawakubo for Comme des Garçons presented in Paris a now iconic piece of knitwear; a deliberately distressed black sweater with holes in it. In this and her following collections Kawakubo posited the hyper-reflexive question 'can this be fashion?' through her fashionable designs.

Yet probing the limits of fashion in such a way was possible only because the communications of those (traditionally journalists, buyers, editors) who talk and write *about* fashion fostered the prior recognition that Kawakubo's experimental designs were part of the fashion system's communications. Communications *about* fashion recognized her communications *through* the distressed sweater as *within* the system. Hence, communications *through* fashion, where interpretation is contingent on the degree that it could be read and interpreted otherwise, do not gain meaning independent of communications *about* fashion. The latter communications thus need to be conceptualized as part of the subsystem.

Finding that fashionable dress is indeed an autopoietic subsystem of modern society implies a forceful argument against critics who think of fashion as immersed in a hierarchical relationship with other cultural formations. Recall that in the Luhmannian framework, there is no bird's eye perspective from which to observe the entire system. In other words, the fashion system does not operate hierarchically, as it appears to in other sociological perspectives of fashion production. For instance, working within a Marxist tradition that prioritizes the economic system, Bourdieu sees fashion as caught between the artistic and economic fields (Bourdieu and Delsaut, 1975: 22). Financial considerations (particularly in the case of fashion at a high price point) are thought to debase the status of fashion as a valorized cultural or artistic practice. When fashion seeks to climb the ladder of cultural valorization, it thus misrecognizes its market liaisons in a *reversed economy*. As it aligns itself more closely with fine arts, we speak of *artification* (Shapiro, 2007), meaning that fashion becomes 'artful' or an art 'more or less'. This idea is embedded, for instance, in the widespread assumption that fashion is not a 'pure art', but an 'applied art' or part of the 'decorative arts'. Yet when thinking of fashion as a functional subsystem neither scholars, nor politicians, nor artists can decide what the next fashion will be, which implies that the communications that constitute the fashion system have to be regarded in and for themselves, rather than as being located on a comparative scale with other cultural formations, such as the fine arts and literature. Thinking of fashion through the Luhmannian framework goes beyond the idea of a cultural hierarchy between fashion and art. Fashion communications simply pertain to the fashion system and art communications to the system of art.

Nonetheless, several fashion scholars have noted that fashionable dress soaks up developments and changes in the economy, politics and the arts (Blumer, 1969: 283; Schiermer, 2010: 30), suggesting that fashionable dress is not completely self-producing and thus not a modern functional subsystem, as Schmidt and Loschek claimed it to be. Elena Esposito (2004) and Bjorn Schiermer (2010) have developed this line of thought, with two key elements. First, scholars have hitherto insufficiently theorized the exclusive task fashionable dress fulfils in modern society. Recall that in the Luhmannian framework all subsystems offer society something only they can deliver. Despite the insightful contributions to this question from the theory of social ambivalence (Kaiser et al., 1995), the academic debate has not considered fully whether fashionable dress has something unique to offer modern society. Second, we may raise serious objections to the idea of Fashionable and Old-fashioned as the binary code of the subsystem. When Kawakubo drew on this distinction, such communications through the materiality of design must have been possible by an autonomous code different from the one Kawakubo played with to observe the difference between fashionable dress and its environment. Ultimately we may therefore wonder whether fashion has a binary code and is a functional subsystem of modern society after all. Although future research may conclude that we cannot theorize fashionable dress as a Luhmannian system (which blocks the route to a non-hierarchical reading of the cultural worth of fashion), the power of fashion remains beyond dispute. It manifests itself in the frivolous and transient character of fashion, which is mired in paradoxes regardless of it being a functional subsystem of society.

CONCLUSION: NIKLAS LUHMANN IN FASHION STUDIES

This chapter has sought to offer a first introduction to the comprehensive framework Niklas Luhmann developed in social systems theory in light of its potential wider application to fashion studies. Hitherto few fashion scholars have adopted a Luhmannian perspective. The chapter took up the question of whether we may regard fashionable dress as a functional subsystem of modern society, on which scholars have not yet made up their minds. Future research will have to examine in greater detail whether and to what extent the necessary conditions to make such an assertion apply to fashionable dress. In this respect I proposed a key element for further consideration: communications *about* fashion have to be considered as part and parcel of the system of fashion. This argument offers a stepping stone to understanding 'the fashion system', if we find it to be in place, as interlaced with insights from Bourdieusian field theory.

Before I point out some promising courses Luhmann's framework might take in the academic debate on fashion, let me note an important shortcoming of his work. Scholars interested in the materiality of fashion and dress will find little value in Luhmann's framework. He explicitly wrote regarding art that its material aspects are not part of the system (Luhmann, 2000). Luhmann would not be interested in the material grounds of fashion: its fabrics, cuts, silhouettes and connection to the living body. Surely such an observation proves problematic when applied to fashion, which cannot do away with its material roots nor with its embodied nature. Many contemporary designers communicate their ideas through the stuff of fashion. To them the material of the dress is meaningful. Despite this shortcoming, Luhmann's comprehensive framework offers fashion studies an important pathway for further exploration.

A better understanding of the paradoxical nature of fashion will benefit the theoretical advancement of the academic debate, because the analysis of second-order observations allows us to unravel what remained unseen before: its various strategies to dismantle paradoxes. In my own research I examine the notion of paradox in the historical relation between change and continuity in fashionable dress. In any paradox or Luhmannian observation, one pole cannot do without the other. Yet in the current academic debate this mutual dependence tends to be denied, owing to plentiful definitions of fashion essentially predicated on change (e.g. Kawamura, 2004; Lipovetsky, 2002; Wilson, 2003). Furthermore, this conception is sometimes granted a transhistorical component. Fashion has always been about change, irrespective of the time period (Kawamura, 2004: 5). Yet bearing in mind the Luhmannian paradoxes discussed, such tendencies to essentialism obviously do not fall into place. Just as fashion is not all-concerned with mimesis or individuality, it is neither all-concerned with change. The fact, however, that both actors in the current high-fashion industry and scholars of fashion are prone to work with such a one-sided vision merits our attention. It begs the question how we and they have grown to take for granted the idea that fashion is immersed exclusively in constant change. I would thus like to propose for the future study of the paradoxes of fashion a thorough historicization of the performative aspects by which many involved in the production of fashion and its study have aligned themselves to just one side of the distinction. Moreover, a thorough analysis of the various paradoxes of fashion would contribute to an improved comprehension of the power of fashion. Referring to the citation that opened this chapter, I would argue that critics can oppose fashion as much as they want, 'but don't think for a moment that you have dodged the fickleness of dress codes, aka fashion' (Tuck, 2013).

REFERENCES

Blumer, H. (1969) 'Fashion: From Class Differentiation to Collective Selection' in *Sociological Quaterly*, 10 (3): 275–91.

Borch, C. (2011) *Niklas Luhmann*, London: Routledge.

Bourdieu, P. (1996) *Distinction: A Social Critique of the Judgement of Taste*, London: Routledge.

Bourdieu, P. and Delsaut, Y. (1975) 'Le Couturier et sa Griffe: Contribution à une Théorie de la Magie' in *Actes de la Recherche en Sciences Sociales*, 1 (1): 7–36.

Derrida, J. (1974 [1967]) *Of Grammatology*, G.C. Spivak (trans), Baltimore, MD: Johns Hopkins University Press.

———(1978 [1967]) *Writing and Difference*, A. Bass (trans), Chicago: University of Chicago Press.

Esposito, E. (2004) *Die Verbindlichkeit des Vorübergehenden: Paradoxien der Mode*, Frankfurt am Main: Suhrkamp.

———(2011) 'Originality through Imitation: The Rationality of Fashion' in *Organization Studies*, 32 (5): 603–13.

Kaiser, S., Nagasawa, H. and Hutton, S. (1995) 'Construction of an SI Theory of Fashion: Part I: Ambivalence and Change' in *Clothing and Textiles Research Journal*, 13 (3): 172–83.

Kawamura, Y. (2004) *The Japanese Revolution in Paris Fashion*, Oxford: Berg.

Lipovetsky, G. (2002) *The Empire of Fashion: Dressing Modern Democracy*, Princeton, NJ: Princeton University Press.

Loschek, I. (2009) *When Clothes become Fashion: Design and Innovation Systems*, Oxford: Berg.

Luhmann, N. (1984) 'Udo H.A. Schwarz, Das Modische' in *Soziologische Revue*, 7: 73–74.

———(1989) 'Individuum, Individualität, Individualismus' in *Gesellschaftsstruktur und Semantik: Studien zur Wissenssoziologie der modernen Gesellschaft*, Band 3, Frankfurt am Main: Suhrkamp.

———(1990a) 'Meaning as Sociology's Basic Concept' in *Essays on Self-Reference*, New York: Columbia University Press.

———(1990b) 'The Improbability of Communication' in *Essays on Self-Reference*, New York: Columbia University Press.

———(1990c) *Die Wissenschaft der Gesellschaft*, Frankfurt am Main: Suhrkamp.

———(1993) 'Deconstruction as Second-Order Observing' in *New Literary History*, 24: 763–82.

———(1995a [1984]) *Social Systems*, J. Bernarz Jr (trans), Stanford, CA: Stanford University Press.

———(1995b) 'The Paradoxy of Observing Systems' in *Cultural Critique*, 31: 37–55.

———(1998 [1992]) *Observations on Modernity*, W. Whobrey (trans), Stanford, CA: Stanford University Press.

———(1999) 'The Concept of Society' in A. Elliott (ed), *Contemporary Social Theory*, Oxford: Blackwell.

———(2000 [1995]) *Art as a Social System*, E. Knodt (trans), Stanford, CA: Stanford University Press.

———(2002a) 'What is Communication?' in W. Rasch (ed), *Theories of Distinction: Re-describing the Descriptions of Modernity*, Stanford, CA: Stanford University Press.

———(2002b) *Einführung in die Systemtheorie*, D. Baecker (ed), Heidelberg: Carl-Auer-Systeme Verlag.

———(2012 [1997]) *The Theory of Society*, R. Barrett (trans), Stanford, CA: Stanford University Press.

Parsons, T. (1951) *The Social System*, London: The Free Press of Glencoe.

Schiermer, B. (2010) 'Mode, Bewusstsein und Kommunikation' in *Soziale Systeme, Zeitschrift für Soziologische Theorie*, 16 (1): 121–49.

Schinkel, W. (2010) 'The Autopoiesis of the Artworld after the End of Art' in *Cultural Sociology*, 4 (2): 267–90.

Schmidt, D. (2007) *Die Mode der Gesellschaft: Eine systemtheoretische Analyse*, Baltmannsweiler: Schneider Verlag.

Schwarz, U.H.A. (1982) *Das Modische: Zur Struktur sozialen Wandels der Moderne*, Berlin: Duncker & Humblot.

Shapiro. R. (2007) 'Art et Changement Social: l'Artification' in P. Le Quéau (ed), *Vingt Ans de Sociologie de l'art: Bilan et Perspectives*, Paris: L'Harmattan.

Spencer-Brown, G. (1969) *Laws of Form*, London: Allen & Unwin.

Tuck, A. (2013) 'When Fashion is no Longer Fashionable' in *Monocolumn*, retrieved from http://monocle.com/monocolumn/design/when-fashion-is-no-longer-fashionable on 2 March 2013.

Wilson, E. (2003) *Adorned in Dreams: Fashion and Modernity*, London: I.B. Tauris.

13

JEAN BAUDRILLARD
Post-modern Fashion as the End of Meaning

Efrat Tseëlon

INTRODUCTION

Jean Baudrillard (1929–2007) is considered one of the major thinkers of the post-modern age. Trained as a sociologist at the University of Paris-Nanterre, he emerged on the French intellectual scene of post-May 1968 to challenge orthodoxies and conventional wisdoms of the disciplines, methods, theories, styles and discourses of the academic intellectual establishment. His work spans philosophy, social theory, his own blend of critical cultural analysis and metaphysics of appearances. He addresses consumption in a media-saturated age as a cultural and signifying process.

Although in his writings he did not theorise fashion, except for *Symbolic Exchange and Death* (1993 [1976]), where he devotes a chapter to the subject, fashion by virtue of being an example of consumer object is never absent from his work. In fact he refers to them as interchangeable when he says in an earlier work on consumer culture that 'consumption is inseparable from fashion' (1981 [1972]: 50). In this chapter I apply Baudrillard's theorizing of consumption more broadly to the understanding of the meaning of fashion in consumer culture. I thus hope to show that his writing on consumption is invaluable to thinking through fashion.

FROM SIGNIFICATION TO SIMULATION

With the advent of consumer culture, forms of commodification and consumption, and the prominence of the image in mass media and advertising, Baudrillard appropriated neo-Marxist social theory as a dominant critical discourse. He rejected the idea that consumption is based on the fulfilment of needs or the experience of personal pleasure. Rather, he developed a theory of consumption that analyses our relation to objects as a discursive system. Objects, such as clothes, become elements in a system of signification that has the simplicity and effectiveness of a code. They are not material goods but rather 'signs'. Consumption is a systematic act of the manipulation of signs driven by the logic of desire. To develop this approach, Baudrillard engaged with some of the ideas underpinning psychoanalysis, which were developed in the twentieth century (see also chapter 3 on Freud). He dispensed with psychological motives but retained the psychoanalytic distinction between 'object' and 'aim', where aim is a specific motivation that can be fulfilled by a variety of non-specific objects. A forerunner for the notions of leisure fashion and shopping for clothes as a pleasurable pastime, he shows that 'pleasure' is as much an obligation as a 'duty'. Thus, in his work consumption has the character of desire 'which is insatiable because it is founded on a lack. And this desire, which can never be satisfied, signifies itself locally in a succession of objects and needs' (Glickman, 1999 [1970]). The desire is not motivated by any need that objects can fulfil. Rather, it is a desire for its own image (Baudrillard, 1993 [1976]). This observation explains, for example, why consumers of fashion keep buying, are never satisfied, and forever feel that they have nothing to wear even in front of a closet full of clothes.

Baudrillard's work was also influenced by the structural linguistics of Ferdinand de Saussure and the science of signs – semiology or semiotics – he developed within this framework (also influential on the work of Barthes; see chapter 8). In structural linguistics the process of signification is performed through a system of signs. A sign, according to Saussure, is made up of a signifier and a signified. The signifier (sound-image) indexes the signified (concept). The signifier is a container for the signified and the two unite in creating a sign and its meaning. The real thing out there, to which a sign is attached and refers to, is called a referent. The sign of a human silhouette whose body resembles two opposite triangles (see figure 13.1) symbolizes a woman, on public toilets. This triangle silhouette is the signifier, the idea of the woman (symbolized by the skirt wearing figure) is the signified, and the real woman is the referent. Moreover, signs do not have inherent meaning but gain their meaning through their relation to other signs. For example, in the toilet signs, the solid triangle mounted on a triangle with a narrow base

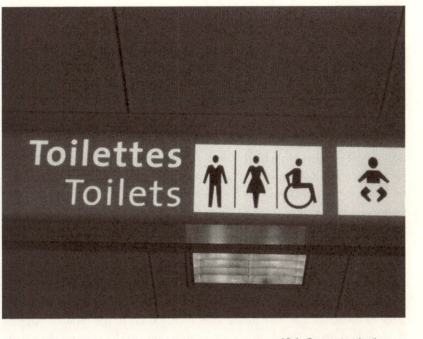

13.1 Conventional toilet signs. The female figure is often positioned on a narrower base.

(balanced on the apex) gains the meaning of a woman against the silhouette of the man which is an outline triangle balanced on its base, has a firm base on the ground, and has trousers instead of a skirt.

Baudrillard applied the structuralist linguistic methodology of Saussure and Barthes to a semiotic system in a post-modern framework. His analysis is post-semiotic because he claims that in post-modernism signs no longer signify. According to him, we have now entered a non-signifying post-modern age where signs refer only to other signs and the system is short-circuited by having no more signifieds. Whereas in the pre-modern and modern stages signifiers still had signifying referents or underlying meanings, in the simulation stage of post-modernism there is no longer depth but everything has become self-referential. Fashion is therefore more about carnival and artifice than form and style.

My analysis of the history of dress signification using Baudrillard's approach would see the meaning of clothes as a transition from (1) a semiology where meaning resides in natural signs, through (2) a structuralist semiology where meaning resides in arbitrary signs, to (3) a new post-structuralist semiology where signs transcend meaning. It is a change from *dress* whose function is to regulate ceremonial distance between bodies, that is to create discrimination from nature, to *fashion* which creates social distinctions, to *post-fashion* which is 'a deconstruction of both the form of the sign of fashion and the principle of signification itself' (1993 [1976]: 133). Baudrillard's genealogy of sign structures thus consists of three orders. The first order, founded on imitation characterizes the pre-modern period. It presupposes dualism in which appearances *reflect* reality. In the second order, founded on production, appearances *mask* reality. In the third order, founded on simulation, appearances *invent* reality. No longer concerned with the real, images are reproduced from a design model. This lack of a reference point blurs the distinction between true and false.

As I have argued elsewhere (Tseëlon, 1994, 1995, 2012a, 2012b) an examination of Baudrillard's historical theory of sign structures shows it to correspond to the historical theorizing of European sartorial representation, as I discuss below. The order of imitation corresponds to the pre-modern stage of dress, the order of production corresponds to the modern stage of fashion, and the order of simulation corresponds to the post-modern stage of post-fashion.

THE THREE STAGES OF SARTORIAL REPRESENTATION

Pre-modern Stage

Throughout European history dress has divided people along the lines of class. From the Greek and Roman periods, through Byzantine and medieval eras, but particularly since the fourteenth century, which marks the beginning of European fashion (e.g. Laver, 1985 [1969]; Wilson, 2013 [1985]), the costliness of materials or workmanship involved in the production of garments distinguished courtly from common. The history of dress is characterized by the principle of scarcity of resources that symbolized rank in dress. Natural scarcity provided a 'guarantee of exclusivity' (Goffman, 1951). Scarcity took either the form of rarity in nature (as in the case of the furs of certain animals, or of gold and precious stones), or in man-made resources (as the case of silk which up to the fifteenth century was imported from the East). All the above meant that economic constraints effectively maintained the social order since those expensive materials were only within reach of the nobility. Servants and workmen wore more wool, no silk or dyed cloth, and less ornamentation than their masters (Black and Garland, 1975). Coarse and common furs were used by the lower classes, while finer, smaller and more rare ones were worn by the wealthy (Ewing, 1981). Contemporary examples of distinction include sales of 'limited edition' items, excessive consumption or entry requirements to shopping venues that are not commonly available such as 'by invitation only'.

During the fourteenth century the expansion of trade and the prosperity of the wool and weaving industries made previously expensive materials affordable by the rising urban middle classes. This development threatened the hierarchy of feudal society where class order was as rigid as if it were ordained by a divine power. As long as the class system was stable and undisturbed, there were few fashion changes among the lower classes. The system got challenged when 'the urban patricians began to manoeuvre into positions of equality with the old feudal nobility' (König, 1973: 111). This challenge triggered the legislation of sumptuary laws that began in the thirteenth century throughout Renaissance Europe. They were an attempt to regulate clothing practices along status lines, and did so by defining precisely the type and quality of fabrics that various classes were allowed to wear.

Until the fourteenth century the shape of garments remained almost unchanged. Since styles were not sanctioned by law, towards the end of the fourteenth century clothes began to take on new forms. This tendency set in motion a process of differentiation whereby the aristocracy could distinguish itself by the speed of adopting new styles. The new styles which were not within reach of lower classes were adopted by them only later, in less luxurious materials, or using their masters' cast-off garments. This dynamic was captured in Simmel's (1904) 'trickle down theory': as soon as a new style was copied by the lower classes, the upper classes moved on to a new one (see also chapter 4 on Simmel).

Modern Stage

The technological developments that characterized industrial capitalism since mid-eighteenth-century England, such as the invention of the sewing machine and wash-proof dyes, increased the democratization of fashion. They reduced the price of materials and made coloured fabrics – once an aristocratic preserve – available to the mass market. The industrial revolution created the distinction between public and private zones unknown in the Middle Ages. Technological advances increased mobility and the pace of life, and multiplied social roles. A new order was created in which work (an achieved status) rather than lineage (an ascribed status) determined social positioning. Uniforms were introduced in the work place to denote rank, as dress no longer reflected rank but instead defined time of day (daywear, eveningwear), type of activity (work, leisure), type of occasion (formal, informal), gender and even an individual's mood.

In the nineteenth century, fashion kept pace with the increasingly compartmentalised, multi-role life of the bourgeoisie. These threats to the traditional social order contributed to the development of an alternative system of demarcation. Thus when clothes ceased to indicate status due to the homogeneity of styles, a subtle expert system evolved that differentiated status between the aristocracy and new money (e.g. Sennett, 1976). This system coded the minutiae of appearance and was accessible only to initiates. It attributed symbolic meanings that reflected a person's character or social standing. It also anchored certain sartorial practices to moral values. For example, the concept of gentility, developed in the nineteenth century by the landed gentry to distinguish the genuine from the pretence, encapsulated the code of ethics of 'noblesse oblige'. This code defined for a lady or a gentleman a standard of conduct which included rules of etiquette, appearance, subtlety and propriety.

Post-modern Stage

In the 1960s post-modernism created a radical break with the dominant culture and aesthetics. In architecture it represented romantic subjectivity, plurality of forms, fragmentation of styles and diffuse boundaries. Thus it substituted disunity, subjectivity and ambiguity for the modernist unity, absolutism and certainty. In the sciences it was evidenced in a Western 'crisis in representation', its authority and its universal claims. This epistemological challenge resulted in replacing universalist explanations about human nature with contextualized ones pertaining to specific times or places. Thus totalizing 'grand narratives' gave way to a plurality of 'narrative truths' that reflected, instead, the conventions of discourse (see, for further details on post-modern thinking, Bauman, 1999; Burr, 2003; Drolet, 2004; Jencks, 2011). The post-modern cultural shift has left its mark on the fashion world through its rejection of tradition, its relaxation of norms, its emphasis on individual diversity and its multiplicity of styles. The result was diminished shared meanings of styles.

In my work I have transposed Baudrillard's analysis of the nature of signification to the three stages of sartorial representation (Tseëlon, 1994, 1995, 2012b), which has produced the model outlined in Table 13.1.

Table 13.1 Baudrillard's orders of simulacra adapted to fashion signification

Order of simulacra	Metaphor	Corresponding stage of European fashion	Metaphysical analogy	Signification order
Imitation	Counterfeit	Pre-modern stage	Metaphysics of depth	Direct signifier–signified links
Production	Illusion	Modern stage	Metaphysics of depth	Indirect signifier–signified links
Simulation	Fake	Post-modern stage	Metaphysics of surface	Signifier–signifier links

In terms of signification the three orders can be understood as follows. First, the order of *imitation* involves direct signifier–signified links. In the order of *imitation*, which characterized the pre-modern stage, clothes refer unequivocally to a status. They signify 'the order of things' without ambiguity. Thus, for example, medieval dress recreated the social order by assigning the more elaborate and rich garments to the elite. Second, the order of *production* involves indirect signifier–signified links. It is characterized by the modern stage where technological and social developments such as mechanization and urbanization enabled the production of mass-produced clothes made available to all classes simultaneously. These developments detached sartorial meaning from its inevitable link to a particular signified, and opened it to a struggle for meaning. For example, luxury materials or dyes previously only within reach of the elite become accessible to the masses, or downmarket second-hand clothes shops are re-cast as upmarket vintage boutiques. The development of the city encouraged a taste for anonymity in cosmopolitan life. The cosmopolitan city was a world in which the meanings of physical appearance were uncertain. For this reason it became important to establish whether people were what they claimed to be. A new status differentiation system evolved to accommodate the new developments. In Baudrillard's vocabulary, the transition from 'products' to 'objects' is 'a process transforming use value into exchange value [...] according to an arbitrary code of differences' (1981 [1972]: 91). Baudrillard argues here that consumer goods moved from utility to symbolism. Originally appreciated and enjoyed as a function of their practical value (use value), they transformed this for exchange value (symbolic or emotional meaning) (1981 [1972]) (see chapter 2 on Marx).

Third, the order of *simulation* involves signifier–signifier links, that is links between signs (signifiers) that are divorced from the objects they represent

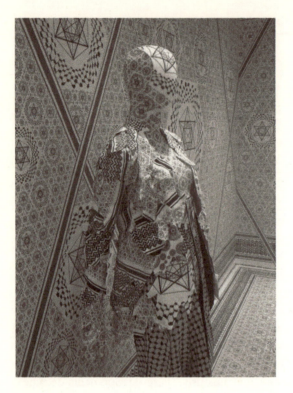

13.2 From *Insalaam, Inshalom.* By threeASFOUR, a New York based fashion and art collective, from their exhibition at Beit Hair Center for Urban Culture, Tel Aviv, 2011–2012.

(signified). These links subvert signification in favour of a play of signs. In both the orders of *imitation* and *production* the signifier indexes an underlying meaning, either inherent or constructed. By contrast, the order of *simulation* refers to the principle of the post-modern dress which is indifferent to any traditional social order, and is completely self-referential; we are now looking at 'fashion for its own sake'. Baudrillard's analysis of the order of simulation, or post-modernism, problematises the notion of a correspondence theory of representation, and is based on coded similarities and differences. Since fashion makes no reference to an outside reality, it invites a reading of a different order: a perpetual re-examination of the code.

Baudrillard views fashion as a transition from a purely referential function that encodes symbolic meaning to a purely self-referential function that marks the end of meaning. In his analysis simulation replaces signification: fashion is a playful spectacle, a carnival of appearances. It empties signs of their traditional meaning. Take, for example, the way in which fashion design can empty religious symbols (e.g. the cross), ethnic symbols (e.g. keffiyah,

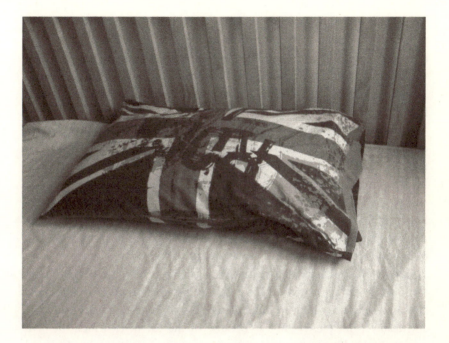

13.3 A British national flag is reduced to its ornamental features, to decorate functional domestic objects like pillow cases, or towels.

see figure 13.2), or national symbols (e.g. national flag, see figure 13.3) of their original meaning. Instead, it fetishizes them for their aesthetic quality. For Baudrillard, the effacing of real history as referent leaves us nothing but empty signs, marking the end of signification itself.

FROM COMMUNICATION TO SEDUCTION

In his latest books, Baudrillard characterized post-modern fashion by a shift from the modern order of production to the post-modern order of seduction. The principle of seduction 'which is the order of sign and ritual' (elaborated in *Seduction*, 1990 [1979] and *Fatal Strategies*, 1990 [1983]) is the anti-thesis to the order of production in that it replaces the values of instrumental rationality, utility and functionality. It is a strategy of superficial appearances involving the charms of games and artifice, and negating the seriousness of reality, meaning, morality and truth. Thus, seduction derives pleasure from excess. It is a sumptuary and useless consumption of surplus, as for example displayed by celebrities. The heroes of production, such as the factory workers, self-made men, entrepreneurs, pioneers and explorers, have been replaced by idols of consumption, such as movie stars, sports heroes, royals and celebrities.

As opposed to modern fashion which is governed by rules of style, colour and product combination, post-modern fashion is ruled by artifice for the sake of artifice. It allows for more disordered and non-systematic combinations mixing clothes, styles and looks and the rest from various periods, subcultures, classes and so forth into a form of eclectic fashion pastiche. Marking the end of the structuralist principle of an opposition between signs as a basis for meaning, it replaces the psychoanalytic economy of drives and desires with a playful spectacle and a carnival of appearances.

Seduction functions as a metaphysics for Baudrillard. It is an attempt to postulate an alternative to the mode of production and to delineate a sphere of practice, which would undermine and reverse the dominant logic and reality principle. He notes: 'Because of the extent to which the economic shackled to the functional, has imposed its principle of utility, anything which exceeds it quickly takes on the air of play and futility' (1990 [1979]: 94–95). In other words, his theory replaces rationality and delayed satisfaction that were the hallmark of the Protestant ethic, with instant gratification that is based on an immediate fulfilment of desires. The essence of his argument is that fashion as a form of communication has been usurped by fashion as a form of pleasure. As simulation substitutes for production it replaces the linear order with a cyclical order, and frees the signifier from its link to the signified. This, in turn, results in subverting the visual code from a language to a spectacle (1993 [1976]). Regarding both language and fashion as social discourses, Baudrillard also contends that, while language aims for meaning, fashion aims for 'theatrical sociality' which 'delights in itself' in 'aesthetic pleasure', turning the game into 'signification without a message' (Baudrillard, 1993 [1976]: 94).

BAUDRILLARD AND FASHION THEORY

So far we have seen how Baudrillard advances a radical position about the 'end of signification' which is the 'end of meaning'. His overview of fashion signification charted a path from pre-modern to post-modern societies.

In pre-modern societies the presentation of signs mirrors the social order. In modernity, excess of signs whose function is both ornamental and representational facilitates a pretence of the social order. In post-modernity, the transgression of signs makes the social order irrelevant: 'the passion for futility and the artificial [...] plays the role of transgression and violence, and fashion is condemned for having within it the force of the pure sign which signifies nothing' (Baudrillard, 1993 [1976]: 129).

Thus the post-modern world according to Baudrillard is a collage of absences: of signification that existed but disappeared in the course of history. It is a critique of consumer culture where images first linked to objects, then replaced them, and finally have become unmoored from them in a world of meanings where images have no reference in reality. Baudrillard's post-modernity, says Bauman, is more than just a change, a disappearance of the old order of signification. It is 'a change to put paid to all changes'(Bauman 1992: 149). It is a world of hyperreality. 'Reality is "more real than the real", in that it no longer sets itself against something else which unlike itself is phoney, illusionary or imaginary [...]. In hyperreality, everything is in excess of itself' (Bauman 1992: 151). In the world outlined by Baudrillard's post-modernity, criteria such as golden standard or ideal do not seek to establish which account is more true than another. Since we live in hyperreality, where the real and the illusory or imaginary are indistinguishable, it is hard to tell reality TV from fiction, fake Venice in Las Vegas from historical Venice in Italy, truth from falsity. And when we cannot distinguish the reality of Los Angeles from Disneyland (as Baudrillard implies in *America* (1989 [1986]), 'truth has not been destroyed. It has been made irrelevant' (Bauman, 1992: 149–51). This is a radical vision, which negates every certainty and solidity of everything we know and take for granted. This is also not unlike Goffman's notion of backstage and frontstage (see also chapter 9 on Goffman), which separates not the authentic and the act, but different kinds of acts played to two different audiences each with their presentational requirements.

Similarly, Baudrillard's vision pulls the plug on notions of solid well defined entities like 'identities' and 'communication' through objects. Elsewhere I have argued (Tseëlon, 2010) that identity is no longer a useful critical concept. I have also demonstrated empirically (Tseëlon, 1989, 1994, 1995, 2012a) that the discourse of fashion and personal appearance is not nearly as accurate as is often claimed in simplistic models of fashion communication (for example Barnard, 2002). Further, there is evidence of 'semiotic fatigue', where the motivation to identify the meaning of fashion, in particular that of the 'stereotype approach' to fashion, is driven by popular culture and academic theory more than it is justified by the views of the users of fashion themselves.

Can we then claim that fashion signification is more a myth than a reality? By way of answer, let's examine fashion theories which suggested that post-industrial production contributed to a process of democratization where styles that were previously only available to the upper classes then trickled down, and are now available to all classes simultaneously. Has this been a trigger for erosion of fashion symbolism? Baudrillard's position is antithetical to such fashion theorizing (e.g. Blumer, 1969; Crane, 2000; Simmel, 1957 [1904]). He views the democratization thesis as an ideology that creates the illusion of democratization by confusing the ideology of consumption with consumption itself. Such ideology promotes the myth of the universal meaning of fashion all the way down the social scale, and masks the social inequalities behind a democracy of leisure that is only available to the privileged classes and not across the board. Giddens, for instance, in his discussion of post-modern identity, emphasises that the idea of life-style choices does not apply to those whose economic deprivation and other external constraints limit their choices.

'To speak of multiplicity of choices', he writes, 'is not to suppose that all choices are open to everyone, or that people take all decisions about options in full realization of the range of feasible alternatives' (Giddens, 1991: 82). Diana Crane (2000), too, qualified her discussion about twentieth-century fashion by saying that post-modern attitudes toward identity are confined to certain segments of the population.

From the perspective of fashion theory, post-modern fashion with all its playful nihilism and cannibalization of styles, still alludes to a reality of signification. This can be illustrated by two paradigmatic features of post-modern fashion: fake jewels and vintage clothes. In the world of jewellery a conscious and deliberate use of non-precious materials is made without the low status connotations associated with such materials; quite the contrary. One of the hallmarks of current luxury fashion is the irreverent mixing of precious and simple materials. Designer jewellery, even when made of recycled or common materials is no less prestigious or pricy.

Another hallmark of post-modern fashion is the imitation and integration of an eclectic mixture of styles and periods into a new discourse of vintage fashion. It has become a major trend, partly due to its added layer of sustainable credentials and partly because it is invested with yearning for the age of craftsmanship, authenticity and simplicity. Despite its seeming up-rootedness such nostalgic fashion need not be taken at face value.

Instead, it can indicate that fashion does not cease to signify even when it removes itself from market forces. For Jameson, imitation of bygone styles lends historical depth to a world of surface signifiers, and shows 'a desperate attempt to appropriate a missing past' (1984: 19). For Baudrillard (1981 [1972]), bygone objects derive their value from affirmation of craft-value and repudiation of the stigma attached to industrial production. Angela McRobbie (1989) argues that second-hand fashion is used by those who can risk looking poor in a stylised way that marks out their distance both from conventional dress and from real poverty. The current trend for vintage fashion, albeit under the banner of sustainability, shows how repudiation of the stylistic values of representation expresses yearning for these same values.

FASHION AND THE END OF SIGNIFICATION

Baudrillard's notion of fashion as the end of signification is not without limits, and in the final section I would like to take issue with it. Most of the discussion is based on the chapter on 'Fashion or the Enchanting Spectacle of the Code' from *Symbolic Exchange and Death* (1993 [1976]). Baudrillard articulates in a single stroke two contradictory accounts of fashion: modern fashion hides a myth of change that reproduces the power relations of industrial capitalism; and post-modern fashion marks an end-point in the relationship between signs and meaning. As we have seen before, post-modern fashion is a stage 'beyond meaning' where 'fashion is a pure speculative stage in the order of signs. There is no more constraint of either coherence or reference' (1993 [1976]: 125).

The two accounts not only represent two stages of development, but they are structurally different. Baudrillard's account of modern fashion regards fashion as a signifier of a wider social process within industrial capitalism. He argues that 'modernity is a code, and fashion is its emblem' (1993 [1976]: 122). His account of post-modern fashion, however, falls into the same trap of self-referentiality that he attributes to post-modern fashion itself. This account falls short of acknowledging that whatever happens inside fashion does not necessarily affect its signifying function as an emblem of a social process. It also confuses fragmentation of the code with its disappearance. Diana Crane (2000) explains that the shift from a production-oriented class society to a consumption-oriented lifestyle society created such a multiplicity of codes that one can better refer to it as a set of dialects rather than as a language. Importantly, she also points out that fragmentation such as characterises contemporary society is not the same as chaos: 'enormous variety and incongruity of styles and codes are not inherently meaningless or ambiguous: they are understood primarily by those who share identities and are opaque to outsiders' (Crane, 2000: 244).

In discussing post-modern fashion, Baudrillard builds on a number of assumptions in a way that is not always justified, and is not always compatible with his own argument. First, his assumption of the indeterminacy of the code and the instability of the signifier–signified relationship leads him to doubt the possibility of a referential function. This predicament is neither logically necessary nor based on actual behaviour. From a theoretical viewpoint, looser signifier–signified relationships may simply mean fragmentation of society into smaller units of relevant frames of reference, with less rigid boundaries, rules and membership requirements. It may also imply shorter and faster cycles of change of what a relevant reference group regards as the appropriate code, but it does not necessarily indicate the abolition of a code. From an empirical viewpoint there is ample evidence, both experimental and anecdotal, to suggest that signification in fashion is far more resilient than some post-modern thinkers would have us believe. (For a review and critique see Tseëlon, 1989, 2012a.)

Second, another assumption, that of self-referentiality – the fact that fashion is referent-free and does not represent anything – does not in itself herald the end of meaning altogether. In some sense the catwalk is the quintessential self-referential ritual of the fashion world where top designers showcase their new collections to a carefully chosen and well-connected privileged and limited audience of fashion editors, fashion buyers and distinguished clients. The cycle of competition, prestige, ingratiation and glamour that is set in motion by such events testifies to its ceremonial qualities and signifying function, which are not confined to the fashion world alone. The participants of the fashion shows keep re-inventing themselves by creating or editing a real or invented tradition. As the logic of branding illustrates, recycled heritage stories or re-invented myths of origin can be produced and added on and incorporated into the ethos of a group. Recent examples include labels such as Louis Vuitton, repositioning itself as the brand of the traveller harking back to its origins as a manufacturer of travelling cases; Ralph Lauren, the son of Jewish immigrants whose own sense of displacement was leveraged into inventing the established aristocratic look for the New World, is polishing his credentials as a house of classic heritage. Even a high street store like M&S is launching a 'Best of British' line of its wool and checks, capitalizing on a successful tradition that Burberry so successfully appropriated, by going back to its own archives and resurrecting successful styles.

Third, Baudrillard himself points out that even resistance to fashion is still defined within the order of fashion, but fails to acknowledge that fashion as a whole is locked into a broader signification system. In other words, the very participation in the playful carnival of fashion with its floating signs is already inscribed in signification. Paradoxically, the act of subverting signification itself becomes a signifier. It is a status marker of the rich and famous, those powerful enough or distinguished enough to flaunt conventions, those creative enough and confident enough to invent, or those marginalized enough not to care. There is a sense in which even globalized postmodern fashion is subject to a meta narrative of meaning. In his book *Globalization: The Human Consequences*, Zygmunt Bauman (1998) argues that globalization of markets and information redistributed privileges and deprivations, and re-stratified people on a world-wide scale. The hallmark of the new elite is 'exterritoriality' and it is characterized by the compression of space and time. In this new landscape mobility has become the most coveted stratifying factor. The freedom to move is a perpetually scarce and unequally distributed commodity. 'Being on the move', Bauman suggests, has radically different meaning for those at the top and the bottom of the new hierarchy. For the top it implies freedom from the constraints of space. For the bottom it signals existential uncertainty, anxiety and fear. The criterion of mobility shares a fundamental insight with Baudrillard's view of fashion in one of his earlier books. In *For a Critique of the Political Economy of the Sign* (1981 [1972]), he articulates his theory that consumption, including fashion, is a function not of a need for the objects themselves, but for the signifying value. He writes: 'since objects play a role of exhibitors of social status, and since this status has become potentially mobile, the objects will always simultaneously give evidence of acquired situation (inertia) and of the potential mobility (fast circulation of objects)' (1981 [1972]: 50).

Finally, on another level, Baudrillard's paradigm of seduction suggests that even what is habitually considered 'loss of meaning' is still contained within the sphere of meaning. Here, Baudrillard is articulating the memory function of clothes, and its defensive quality. Almost like the Freudian fetish, the seduction of absence of meaning by presence of artifice is 'the only existing form of immortality', turning even death into 'a brilliant and superficial appearance' (1990 [1979]: 97). As Baudrillard writes: 'This is the despair that nothing lasts, and the complementary enjoyment of knowing that, beyond this death, every form always has the chance of a second coming'

(1993 [1976]: 119). Thus, contrary to what one might expect, death is not interpreted as the end of meaning. Rather, post-modern fashion reflects at least one level of meaning: that of countering death. Later in *The Transparency of Evil: Essays on Extreme Phenomena* he refers to fashion with the analogy of an epidemic that flares up and fades away so fast without being mediated by meaning (1993 [1990]: 70). It can be argued that the trajectory of fashion has moved from uncontested meaning to contested (or no) meaning on the micro level. Yet, on the macro level the very ability to engage with the mobility that is inherent in fashion is still meaningful in the sense that is outlined by Bauman and by early Baudrillard himself. Objects may not signify in themselves, and the speed of change of 'fast fashion' may not be signifying acts in themselves. However, the very ability to engage with a fast changing world has become a status marker of those who live on the fast lane.

Variety and diversity of styles are evidence of the change in fashion that Baudrillard postulates, from representational signs to self-referential signs indicating that there is no other reality, just a questioning of the code. Baudrillard sees signification as being totally annulled and being replaced by simulation with historical references emptied of all their meanings. In contrast to his radical negation of any signification, I argue that even in a system that appears to have repudiated meaning in favour of the playful use of signs and historical styles, there are micro and macro ways to index status to maintain meaning. While fashion continues to serve as a form of expression, it functions less as a form of communication which is widely shared and understood by masses.

CONCLUSION

William Golding once said that myth is truth that can only be told in a story (in *Arena* documentary on BBC TV, *The Dreams of William Golding*, 17 March 2012). For me this is the value of Baudrillard's insights. Their sign-value is given not in their accurate depiction but in their mythical perceptiveness encased in a poetic format. And like that of any complex thinker, Baudrillard's theory is not woven of a single thread, but with various, sometimes dissonant, ones.

Baudrillard's analysis of the total disappearance of any signification, which negates every certainty and solidity of everything we know and take for granted, is a radical vision. It is an extreme view which is best understood as a heuristic rather than a literal description of a process. Clothes carry meaning in some form, even if it is harder to identify. Traditional, signifying stereotypes may be used seriously or ironically to reinforce or subvert. Clothes continue to project meaning, but not in a dictionary-like manner. Their meaning is contextual and ephemeral or varies from one stylistic tribe to another. Our challenge as researchers is to trace the line between what I call the stereotype approach and the wardrobe approach: between what clothes really signify, and what we imagine they do.

REFERENCES

Barnard, M. (2002) *Fashion as Communication*, Hove: Psychology Press.

Baudrillard, J. (1981 [1972]) *For a Critique of the Political Economy of the Sign*, C. Levin (trans), St. Louis, MO: Telos.

———(1983) *Simulations*, P. Foss, P. Patton and P. Beitchman (trans), New York: Semiotext(e).

———(1989 [1986]) *America*, C. Turner (trans), London: Verso.

———(1990a [1979]) *Seduction*, B. Singer (trans), New York: St. Martin's Press.

———(1990b [1983]) *Fatal Strategies*, P. Beitchman and W.G.J. Niesluchowski (trans), New York: Semiotext(e).

———(1993a [1976]) *Symbolic Exchange and Death*, I. Grant (trans), London: Sage.

———(1993b [1990]) 'Prophylaxis and Virulence' in *The Transparency of Evil: Essays on Extreme Phenomena*, J. Benedict (trans), London: Verso.

Bauman, Z. (1992) *Intimations of Postmodernity*, London: Routledge.

———(1998) *Globalization: The Human Consequences*, Cambridge: Polity.

———(1999) *Liquid Modernity*, Cambridge: Polity.

Black, A.J. and Garland, M. (1975), *A History of Fashion*, London: Orbis.

Blumer, H. (1969) 'Fashion: From Class Differentiation to Collective Selection' in *Sociological Quarterly*, 10: 275–91.

Burr, V. (2003) *Social Constructionism*, London: Routledge.

Crane, D. (2000) *Fashion and its Social Agendas: Class, Gender, and Identity in Clothing*, Chicago: Chicago University Press.

Drolet, M. (ed) (2004) *The Postmodernism Reader: Foundational Texts*, London: Routledge.

Ewing, E. (1981) *Fur in Dress*, London: Batsford.

Giddens, A. (1991) *Modernity and Self Identity*, Cambridge: Polity.

Glickman, L.B. (ed) (1999 [1970]) *Consumer Society in American History: A Reader*, Ithaca, NY: Cornell University Press (reprinted from M. Poster (ed) (1988) *Jean Baudrillard: Selected Writings*, Palo Alto, CA: Stanford University Press).

Goffman, E. (1951) 'Symbols of Class Status' in *British Journal of Sociology*, 2: 294–304.

Jameson, F. (1984) 'Postmodernism or the Cultural Logic of Late Capitalism' in *New Left Review*, 146: 53–92.

Jencks, C. (2011) *The Story of Post-modernism: Five Decades of the Ironic, Iconic and Critical in Architecture*, Hoboken, NJ: John Wiley.

König, R. (1973) *The Restless Image: A Sociology of Fashion*, F. Bradley (trans), introduced by T. Wolfe, London: George Allen & Unwin.

Laver, J. (1985 [1969]) *Costume and Fashion: A Concise History*, Oxford: Oxford University Press.

McRobbie, A. (1989) 'Second-Hand Dresses and the Role of the Ragmarket' in A. McRobbie (ed), *Zoot Suits and Second Hand Dresses: An Anthology of Fashion and Music*, London: MacMillan.

Sennett, R. (1976) *The Fall of Public Man*, London: Faber and Faber.

Simmel, G. (1957 [1904]) 'Fashion' in *American Journal of Sociology*, 62: 541–58.

Tseëlon, E. (1989) *Communicating Via Clothes* [PhD Thesis], Oxford: University of Oxford.

———(1994) 'Fashion and Signification in Baudrillard' in D. Kellner (ed), *Baudrillard: A Critical Reader*, Oxford: Blackwell.

———(1995) *The Masque of Femininity: The Presentation of Woman in Everyday Life*, London: Sage.

———(2010) 'Is Identity a Useful Critical Tool?' in *Critical Studies in Fashion & Beauty*, 1 (2): 151–59.

———(2012a) 'How Successful is Communication via Clothing? Thoughts and Evidence for an Unexamined Paradigm' in A.M. Gonzalez and L. Bovone (eds), *Identities through Fashion: A Multidisciplinary Approach*, Oxford: Berg.

———(2012b) 'Fashion and the Orders of Masking' in *Critical Studies in Fashion & Beauty*, 3: 3–9.

Wilson, E. (2013 [1985]) *Adorned in Dreams: Fashion and Modernity*, London: I.B. Tauris.

14

PIERRE BOURDIEU
The Field of Fashion

Agnès Rocamora

INTRODUCTION

When in 1975 Pierre Bourdieu and Yvette Delsaut published 'Le Couturier et sa Griffe', an article devoted to postwar French couture, the work came in continuation with Bourdieu's interest in analysing the consumption and production of culture. As well as his ethnography of Kabylia (Bourdieu, 2000a) the French sociologist had started interrogating everyday cultural practices such as amateur photography (1965: 17) or art gallery visits (1966). This approach was to culminate in his celebrated 1979 book *Distinction*, where he investigates French people's tastes in goods such as food, fashion, music and art. Condemning the 'hierarchy of legitimate objects of study' (Bourdieu, 1965: 17) that, he argued, informed academic enquiry he insisted that 'any cultural asset from cookery to dodecaphonic music by way of the Western movie, can be an object for apprehension ranging from the simple, actual sensation to scholarly appreciation' (Bourdieu, 1993a: 220). Thus, by looking at objects which are less 'noble', or as he puts it, are seen as 'unworthy' (Bourdieu, 1993b: 132), such as fashion and photography, Bourdieu distinguished himself from an academic field focused on more 'legitimate' subjects of sociological enquiry such as the state and work, placed high in 'the hierarchy of objects regarded as worthy or unworthy of being studied' (Bourdieu, 1993b: 132).

Although Bourdieu devoted two articles to fashion (Bourdieu and Delsaut, 1975; Bourdieu, 1993b) and discussed it in *Distinction*, his attention to this field has been given comparatively less space in the many texts that engage with his work (see, for instance, Brown and Szeman, 2000; Calhoun et al., 1995; Pinto, 1998; Swartz, 1997); witness also the absence of an English translation of 'Le Couturier et sa Griffe' when most of his writing is available in that language. This is also at odds with Bourdieu's acknowledgement that the field of haute couture has been key to his understanding and theorizing of the logic of the field of cultural production more generally. He puts it thus: 'the field of haute couture has introduced me more directly than any other universe to one of the most fundamental properties of all the fields of cultural production, the properly magical logic of the production of the producer and of the product as fetishes' (Bourdieu, 1992: 300).

The following chapter focuses on Bourdieu's writing on fashion. I first present an overview of his key concept of 'field' to then discuss it in the light of his work on fashion and as a way of further exploring his theoretical framework. Although I draw attention to some of the limits of Bourdieu's work, in the final section I also point to its relevance for interrogating the contemporary rise of fashion bloggers in the field of the fashion media.

FIELD THEORY

Pierre Bourdieu (1930–2002) used the notion of field as early as 1966 but it is really in later work such as The Field of Cultural Production (1993a),[1] Sociology in Question (1993c [1984]) and especially The Rules of Art (1992) that what became known as field theory came to be fully defined (see Bourdieu, 1992: 298–99 and Bourdieu 2005: 29 for an 'intellectual genealogy' of the term).

A field is a 'structured space of positions' and forces (Bourdieu, 1993c: 72; Bourdieu, 2004: 33). It is a 'social microcosm' (Bourdieu and Wacquant, 1996: 97) informed by specific rules of functioning which shape the trajectories and practices of the agents that belong to it. There, agents' and institutions' positions are dependent on and determined by 'the other positions constituting the field' (Bourdieu, 1993a: 30). In fields, then, meanings and values are not inherent in things, they are relational, and Bourdieu developed the concept of field to capture this primacy he gives to the role of the relational in the formation of social spaces (Bourdieu, 1998: vii).

There are 'general properties of fields' (Bourdieu, 2005: 36), amongst which is the struggle for the definition of their dominant values. Indeed, a field is always made of established players and newcomers who fight for the power to define what can be acknowledged as legitimate practice, aesthetic, taste or norm. A field, then, is a microcosm structured by the power relations between forces of conservation and forces of transformation, and the state of these power relations at a particular historical time determines the structure of the field at that time (Bourdieu, 1993c; Bourdieu, 2004).

Bourdieu also conceived of the notion of field as a methodological tool that informs empirical work:

It forces the researcher to ask what people are 'playing at' in the field [...] what are the stakes, the goods or properties sought and distributed or redistributed, and how they are distributed, what are the instruments or weapons that one needs to have in order to play with some chance of winning, and what is, at each moment in the game, the structure of the distribution of goods, gains and assets.

(Bourdieu, 2004: 34)

The notion of field then helps us understand the collective dimension of practices and their interrelated constitution, and forces us to see that it is not just one institution or just one critique which makes the work of art, but the field of production itself, that is the system of relations which exist between all the agents and institutions of consecration which compete for 'the monopoly of the power to consecrate' (Bourdieu, 1993a: 78). Thus the artwork, Bourdieu points out, is made 'a hundred times, by all those who are interested in it, who find a material or symbolic profit in reading it, classifying it, deciphering it, commenting on it, combating it, knowing it, possessing it' (Bourdieu, 1993a: 111), amongst which are a variety of institutions whose role is to institute reality and create the value of an object by talking about it.

Thus Bourdieu reminds us that culture is both material and symbolic. This is why he writes:

The sociology of art and literature has to take as its object not only the material production but also the symbolic production of the work, i.e. the production of the value of the work or, which amounts to the same thing, of belief in the value of the work. It therefore has to consider as contributing to production not only the direct producers of the work in its materiality (artist, writer, etc.) but also the producers of the meaning and value of the work – critics, publishers, gallery directors and the whole set of agents whose combined efforts produce consumers capable of knowing and recognizing the work of art as such.

(Bourdieu, 1993a: 37)

Through 'their symbolic sanctions', all such producers 'consecrate a certain type of work and a certain type of cultivated person' (Bourdieu, 1993a: 121).

In the same way that the value of a cultural object has to be sought in the structure of the field itself, so has the value of the words attached to it. Bourdieu and Delsaut put it thus:

> The power of words does not lie in the words but in the conditions that give power to the words by producing the collective belief, that is, the collective misrecognition of the arbitrariness of the creation of value that is accomplished through a determined use of words.
>
> (Bourdieu and Delsaut, 1975: 23)

The value of a thing, be it a work of art, a word or a sentence, is not to be found in the thing itself or in its author, but in the field it belongs to, in the interplay between the forces of opposition and conservation that structure the field and give its agents the power to speak and be listened to; the power to consecrate.

It is in the field of fashion Bourdieu argues that this power to consecrate is most clearly at play. Bourdieu and Delsaut write: 'If there is a case where one does things with words, as in magic, and even better than in magic [...] it is in the universe of fashion' (1975: 23). In the following section, and to further explore Bourdieu's theoretical framework I turn to his writing on fashion.

THE FIELD OF FASHION

Bourdieu's most extensive discussion of the field of fashion can be found in the 1975 article he co-wrote with Yvette Delsaut, 'Le Couturier et sa Griffe' (hereafter 'Le Couturier'), published in the academic journal he founded: *Actes de La Recherche en Sciences Sociales*. A 1974 text, 'Haute Couture and Haute Culture', published in *Sociology in Question*, prefigures some of its points. In 'Le Couturier' Bourdieu and Delsaut look at the structure of the French field of high fashion in the 1970s, discussing its instances of consecration, its newcomers and established players, their position, strategies and values, and the rules and struggles it is underpinned by. (See also Rocamora, 2002a for an account of this discussion.) They argue that the field of fashion is 'a field ruled by the competition for the monopoly of specific legitimacy, that is, for the exclusive power to constitute and impose the legitimate symbols of distinction in regards to clothing' (Bourdieu and Delsaut, 1975: 15).

By focusing on haute couture, Bourdieu and Delsaut are in effect focusing on one subspace only of the field of fashion, what Bourdieu calls a subfield. Indeed, in his work, he makes a distinction between two subfields: one – 'the field of restricted production' – is a field of producers, for producers, where the values of art for art's sake dominate practices and aesthetic judgements; the other – 'the field of large scale production'– is a field dominated by the principles of commerce and profit (see Bourdieu, 1993a).

Fields' ability to resist external forces such as those of commerce or of the media is an indicator of their independence and of their ability to set their own criteria of functioning. The more autonomous a field, the more able it is to establish its own rules, as is the case for instance, following Bourdieu, with the field of restricted production. In contrast, the field of large scale production is a heteronomous field, dependent on the pressures of commerce and the media. In the hierarchy of the field of fashion, the field of haute couture is akin to a field of restricted production whilst mass fashion belongs to the field of large scale production. In 'Haute Couture and Haute Culture' Bourdieu even draws a homology between high culture and high couture to argue that 'when I speak of *haute couture* I shall never cease to be speaking also of *haute culture*' (Bourdieu, 1993b: 132).

The distinction between subfields draws attention to the hierarchies that exist between fields of culture, with the subfield of restricted production being often given a higher status and legitimacy than that of large scale production. Thus, although Bourdieu argues that the field of haute couture and the field of haute culture are homologous fields in that their functioning is informed by homologous rules, these fields occupy different positions in the hierarchy of culture. Indeed Bourdieu and Delsaut refer to fashion as an 'art moyen', and an 'art mineur' to indicate that it is situated at an intermediary position (Bourdieu and Delsaut, 1975: 16).

Thus in an attempt to elevate their status and consecrate fashion, members of the field of fashion, they argue, will mobilize references to high culture when discussing their work. They note:

> The references to the legitimate and noble arts, painting, sculpture, literature, which give most of its ennobling metaphors to the description of clothing, and many of its themes to the evocation of the aristocratic life which they are supposed to symbolise, are as many homages that the 'minor art' [art mineur] makes to high arts [arts majeurs]. [...] It is the same

with the eagerness which couturiers are keen to demonstrate on the topic of their participation in art or, by default, in the artistic world.

(Bourdieu and Delsaut, 1975: 16)

Indeed, in her study of British fashion designers, Angela McRobbie (1998), drawing on Bourdieu's theoretical framework, discusses the strategies the trainee designers she interviewed developed to legitimate and ennoble their art. She cites a fashion design student: 'Having been inspired by a Matisse exhibition entitled "Jazz" I aim to continue his collage technique through to appliqué details for beachwear' (cited in McRobbie 1998: 61). Her respondents' strategies of consecration of fashion, she argues, are articulated through a rejection of the idea of commerce (McRobbie, 1998: 13). As Bourdieu notes:

> The opposition between art and money (the 'commercial') is the generative principle of most of the judgements that, with respect to the theatre, cinema, painting and literature, claim to establish the frontier between what is art and what is not, between 'bourgeois' art and 'intellectual' art, between 'traditional' art and 'avant-garde' art.

(1996c: 162)

Similarly, in my study of fashion in Le Monde (Rocamora, 2002b) and in Vogue (2006) I discuss the way the references to high culture that both titles draw on when reporting on fashion serve their interest in constructing fashion, and themselves, as spaces of high culture.

In 'Le Couturier', Bourdieu and Delsaut also refer to the idea of 'fashion discourse' ('le discours de mode') (1975: 23), the discourse of fashion insiders, the members of the field of fashion such as designers and fashion journalists, and a notion useful for unpacking 'fashion media discourse' (Rocamora, 2009: ch.3). Thus they argue that the adjectives designers use to describe their products are an illustration of the homology between their aesthetic position and their position in the field of fashion. The language of 'exclusivity, authenticity and refinement' of the dominant designers is opposed to the rigorous and audacious language of avant-garde designers (Bourdieu and Delsaut, 1975: 12). The former is the language of 'sobriety, elegance, balance and harmony' whereas the latter is that of 'liberty, youth and fantasy' (ibid.). In drawing attention to the role of fashion discourse, Bourdieu and Delsaut once again remind us of the importance of the symbolic production of culture, a type of production I also unpack in my analysis of the discursive production of fashion as pop culture in the *Guardian*, and as high culture in *Le Monde* (Rocamora, 2001).

Words that are used in fashion writing do not simply describe the value of objects they are related to, they make it (Bourdieu and Delsaut, 1975: 23), and that is where Bourdieu and Delsaut distinguish their approach to fashion discourse from that of Barthes (1990 [1967]). Because Barthes' semiotic analysis concentrates solely on an internal reading of the fashion discourse (see chapter 8), it leaves aside, they argue, 'the question of the function of the fashion discourse in the process of the production of fashion goods' (Bourdieu and Delsaut, 1975: 23). Both Barthes and Bourdieu are interested in the system of words which are interposed between the object and its user, which Barthes calls a 'veil' (1990 [1967]: xi) and Bourdieu a 'screen' (1993b: 138), and for Barthes, as for Bourdieu, fashion exists not only through clothes but also through discourses on them. But whereas Bourdieu and Delsaut look at the system of words as one part only of a wider system of production, the field, and therefore external to the discourse itself, Barthes focuses on the internal system, its linguistic structure. This is why Barthes, Bourdieu and Delsaut argue, fails to understand the function of fashion discourse and its relevance as a specific instance of the structure of the field in which it is situated (1975: 23).

The oppositions between designers, their styles and their lifestyles objectified in the discourses of these same designers, Bourdieu and Delsaut point out, also inform the different styles of discourse of the different fashion magazines, discourses which are, according to Bourdieu 'the privileged site for the affirmation of differences' (1996b: 63). These differences also oppose the readers of those magazines. The higher a specific magazine is in the hierarchy of magazines, the more sober its descriptive style, corresponding to the high social position of its readers.

Bourdieu's theoretical framework, and more particularly his notion of field, is useful for making sense of the discourse of fashion magazines in the field of the fashion media, but it is also useful to interrogate the places and spaces where fashion is acted out. This is what Joanne Entwistle and I aimed to demonstrate when applying Bourdieu's theoretical framework to the particular case of London Fashion Week as staged on London's King's Road in 2002 and 2003 (Entwistle and Rocamora, 2006). We draw attention to the importance of the idea of field as both a conceptual framework and a lived reality. The field of fashion, we argue, is captured, and reproduced – materialized – in the layout of the London Fashion Week enclosure as well as in the layout and sitting hierarchies of the catwalk shows.

In that article we also mobilize the key Bourdieuian concept of capital (see, for instance, Bourdieu, 1993a). One's position in a field, Bourdieu argues, is determined by one's capital, and field struggles are also struggles to determine the legitimate forms of capital and their composition. Thus he makes a distinction between four forms of capital: economic, social, symbolic and cultural. Where economic capital refers to the financial assets of an institution or agent, social capital refers to the strength of their contacts and their network, symbolic capital to the amount of status they hold, and cultural capital – renamed 'information capital' in *An Invitation to Reflexive Sociology* (Bourdieu and Wacquant, 1996) – to the set of cultural resources, whether embodied, in bodily manners for instance, objectified, such as in books or works of art, or institutionalized, in diplomas for instance, which allows one to gain social power and distinction (see, for instance, Bourdieu and Wacquant, 1996: 119; Bourdieu, 1997: 124–25; Bourdieu, 1986: 47).

Whilst 'economic capital is at the root of all the other types of capital' (Bourdieu 1986: 54), all three forms – social, symbolic and cultural – can be converted into one or more of the other forms. Capital is unequally distributed amongst a field and this unequal distribution participates in the structuring of the field whilst in turn a particular field determines the force or value of the kinds of capital that may circulate in it and be drawn on and accumulated to establish one's position (1986: 49). Thus, in 'Le Couturier', Bourdieu and Delsaut (1975) argue that while established players such as Dior have high symbolic and economic capitals, newcomers such as Paco Rabanne have to deploy strategies of subversion to develop their capital and become consecrated both symbolically and economically. At the same time, newcomers are dependent on their experience at established couture houses to generate an 'initial capital of authority' (Bourdieu and Delsaut, 1975: 15). Similarly Entwistle and I discuss the symbolic, social and cultural capitals fashion players must deploy to belong to the field of fashion as materialized during London Fashion Week. Cultural capital displayed through appropriate, in-the-know outfits, itself dependent on economic and social capitals, is key to one's membership of the field of fashion.

Bourdieu's point that capital can be embodied reflects his attention to the incorporated logic of practices, captured in his key notion of habitus. Indeed, embodied capital, he writes, is 'external wealth converted into an integral part of the person, into a habitus' (1986: 48). Most systematically discussed in his *Logic of Pratice* but a recurring notion in his work, 'habitus' is defined as 'limited conditioned spontaneity', a 'practical sense' (Bourdieu, 2000b: 260, 262) as well as 'a set of historical relations "deposited" within individual bodies in the form of mental and corporeal schemata of perception, appreciation, and action' (Bourdieu and Wacquant, 1996: 16).

Like the concept of field, the notion of habitus is aimed at bypassing the opposition structure/agency: 'situated beyond the dualism of the subject and the object, of activity and passivity, of means and ends, of determinism and freedom, the relation of habitus to field, through which the habitus determines itself by determining what determines it, is a calculation without calculator, an intentional action without intention' (Bourdieu, 2000b: 262). Structured by their habitus, agents always seek to maximise their profit and follow the strategy most appropriate to their interest. It is a strategy, however, without a conscious strategist as it is the habitus itself that shapes agents' positions and position takings. Their feel for the game is an incorporated disposition dictated by their habitus. Thus in 'Le Couturier' Bourdieu and Delsaut argue that Courrèges' habitus, in being distinct from that of established players such as Balmain and Givenchy but aligned with that of the new 'modern' and 'dynamic' French bourgeoisie of the time could only yield him success amongst this social group.

DISTINCTION

Whilst Bourdieu devoted two articles to the field of fashion, this is a topic largely absent from his other writings, except for *Distinction* (1996a), probably his most famous work. There, as in *Photography* (1996b), Bourdieu argues that it is the Kantian aesthetic which organizes judgements on cultural objects and practices. These judgements are split between a set of dichotomies at the basis of Kant's opposition between a pure aesthetic, that of the dominant class, following Bourdieu, and a popular one, that of the working class, which, he notes 'is the exact opposite of the Kantian aesthetic' (1996a: 5). The dominant aesthetic is informed by the notions of form, mind, distance and disinterest, whereas it is the ideas of content, the body, immediacy and interest which inform the working class' engagement with cultural objects.

Bourdieu aims to show that aesthetic judgements must be socially and historically situated. For Bourdieu, and unlike Kant, aesthetic experience cannot be explained as an independent expression of the mind, an autonomous and universal spiritual life, but as a socially and historically constituted disposition. This is why tastes, Bourdieu writes, are 'markers of "class"' (1996a: 2).

The contemplative distance valued by the aesthete is nothing but a distance from financial needs, made possible by the privileged social position of the agent (Bourdieu, 1996a: 56). It can only be achieved through the possession of economic capital, which keeps the aesthete at 'distance from necessity' (53). It is because, Bourdieu argues, the working class lacks economic capital that its taste is a 'taste for necessity' (374) which seeks in all cultural objects '"value for money"' (378). It is a taste which condemns them to like *only* what they can *afford* to like. In contrast, the bourgeoisie's tastes are 'tastes of luxury (or freedom)' (177) enabled not only by one's possession of economic capital but also by that of cultural capital. Bourdieu's approach of taste as a marker of class is captured in this well-known statement: 'Taste classifies, and it classifies the classifier' (6).

In *Distinction*, then, Bourdieu sets out to de-essentialise the idea of taste and to expose the social arbitrary that informs cultural practices. In doing so he showed the importance of culture as a vector of social distinctions. The dominant culture is the culture of the dominant class, whose interest is to maintain this dominance by producing and reproducing its values and by naturalizing its taste as good taste. Cultural practices are the product of, and reproduce, class antagonisms; culture is an object of power relations and class distinctions.[2] Thus, for instance, in her discussion of popular British TV shows such as *What Not To Wear*, McRobbie (2005) argues, drawing on the work of Bourdieu, that by promoting middle class standards in appearance such programmes produce and legitimate class distinctions and struggles, particularly amongst women.

In *Distinction*, Bourdieu uses the example of dress to capture the idea of the class structuring of taste and of the related practices of distinction. He writes: 'fashion is the latest fashion, the latest difference. An emblem of class (in all senses) withers once it loses its distinctive power. When the miniskirt reaches the mining villages of northern France, it's time to start all over again' (Bourdieu, 1993b: 135). Here Bourdieu's idea recalls that of Simmel (1971 [1904]), for whom, as discussed in chapter 4, trends emanate at the top of social hierarchy to then trickle down classes. In this model – known as the trickle down theory – fashion is explained in terms of class distinctions and class emulation.

The limits of the trickle down theory have been discussed by various authors (see, for instance, Crane, 2000; Edwards, 2010; Rocamora, 2002a), which points to one of the shortcomings of Bourdieu's work. Indeed, whilst he is regularly identified as one of the most influential thinkers of the twentieth century (e.g. Silva and Warde, 2010: 157), his theoretical framework

has also been criticized by many, a fact that is testament to the very popularity of his writing and a logical outcome of the close reading it has been
subject to. There is no space in this chapter to cover all the arguments and
points of contention (but see Swartz, 1997 for an impressive discussion of
the strengths and shortcomings of Bourdieu's theoretical framework) but
amongst the recurring critiques are the following.

Although he developed the concept of habitus partly to bypass the structure versus agency dichotomy that informs much of the social sciences, his
analysis ends up veering somewhat to the structuralist and deterministic side
of the opposition, with habitus a conduit for reproduction rather than agent-
ive transformative power (Devine, 2010: 152; Lamont, 1992; Reay, 2010;
Rocamora, 2001). As Bourdieu himself notes, 'the practices that the habitus
produces [...] always tend to reproduce the objective structures of which,
in the final analysis, they are the product' (Bourdieu, 2000a: 257). Thus as
Swartz puts it, 'rather than effectively transcend this opposition, Bourdieu's
work seems paradoxically plagued by it' (1997: 54). Bourdieu's notion of
habitus also reveals agents fuelled by the quest for profit, strategic players
solely interested in maximizing their game (albeit unconsciously, as mentioned earlier), an approach which has been criticised as reducing agents to
calculative strategists, with little room made for disinterested practice and
affects such as emotion or pain (see, for instance, Devine, 2010: 153; Skeggs,
2004).

Moreover, although his work has been appropriated to interrogate
various forms of cultural capital such as the subcultural capital of club-
bers (Thornton, 1997), it is an approach Bourdieu himself could not have
embraced as in his work culture means high culture and cultural capital,
high cultural capital (Rocamora, 2001; Skeggs, 2004). Thus various authors
have parted with his views to insist on the different forms cultural capital can
take (see, for instance, Lamont, 1992, 2010; Skeggs, 2004), also drawing
attention to the particularism of his theoretical framework. Lamont (1992),
for instance, has commented on its inability to account for American cultural practices. She also notes that in *Distinction* he 'tends to generalize about
the culture that prevails in the intellectual milieu in which he lives – arguing that it pervades the French population at large' (Lamont, 1992: 186,
see also Jenkins, 1996: 148; Shusterman, 2000: 197). Thus statements such
as that the working classes are 'deprived of culture' (Bourdieu and Darbel,
1997: 88) have left him open to the accusation of miserabilism (Grignon
and Passeron, 1989). In a similar vein Frow observes that 'the concept of
"deprivation" is itself unsatisfactory because it accepts as given the norms

of high culture. Cultural disadvantage is, in fact, operative only *on the ground of high culture*' (Frow, 1987: 65).

Finally, having focused mostly on the idea of class, Bourdieu has paid comparatively less attention to the role other social categories such as gender[3] and ethnicity play in formations of tastes, habitus and fields.

In spite of these limits, Bourdieu's theoretical framework remains highly influential and has been appropriated or reworked to interrogate a vast range of issues (see, for instance, Adkins and Skeggs, 2004 for a discussion of 'feminism after Bourdieu'). In the remaining section I point to further avenues for research by outlining the value of field theory for engaging with the contemporary phenomenon of fashion bloggers' entry in the field of the fashion media.

BLOGGERS AND THE FIELD OF THE FASHION MEDIA

The field of the fashion media is a social space made of a range of institutions and agents – magazines, newspapers, journalists, photographers, stylists, makeup artists and so on – all involved in the definition of its norms and values. This includes the definition of what constitutes good, tasteful, valuable or innovative fashion (see Rocamora, 2001; Ane Lynge-Jorlén, 2012). Titles such as *Vogue* or *Marie-Claire* are part of its established players whilst more recent creations such as *The Gentlewoman* are amongst its newcomers. Included in the latter category also are fashion bloggers, although the popularity of sites such as The Sartorialist or Garance Doré is fast turning their creators into established players of the field of fashion.

Fashion blogging emerged at the beginning of the twenty-first century (see Rocamora, 2011). At first independent bloggers were excluded from the field of fashion, with two key openings through its boundaries – entry to the fashion shows and access to public relations officers – the preserve of the legitimate players of traditional print magazines and newspapers. Indeed a common complaint on blogs has been brands' reluctance to engage with fashion bloggers. Bourdieu notes that:

> Within the field of journalism, there is permanent competition to appropriate the readership, of course, but also to appropriate what is thought to secure readership, in other words, the earliest access to news, the 'scoop', exclusive information, and also distinctive rarity, 'big names', and so on.
> (Bourdieu, 2005: 44)

In the field of fashion, access to such news and big names is premised on one's ownership of a fashion capital (Rocamora, 2001; Entwistle and Rocamora, 2006) consequent enough to secure access to key events such as the shows (Entwistle and Rocamora, 2006: 740), an access which in turn allows one to consolidate one's capital and further settles one's position in the field.

If fashion bloggers were first ignored by brands, they are increasingly becoming consecrated, the symbolic capital of some such as Susie Lau (Style Bubble), arguably as valuable as that of celebrated fashion journalists such as Cathy Horyn. In 2013, for instance, Lau featured alongside Anna Wintour (editor of US *Vogue*) in an *Observer* 'fashion students' power list' (Fisher, 2013). Thus, fashion bloggers are now a common sight at the shows, whilst many fashion brands have developed social media campaigns aimed at wooing the fashion blogosphere. In 2012 H&M, for instance, commissioned Elin Kling (Style by Kling) to design and model a collection for the Swedish market, whilst in 2013 Susie Lau styled their Oxford Circus shop windows in London. This consecration is undeniably the outcome of the bloggers' success in appealing to a wide readership, but it is also that of the legitimating role of established fashion media players. Indeed fashion bloggers have become a regular object of attention and praise in the traditional print media. It is not uncommon, for instance, for a glossy to report on the fashionable style of bloggers and therefore construct them as trendsetters and influential 'cultural intermediaries' (Bourdieu, 1996a). Some bloggers have even made it to the cover of established titles such as *Pop* (Autumn–Winter 2009) and *L'Officiel* (October 2011) in the case of Tavi Gevinson, or *Company* (January 2013) in that of Susie Lau, whilst various bloggers contribute to print media, as is the case with Garance Doré's column for *Vogue Paris* and Tommy Ton's photographic work for Style.com.

This consecration, however, has not been embraced by all. In February 2013, for instance, an article written by established fashion journalist Suzy Menkes rapidly became an object of debate in the fashion blogosphere. There Menkes (2013) wrote that 'only the rarest of bloggers could be seen as a critic in its original meaning of a visual and cultural arbiter'. She is not alone in having voiced such an opinion. Robert Johnson, for instance, the associate editor of men's magazine *GQ*, wrote that bloggers 'don't have the critical faculties to know what's good and what's not' (cited in Mesure, 2010). A more systematic and in-depth analysis of the discourses of both print journalism and bloggers as well as of their respective position in the field of the fashion media would have to be conducted to fully ascertain the range of values and meanings they attribute to fashion journalism, but the above quotes draw attention to one of its key stakes: the definition of what constitutes (good, valuable) fashion journalism. Indeed two visions seem to be opposed: on the one hand that of established players such as Menkes and Johnson, who see 'true' fashion journalists as those cultural arbiters endowed with the critical skills to identify good or bad fashion, that is, informed objective judges of fashion; on the other hand that of many bloggers and blog readers, for whom the value of fashion blogging lies in the bloggers' openly personal and subjective take on fashion, together with the valuing of authenticity, truthfulness and independence often praised on the blogosphere. As Yuli Ziv (2011: 26) puts it in her fashion blogging guide: 'Does your blog look authentic and sincere? It must.'

The ideals of authenticity and independence stand in opposition to the issue of journalists' lack of autonomy and of the constraining role of advertising on their writing agenda. By promoting authenticity and independence, bloggers lend themselves to Bourdieu's definition of newcomers, whose strategy, he suggests, is to challenge the values and practices of established players. In some instances this challenging has also been articulated through the promotion of bodily ideals – a full body in the case of The Big Girl Blog or Le Blog de Big Beauty for instance; an ageing body in that of Advanced Style or That's Not My Age; or a black body in that of Street Etiquette – in sharp contrast with the body of glossy magazines – white, thin, tall and young.

However, numerous are the blogs that also conform to the canons of established fashion media and play by their rules. Indeed, amongst the most famous female fashion bloggers are young, conventionally good looking women, whose posts also give a significant amount of space to established brands, often displayed on their model-like body. Some have ventured into modelling, such as Rumi Neely (Fashion Toast) for instance, who has been signed by Next modelling agency, or Gala Gonzalez who modelled in Loewe's 2013 advertising campaign. In the field of fashion one's body – particularly a thin, white, young body – is a capital one can nurture to establish oneself and display field membership (Entwistle and Rocamora, 2006: 746), and some bloggers have been able to capitalize on this to rise to visibility and popularity and further consolidate their symbolic and economic capitals.

Thus one must not fall into the trap of what Mosco (2005) calls 'the digital sublime' whereby mythical celebratory discourses on the internet obscure its many limits. The seemingly democratic virtue of blogging as an activity simply open to all with a computer may veil the key role a privileged capital such as one's model-like body can play in one's successful entry into the field of fashion. Chittenden (2010) and McQuarrie et al. (2013) have drawn on Bourdieu's notion of capital to discuss fashion blogging, Chittenden in relation to teen fashion bloggers and McQuarrie et al. by focusing on the idea of cultural capital, but more research could be conducted into the profile of a broader range and genre of fashion bloggers to obtain a better picture of their socio-economic backgrounds and of the types of capital needed and valued to succeed.

Similarly, *contra* visions of the world wide web as a non-hierarchical space (Bolter, 2001; Landow, 1997), hierarchies have not been erased from the fashion blogosphere – witness the presence at the front row of fashion shows of a select number only of bloggers; witness also the recurrent on and off line top ten lists of best fashion bloggers. Page views also are a sign of capital, which figures bloggers can invoke to demonstrate the popularity and visibility of their blog, their standing out above 'the long tail' (Anderson, 2004) of fashion blogs. Thus, fashion blogging can be seen as a subfield of the fashion media, and as such, as a space itself made of newcomers and established players, with popular, by now veteran, figures such as Susie Lau, Garance Doré, Tavi and Scott Schuman, amongst the latter, and bloggers with lower page views and visibility amongst the former.

CONCLUSION

In this chapter I hope to have shown the value of Bourdieu's theoretical framework for thinking through fashion, and, in particular, the field of fashion blogging. The concepts he developed allow us to capture the forces that underpin the work and practices of the agents that move across it and to make sense of the rapidly changing field of the fashion media. Field, position, capital, habitus, all notions at the core of his work, help us shed light on this field's state of flux.

Bourdieu has insisted, as mentioned in the introduction, on the value of the field of fashion as paradigmatic of the processes at play in all fields. In that respect this chapter is also an encouragement to other researchers to take up Bourdieu's work to unpack the field of fashion, but also for them to embrace fashion – that topic still too often seen as an 'unworthy' object of academic analysis – the better to critically engage with his thought.

NOTES

1   This is a collection of articles published throughout the 1960s, 1970s and 1980s and
    brought together for the first time in that English volume.
2   In that respect, through its attention to the idea of class struggles, Bourdieu's theoret-
    ical framework draws attention to the influence of Marx (discussed in chapter 1) on
    his work (but see also Bourdieu (1993: 180–82) on how he departs from Marxism;
    see also Swartz (1997: 38–40) for a discussion of Bourdieu's relation to Marxist
    theory).
3   See, however, his *Masculine Domination* (2001), although it pays virtually no attention to
    related feminist works. (See Witz, 2004 for a critique of this neglect.)

REFERENCES

Adkins, L. and Skeggs, B. (2004) *Feminism After Bourdieu*, Oxford: Blackwell.
Anderson, C. (2004) 'The Long Tail', retrieved from http://www.wired.com/wired/
    archive/12.10/tail.html?pg=2&topic=tail&topic_set on 2 August 2013.
———(1990 [1967]) *The Fashion System*, Berkeley: University of California Press.
Bolter, J.D. (2001) *Writing Space*, New York: Routledge.
Bourdieu, P. (1965) *Un Art Moyen: Essai sur les Usages Sociaux de la Photographie*, Paris: Minuit.
———(1966) 'Champ Intellectuel et Projet Créateur' in *Les Temps Modernes*, 246: 865–906.
———(1986) 'The Forms of Capital' in J.E. Richardson (ed), *Handbook of Theory of Research
    for the Sociology of Education*, Westport, CT: Greenwood Press.
———(1992) *Les Règles de l'Art*, Paris: Seuil.
———(1993a) *The Field of Cultural Production*, Cambridge: Polity Press.
———(1993b) 'Haute Couture and Haute Culture' in P. Bourdieu, *Sociology in Question*,
    London: Sage.
———(1993c [1984]) *Sociology in Question*, London: Sage.
———(1996a [1979]) *Distinction: A Social Critique of the Judgement of Taste*, London:
    Routledge.
———(1996b) (with Boltanski, L., Castel, R. and Chamboredon, J.C.) *Photography: A
    Middle-Brow Art*, Cambridge: Polity Press.
———(1996c [1992]) *The Rules of Art*, Cambridge: Polity Press.
———(1997) *The Logic of Practice*, Cambridge: Polity Press.
———and Darbel, A. (1997) *The Love of Art*, Cambridge: Polity Press.
———(1998 [1994]) *Practical Reason*, Stanford, CA: Stanford University Press.
———(2000a [1972]) *Esquisse d'une Théorie de la Pratique*, Paris: Seuil.
———(2000b) *Les Structures Sociales de L'Economie*, Paris: Seuil.
———(2001) *Masculine Domination*, Cambridge: Polity Press.
———(2004 [2001]) *Science of Science and Reflexivity*, Cambridge: Polity.
———(2005) 'The Political Field, the Social Field, and the Journalistic Field' in R. Benson
    and E. Neveu (eds), *Bourdieu and the Journalistic Field*, Cambridge: Polity.
———and Delsaut, Y. (1975) 'Le Couturier et sa Griffe: Contribution à une Théorie de la
    Magie' in *Actes de la Recherche en Sciences Sociales*, 1: 7–36.
———and Wacquant, L.J.D (1996) *An Invitation to Reflexive Sociology*, Cambridge: Polity Press.

Brown, N. and Szeman, I. (2000) Pierre Bourdieu: Fieldwork in Culture, Oxford: Rowman and Littlefield.

Calhoun, C., Lipuma, E. and Postone, M. (eds) (1995) Bourdieu: Critical Perspectives, Cambridge: Polity Press.

Chittenden, T. (2010) 'Digital Dressing Up: Modelling Female Teen Identity in the Discursive Spaces of the Fashion Blogosphere' in Journal of Youth Studies, 13 (4): 505–20.

Crane, D. (2000) Fashion and Its Social Agenda, Chicago: University of Chicago Press.

Devine, F. (2010) 'Habitus and Classficiations' in E. Silva and A. Warde (eds), Cultural Analysis and Bourdieu's Legacy, London: Routledge.

Edwards, T. (2010) Fashion in Focus, London: Routledge.

Entwistle, J. and Rocamora, A. (2006) 'The Field of Fashion Materialized: A Study of London Fashion Week' in Sociology, 40 (4): 735–51.

Fisher, A. (2013) 'The Fashion Students' Power List 2013' in the Observer, retrieved from http://www.theguardian.com/fashion/2013/mar/03/fashion-students-power-list-2013 on 2 April 2013.

Frow, J. (1987) 'Accounting for Tastes: Some Problems in Bourdieu's Sociology of Culture' in Cultural Studies, 1 (1): 59–73.

Grignon, C. and Passeron, J.C. (1989) Le Savant et le Populaire: Misérabilisme et Populisme en Sociologie et en Littérature, Paris: Hautes Etudes / Gallimard Le Seuil.

Jenkins, R. (1996) Pierre Bourdieu, London: Routledge.

Lamont, M. (1992) Money, Morals and Manners: The Culture of the French and the American Upper-Middle Class, Chicago: University of Chicago Press.

———(2010) 'Looking Back at Bourdieu' in E. Silva and A. Warde (eds), Cultural Analysis and Bourdieu's Legacy, New York: Routledge.

Landow, G.P. (1997) Hypertext 2.0, Baltimore, MD: Johns Hopkins University Press.

Lynge-Jorlén, A. (2012) 'Between Frivolity and Art: Contemporary Niche Fashion Magazines' in Fashion Theory, 16 (1): 7–28.

McQuarrie, E.F., Miller, J. and Phillips, B.J. (2013) 'The Megaphone Effect and Audience in Fashion Blogging' in Journal of Consumer Research, 40 (1): 136–58.

McRobbie, A. (1998) British Fashion Design: Rag Trade or Image Industry?, London: Routledge.

———(2005) The Uses of Cultural Studies, London: Sage.

Menkes, S. (2013) 'The Circus of Fashion', retrieved from http://tmagazine.blogs.nytimes.com/2013/02/10/the-circus-of-fashion/ on 22 February 2013.

Mesure, S. (2010) 'Fluff Flies as Fashion Writers Pick a Cat Fight with Blogger', retrieved from http://www.independent.co.uk/life-style/fashion/news/fluff-flies-as-fashion-writers-pick-a-cat-fight-with-bloggers-1884539.html on 6 March 2011.

Mosco, V. (2005) The Digital Sublime: Myth, Power and Cyberspace, Cambridge, MA: MIT Press.

Pinto, L. (1998) Pierre Bourdieu et la Théorie du Monde Social, Paris: Albin Michel.

Reay, D. (2010) 'From the Theory of Practice to the Practice of Theory: Working with Bourdieu in Research in Higher Education Choice' in E. Silva and A. Warde (eds), Cultural Analysis and Bourdieu's Legacy, London: Routledge.

Rocamora, A. (2001) 'High Fashion and Pop Fashion: The Symbolic Production of Fashion in Le Monde and The Guardian' in Fashion Theory: The Journal of Dress, Body, Culture, 5 (2): 123–42.

———(2002a) 'Fields of Fashion: Critical Insights into Bourdieu's Sociology of Culture' in Journal of Consumer Culture, 2 (3): 341–62.

———(2002b) 'Le Monde's Discours de Mode: Creating the Créateurs' in French Cultural Studies, 13, 1 (37): 83–98.

————(2006) ' "Over to You": Writing Readers in the French Vogue' in *Fashion Theory: The Journal of Dress, Body, Culture*, 10 (1/2): 153–74.

————(2009) *Fashioning the City: Paris, Fashion and the Media*, London: I.B. Tauris.

————(2011) 'Personal Fashion Blogs: Screens and Mirrors in Digital Self-portraits' in *Fashion Theory: The Journal of Dress, Body, Culture*, 15 (4): 407–24.

Shusterman, R. (2000) *Pragmatist Aesthetics: Living Beauty, Rethinking Art*, Lanham, MD, Oxford: Rowman & Littlefield.

Silva, E. and Warde, A. (eds) (2010) *Cultural Analysis and Bourdieu's Legacy*, London: Routledge.

Simmel, G. (1971 [1904]) 'Fashion', Levine, D.N. (ed.) *Georg Simmel*, Chicago: University of Chicago Press.

Skeggs, B. (2004) 'Exchange, Value and Affect: Bourdieu and "the Self"' in L. Adkins and B. Skeggs (eds), *Feminism after Bourdieu*, London: Routledge.

Swartz, D. (1997) *Culture and Power: The Sociology of Pierre Bourdieu*, Chicago: The University of Chicago Press.

Thornton, S. (1997) *Club Cultures: Music, Media and Subcultural Capital*, London: Polity.

Witz, A. (2004) 'Anamnesis and Amnesis in Bourdieu's Work: The Case for a Feminist Anamnesis' in *Feminism after Bourdieu*, Oxford: Wiley-Blackwell.

Ziv, Y. (2011) *Fashion 2.0: Blogging your Way to the Front Row*, CreateSpace Independent Publishing Platform.

15

JACQUES DERRIDA
Fashion under Erasure

Alison Gill

INTRODUCTION

Jacques Derrida (1930–2004) is probably most renowned for confirming the popular notion that philosophical thought is slippery, difficult to pin down. Derrida is known for having a difficult style that destabilizes and unravels language and arguments to show that the meaning of a word, or a voice in a literary or philosophical text, is undecidable. John McCumber accounts for Derrida's reputation as a difficult philosopher who performs 'guerrilla raids on the French language': 'The best way to read him, as with any highly original writer, is first just to relax and let it wash over you' (McCumber, 2011: 333). I would add that one wash is often not adequate and one needs to rinse and repeat, that is, read Derrida again, to develop an awareness of the questions he poses and how they might be useful to the fashion student. As with many continental philosophers his writing is complex, original in style, and has been translated for English readers from a Romance language, French.

Derrida's philosophy will be remembered for deconstruction as a strategy of close reading of texts, that has come to mean in popular usage the critical dismantling of traditions and modes of thought. The relevance of such a close reading strategy for fashion will be characterized in this chapter as a viability to question fashion's foundations via its potentially multiple texts and what they perform. There are a few steps we must take to understand this point. A deconstructed text questions its ground; more than locating a starting point of operation, the text's governing framework, presuppositions and binding logic are revealed. If this chapter is to be both respectful of Derrida's intentions to re-read the history of Western metaphysics with care, and obedient to the challenges that Derridean philosophy makes on its language of expression, it should not call 'deconstruction' a theory, a method, a critique or even 'his' thinking, so central are the questions of authority, nomenclature, translation, derivation and style to this thought.

Any chapter on 'deconstructive philosophy' in relation to fashion must then be reserved about its own style of thinking and 'put it under erasure', as my title indicates, by using single apostrophes, italics, or ~~strike through~~, until the conditions of its possibility as a name for philosophy and a phil-osophy of fashion are clearly delineated (Wortham, 2010: 1; see examples of 'strike through' in Derrida, 1976: xiv). A characteristic slipperiness or hedging around the naming and diagnosis of Derridean thought as a the-ory is intolerably evasive for critics and profoundly confusing for many, and makes the task of 'thinking through Derrida' about fashion quite complex but hopefully curiously puzzling.

The objective of this chapter is to delineate the moorings of Derrida's thinking, selecting only a handful of relevant ideas from an enormous col-lection of writing that I hope to make less difficult by showing how these ideas can be used to make sense of fashion. Much like Deleuze, a contempor-ary of Derrida (see also chapter 10 on Deleuze), his vast output over a period of six decades includes the intertwining of a large number of concepts and complex terms that jockey for significance and require the assistance of a specialist dictionary or introductory book to untangle (Caputo, 1997; Lucy, 2004; Wortham, 2010).

This chapter identifies examples where fashion designers appear to re-think fashion's practice, and discusses how to put 'under erasure' the enabling conditions of fashion's insistent drive to produce collections in line with a commercial system that prizes the aesthetic idealism of innovation, spectacle and seamlessness at a dizzying seasonal pace and a predictable rela-tionship with time. Derridean thought about textual construction, some of which invokes the language of textiles, as well as subsidiary terms such as the trace, can assist to make sense of fashion design's critical dismantling of the principles of garment design. Indeed, the term 'deconstruction' was associated with fashion in the early 1990s, that evidenced an 'analytics of garment creation' (Martin and Koda, 1993: 94), in the paradoxical appear-ance of clothes that were structurally revealing, disassembled and unfinished. Deconstruction, along with *la mode Destroy*, was a label given to these often difficult and challenging clothes by fashion critics and commentators and not a method embraced or applied by designers (Gill, 1998; Martin and Koda, 1993; Spindler, 1993; Zahm, 1995).

In the first part of this chapter I will outline the key features of deconstruction in philosophy, with a focus on the emergence of concepts such as text, trace and double-thinking that will be shown to be relevant to an alternative thinking about fashion design, one that courts the expression of failure and acts out instability. I will identify instabilities in fashion texts that challenge conventional industry notions of authorship, innovation and fashion history. This occurs in the second part of the chapter in which I explore the deconstructive work of the fashion garment through the example of the Belgian designer at Maison Martin Margiela, whose collections have received much attention as critical, experimental clothes that undo themselves.

DE(CON)STRUCTION IN PHILOSOPHY

In a prolific career as a philosopher, Derrida's many books encompassed the subjects of philosophy, literature, art, film, media, politics, history and autobiography amongst others, and while not about fashion they model a critical mode of reading that has found expression in fashion. In her obituary of Derrida, Judith Butler (2004) proposes that Derrida's legacy is in not only teaching us to read, but in giving the act of reading a new significance and a new promise. Deconstruction is the term initially used in Of Grammatology (1976), which is representative of many of his texts in having both a philosophical and a literary dimension to the deconstruction.

A level of technical difficulty is evident in his primary material because his reading involves a philosophical task of taking apart a text's operational logic, while challenging the language used to explain itself by pointing out alternative meanings and inventing new terms. Although not simply negative, deconstruction was coined for the critical, thorough and transformational readings of the language and logic of selected philosophical and literary texts to question inherent conceptual distinctions or oppositions that affect the whole of Western philosophy (Culler, 2008; Reynolds, s.a.). Deconstruction's challenge to these binary oppositions is not to invert the terms, but rather displace them so that neither term is primary. The point to Derrida's close readings is to transform the logic and relationship of concepts by revealing the inter-dependent traces of meaning and activity, say of one concept in another, on which a text's logic depends. Derrida referred to his work as a philosophy of the margins, positioned at the interstices between philosophy and other literature, which accounts for its influence on many literatures and creative practices as a strategy of close reading and writing, and a hall-mark of post-structuralist interdisciplinarity (Culler, 2008).

Derridean textual analysis was highly influential in philosophy, literary theory, law, psychoanalysis, anthropology, feminism, gay and lesbian studies, political theory, history, film theory and cultural studies in the 1980s and 1990s, including the creative arts, design, and architecture (Benjamin, 1988; Caputo, 1997; *Encyclopedia Britannica*, 2014; Reynolds, s.a.). It was during the late 1980s to the mid 1990s that other design fields, such as graphic design, as well as film-makers and screen media theorists had quite a 'heady' time with French theory, namely post-structuralist, identifiably Derridean philosophy and textual analysis, and developed self-consciously radical, theoretical creative practices (Brunette and Wills, 1989; Byrne and Witte, 1990; Wigley and Johnson, 1988; Wigley, 1993; Lupton and Abbott-Miller, 1996; McCoy and Frej, 1988).

This development is in part explained by the cross-disciplinary consequences of a literary and philosophical analysis able to expose the dominant logic of thought, called logocentrism and a 'metaphysics of presence'. To explain this concept in simple terms, for Derrida Western metaphysics repeats a logocentric practice of essence fabrication where a spoken word (*logos*) names the essential *being* of a thing, consequently equated with full-presence and universal truth as a pure conduit of meaning (Derrida, 1976: 18). Derrida questions the unity of a word to capture the full presence of something or to represent a thought, what he calls the logocentrism of language that upholds traditions of thought. His thinking strives to unsettle the impervious idea of essence or identity as fixed notions (Derrida, 1988: 4; Lucy, 2004: 12). This helps us to understand that 'deconstruction begins, as it were, from a refusal of the authority or determining power of every "is"', not because it is to adopt a position of resistance or opposition, or to refuse simple definition, but rather because of 'the impossibility of every "is" as such' (Lucy, 2004: 11). Derrida's deconstruction includes a criticism of a logocentrism that has pursued the capture of pure presence as the proper passage to knowledge, and that ensures the impossibility of thinking at once those terms positioned oppositionally. This is best explained as Derrida's philosophical undertaking to think about difference and to think 'presence' differently as difference-as-presence.

An example of this undertaking can be illustrated in terms of what has been called 'double thinking' and can be represented in the 'double movement' of deconstructing a text. Lucy explains this notion that seems impossibly difficult because it involves considering the aporias or impasses of oppositional logic, involving the necessity of 'a double movement, which is irreducible to a "two-step programme" or successive "phases" of inter-pretation' (2004: 13). The deconstruction of texts gives expression to think-ing at once these oppositions, that is, the difference of two terms, their relationships, and that which makes them impossible to think differently. Lucy argues this is so very difficult because conventionally one term has been valued more highly than the other and there is resistance to it being otherwise.

An analogy of double-thinking was identified in fashion by Richard Martin and Harold Koda in designs by Rei Kawakubo for Comme des Garçons and Karl Lagerfeld for Chloé that expose their structure through holes and unconcealed seams, whereby 'destruction becomes a process of analytical creation' and they 'work more analytically to prolong an interest in apparel' (Martin and Koda, 1993: 94). By association, fashion design is like Derrida's writing that can underscore an instability in the text or garment to para-doxically express both construction and destruction, making and unmaking. Martin and Koda (1993: 96) ask whether there is any difference between the exposure of the garment's techniques in designs by Vionnet in the 1920s and the deconstructions of Lagerfeld and Kawakubo. The late twentieth-century examples, they conclude, seem to work backwards 'from a finished garment, ravaging its integrity rather than simply showing the process of making' (1993: 94).

When the word de(con)struction is written in this way to highlight two terms in one, it exposes the double-movement that deconstruction locates at work in the text; it can be both, at once, taking a text apart as in *destruct*, destabilize, displace an opposition and the *construction* of a new understand-ing of a text's operations – an understanding of its agency and its limita-tions. Amy Spindler in The New York Times defines deconstruction in fashion as '"the action of undoing the construction of a thing". So not only does that mean that jacket linings, for example, can be found on the outside or sleeves detached, but the function of the piece is re-imagined' (1993: 1). I will show below that Maison Margiela's designs express a double movement, or the bi-directionality of *un*-making, in acknowledgement of the dress-maker's labour (usually concealed in the finished garment) and in remembrance of a history of iconic garments. The privative '*un*' in un-making is italicized to show that its work is to suspend the nexus of making fashion apparel in paradox, as undecidable, so as to acknowledge the double-movement within, and a double-thinking of the fashion garment. Included within this double-movement is the expression of possible failure, or the risk that garments are simply destroyed, left ravaged or misinterpreted as an intentional destruction, a nihilism and an uncompleted text.

UNSETTLING THE TEXT: THE INTERWEAVING OF MEANING AND THE FASHION TRACE

The active qualities that Derrida locates in a close reading of texts can be uncovered in fashion objects – a piece of everyday clothing, a designer garment, a fashioned body, fashion magazines, writing, photographs, films – to understand them as constructed texts with an underpinning logic and an interplay of signs that account for their sometimes contradictory signification. While Derrida did not write directly about fashion, French semiotician Roland Barthes has been influential in developing ways to interpret fashion as a language that communicates meaning (see also chapter 8 on Barthes). Derrida can be seen to continue the close reading of texts akin to a Barthesian passion to decode literary and non-written texts, popular and media culture, in a fertile period of philosophical inquiry in France undertaken by a generation of continental philosophers interested in what culture signifies (see the Introduction to this book). Similar to Barthes' (1967) and Foucault's (1969) questioning of the intentions of the author, Derrida questioned the limits of authorial intention to 'fully govern everything we end up meaning by what we say or write' (Butler, 2004: 32). The shift from a conventional notion of the author or producer of a text being regarded as the origin of a text's meaning to the recognition that a text is intertextual means that it is the product of an interplay of signification coming from multiple sites. In this revised conception of authorship, the reader plays an active role as an interpreter of texts that gain their meaning through reference to other texts. Caroline Evans reminds us that if the fashion garment speaks or communicates, 'it speaks independently of its creators' (2003: 6). The point here is not to simply debunk the entire authority of the creator, author or producer, but to activate the role of the reader, captured by Barthes' phrase 'the birth of the reader', in the interpretive work of the text (Barthes, 1967; Silverman, 1994: 28).

What does Derrida's close reading add to our understanding of text and textuality that might be identified in the fashion object? His description of textuality is suggestive of a way of thinking about fashion objects and images as intricately woven inter-texts, rich with traces of meaning to be decoded.

Using language that evokes the cross-weave of textiles, Derrida refers to the signification of textuality as a potentially infinite interplay of differences between words and circulations through discourses:

> Whether in the order of spoken or written discourse, no element can function as a sign without referring to another element which itself is not simply present. This interweaving results in each 'element' [...] being constituted on the basis of the trace within it of the other elements of the chain or system. This interweaving, this textile, is the *text* produced only in the transformation of another text. Nothing, neither among the elements nor within the system, is anywhere ever simply present or absent. There are only, everywhere, differences and traces of traces.
>
> (Derrida, 1982: 26)

After citing the above by Derrida about the text, Kim Sawchuk (2007 [1988]) briefly expands on the potential suggested by Derrida's analogy between text and textile to explain the intertextuality of the fashioned body as a textured fashion object. 'The "fashioned body" is an embodied subjectivity, constituted in the rich weave of social, historical and cultural inscriptions. At any one time, or historical juncture, the fashioned body is potentially located in multiple discourses on health, beauty, morality, sexuality, the nation, and the economy, to name some of the possibilities' (Sawchuk, 2007: 478). The inscriptions of discourse for Sawchuk do not necessarily act *upon* the body, but work at the level of the body, enclosed in a fabric of intertextual relations.

Silverman (1994) contends that if the task of deconstruction is ultimately a theoretical practice of reading texts, it assists to re-conceive the object of interpretation in slight difference to semiotics' object of analysis. Derrida's reading and writing seeks a way to think differently, doubly, about textual limits and borders as hinges or thresholds that join two terms and trouble binaries. Deconstruction is something that 'happens' to things, as happening already there in the text, rather than something one does to it (Lucy, 2004: 12–14). It is the generation of new terms, the 'irruptive emergence of a new "concept"' that is required to effect the displacement of hierarchically organized terms in deconstructive writing (Derrida cited in Lucy, 2004: 13). There are many terms generated (some newly coined or some reworked older terms) across the collection of Derrida's writing – arche-writing, the supplement, the trace, *différance*, ghost, gram, pharmakon – that on account of their ambiguity unsettle the operational logic of a text by troubling evident binaries with undecidables.

The 'trace' is such a term that announces the text's 'happening' and the distributive production of differences in meaning, as one element in a text refers to another (Derrida, 1982: 26). In fashion, the obvious value of the trace is to the interpretive act of tracing elements of meaning, for example to establish and decode notions of conventional clothing design and use. It is also relevant to decoding physical traces as signs of deviation from convention, like a dressmaker's pencil marking on fabric, 'directly referring to the labour process [...] and traditional dressmaking techniques' on the outside of deconstructed garments: 'one can make out lining, seams, darts, shoulder pads, white basting thread, patterns' (Debo, 2008: 12). These traces of labour would normally be effaced or magically concealed in a finished product, until exposed seams, amongst other elements, changed the game. For Derrida, the trace is the (effaced) origin of difference, 'the opening of [...] the enigmatic relationship of the living to its other and of an inside to an outside' (Derrida, 1976: 70). The related notion of the 'seam' in garment construction is highly suggestive as a productive third term, an undecidable, that has the potential to give further insight. In simple terms, the seam is a trace of garment production that cannot be fully concealed: more interestingly, it functions as a hinge, interface and borderline between two pieces. It is both essential to structure and overall garment shape, and it resides on the surface and below. The seam is an interface holding the inside and the outside, depth and surface together, that can take us to both sides when 'double-thought'. When conceived along these lines, the exposure of a seam is a radical element in the vocabulary of deconstruction fashion to think about the juxtaposition of meanings and materials, for instance the exposed seams by Japanese designers Rei Kawakubo and Yohji Yamamoto (English, 2010: 130).

The trace has also assisted to uncover fashion's relationship with history. By tracking or miming the traces from collective fashion history, it can do more than decipher the meaning of particular elements; it can expose the peculiar logic by which fashion has to efface its past to insist on change and innovation. Warwick and Cavallaro (1998) invoke the notion of palimpsest to describe the fashion text that strives for novelty. These novelties are often grafted 'upon prior narratives [...] neither unadulterated or utterly cancelled'. Fashion's text, then, is essentially a palimpsest, a 'manuscript, the original writing on which has been effaced to make room for a second' (Warwick and Cavallaro, 1998: 153). Using Derrida's notion, the trace activates the evidence of original writing, what is absent and not seen, and at play in the textile of the fashion text, the interweaving of elements in one another.

The trace triggers this interplay between presence and absence, including elements of fashion history and the signature motifs of past designers that are neither fully absent nor present. It is argued that for these novel texts to operate as palimpsests entails an *effacement* of the traces of fashion history rather than their *erasure*, and fashion experiment might find ways of making previous traces translucently visible (Warwick and Cavallaro, 1998: 153). We will see that Martin Margiela refuses the illusion of the innovative fashion text as a tabular rasa, a blank slate, as the only possible mark or recognition of originality and innovation.

DECONSTRUCTION IN FASHION: FASHION UNDER ERASURE

Many fashion scholars have linked selected 1990s fashion designs, exposing the labour and techniques of the dressmaker and couturier, to deconstruction as a mode of thinking (Debo, 2008; English, 2011; Evans, 1998, 2003; Gill, 1998; Martin and Koda, 1993, Lynge-Jorlén, 2010; Vinken, 2005, 2008; Zahm, 1995). As such they associate with a deconstructive writing to unsettle texts that has found its way into fashion design as a different 'writing' in clothing forms that unconventionally lay bare a process and logic that is not straightforwardly critical. In the preceding overview of deconstructive writing, it was emphasised that Derrida's interests in words, texts and arguments encompassed not only what they *mean* but what they *do*, and the active capacity of writing to both hold logic together and to unsettle it by testing limits and generating a promise in new forms of writing.

In the vocabulary of fashion design experiment, we can see a similar interest in visibly testing the limits of structure, form and technique to return our attention to the garment to question what it does. Here, it is argued that this is evidence of questioning fashion's ground and its foundation in the garment; what is its cohering framework, its binding logic, its presuppositions or put more simply, the forces at work? However, this thinking of the element, or the basic unit, involves summoning further thinking of the larger structure or system of which they are a part. Various fashion theorists (Debo, 2008; Gill, 1998; Lynge-Jorlén, 2010; Vinken, 2005, 2008) have outlined how a deconstruction of clothing forms extends to a mode of questioning about the fashion system, its *modus operandi*, the industrial structures and commercial, branding systems, and their consumers from this start in re-thinking fashion garments. There are many other examples of deconstructive fashion that could be discussed as part of this chapter, yet selections from Maison Margiela can clearly explain an 'analytics of construction' and provide further insights organized here as themes – of authorship, innovation and time – that put fashion under erasure by questioning clothing forms and the fashion system.

MAISON MARGIELA: AN ANALYTICS OF CONSTRUCTION

An engagement with clothing's conceptual underpinnings can be illustrated by the insights about structure found in deconstructed fashion forms by Maison Margiela. Caroline Evans' reading of several garments from Margiela draws attention to an analogy between a garment's structure as a cohering framework and what she calls a 'formal logic of dress itself' (2003: 250). In pointing out the indicators of a structural questioning, say about the role of a dress's lining, she provides an example of a destabilizing dress that displaces the formal logic between a dress's inside and outside, and the structural relationship between the internal lining and the external fabric frame of a dress (Figure 15.1).

Margiela 'reproduced the lining of a 1950s cocktail dress as a contemporary dress, and then photographed the original lining of the dress inside out and screenprinted this image onto the new dress' (Evans, 2003: 250). The dress reproduces a lining that becomes 'dress as lining', internal support becomes external frame, revealing a destabilizing movement in the framework that goes further than turning clothes inside-out. In a second example (Figure 15.2), Margiela questions the structural role of a wearer's body as the internal foundation for clothing by adding an extra layer of 'body' – the linen and shape of the usually temporary tailor's dummy – into the worn outcome. Evans observes: 'he […] recreated the tailor's dummy as a linen waistcoat, so that the foundation became underwear, the body became the dress' (Evans, 2003: 250). In another version of this 'dummy' waistcoat it is tacked together with half of the bodice of a silk chiffon dress.

In these readings, Evans locates evidence of a destabilising play within structure as Margiela puts clothing 'structure' under erasure. The toile dress from 1997/8 is a clear indication of the play within the structural framework of fashion as it gives the provisional, make-shift material of the dressmaker's prototype and process to be the product (Figure 15.3). In answer to the question of 'what is fashion's foundation or ground?' Margiela wants

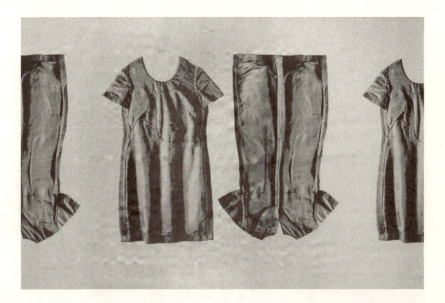

15.1 Lining Dress or 'Dress as (photographed) lining', S/S 1996, Maison Martin Margiela, Photograph by: Guy Voet.

to make visible the conceptual and material framing work that a structure does, its active *structur-ing* of clothed bodies, in delineating the boundaries and surfaces between inside and outside. The foundation includes a moving structure that is not only collapsible but also reconfigurable and transformable, as boundaries can shift and multiply in the layering of surfaces or folds between skin and its outside.

By presenting 'work in progress', garments that are wearable but unfinished like dresses with unfinished hems, tying threads and a waistcoat tacked together with half a dress, this design house seeks to expand the critical fashion vocabulary beyond the ravaging of anti-fashion to include a wide range of possibilities both formal, material and conceptual. Recalling the privative 'un' in *un-*making to signal a double movement, these 'works in progress' add to the design vocabulary the risk of failure, the risk that these garments will never be finished, particularly according to the conventional standards of finish expected of designer fashion. A blatant expression of failure to finish making by Margiela can be seen when he tries to fit sleeves that are too wide into much narrower armholes, and he leaves these unseamlessly juxtaposed to question whether finish is necessary (English, 2010:

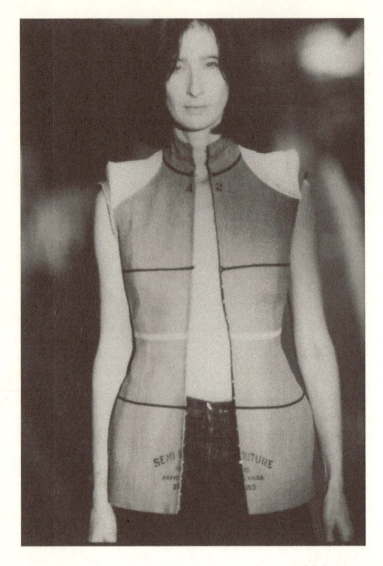

15.2 Dummy waistcoat, S/S 1997, Maison Martin Margiela, Photograph by: Ronald Stoops.

130). Detachable sleeves on a suit jacket are a more obvious invitation to the wearer to be part of a living 'work in progress', perhaps not an unfamiliar invitation to reconfigure identity through an interaction with the garment. In that these examples appear to refuse the notion that fashion magically imparts fashionability to its wearer, Margiela's designs show an interest in

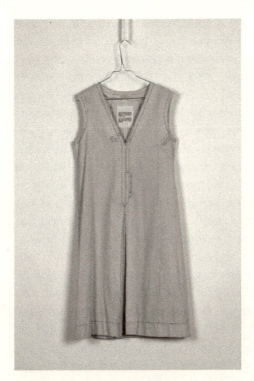

15.3 A cotton dress with label stating 'Toile of a garment after its first fitting: all rectification marks and faults remain apparent.' A/W 1997/8, Maison Martin Margiela, Photograph by: Guy Voet.

expanding beyond the runway to articulate the unfinished nature of much design whose life is only beginning at the point of sale. They engage with the life of everyday use as a field for the wearer to explore with their clothing the various possibilities that fall between unfinished and finished. He offers an invitation to a user to be part of the living work in progress of fashion and clothing, to experiment with use, with what clothes do and what fashion makes possible.

AUTHORSHIP

Martin Margiela has been tagged the 'incognito designer' by ' "disappear[ing]" as much as possible from his own creations' and by refusing to be positioned as the name behind the label (Debo, 2008: 7). Much has been written about Margiela's anonymity in an industry that breeds fascination about the designer's name, celebrity life and personality, as a measure of the brand (Debo, 2008; English, 2010; Lynge-Jorlén, 2010; Vinken, 2005; Zahm,

1995). Debo writes that the use of a blank, white cotton tag, tacked onto the inside of a garment, free of any signature, is like a blind spot, that in terms of marketing is completely useless and waywardly counters the label as a certificate of authenticity (Debo, 2008: 7). Olivier Zahm (1995: 119) observes that this use of a blank label has the effect of bringing one's attention back to the clothes, but of course it has become a signature, a representation of the house's non-superlative approach to making, albeit un-signed. Margiela shuns publicity and interviews and his dual silences on the matter of what his clothes mean and deconstruction as a movement to which he aligns himself are significant in this disappearance. While designer fashion communicates, like all clothes, in the absence of their designer (even as they bear a label of authorship), Margiela's refusal to assume any individual part as lead author, producer or visionary risks debunking the designer's ideas to activate the text. He prefers to disperse authorial agency to the atelier team and respect for their collaborative work (when necessary to go by the house name 'Maison Margiela') (English, 2010: 131–32) and to the wearer who is invited to interpret the challenging clothes. Like Derrida, he refuses the position of the master, the source of a critique of the fashion system, and the experimental agency of the clothes seems to come from them, as the deconstruction 'goes on' between the clothes, their un-making and their invitation to the wearer.

INNOVATION

Related to the deconstructionist refusal of conventional authorship is Maison Margiela's resistance to an idea of fashion innovation coupled to authenticity and originality. By omitting a signature and not claiming the authority of the creator, it disavows absolute innovation (Debo, 2008: 7). Obvious evidence of an effort to uncouple the collections from customary trend setting, see-sawing, game-changing and the view that fashion must reinvent itself each season, are their reproductions of archetypal or iconic second-hand garments from the canon of fashion history and different style periods. Going by the name of 'Replicas', they can be seen as a gesture of conservation because of the inclusion of a label with information about the garment's style, provenance and date, and also a refusal of the idea that innovation must be regarded as entirely new (Debo, 2008: 12).

These are tributes to vintage clothing, reproduced as accurately as possible, clothes that are susceptible to fashion death after a frequently fleeting appearance in the spotlight of an industry that is addicted to moving on. Recognising an authentic pursuit of an innovation that is not entirely new, Debo writes that 'The fashion world is so willing to forget that true innovation is only possible when founded upon a total command of the craft and a rigorous historical knowledge' (2008: 12). While these 'Replicas' are not equivalent to the material recovery of aged fabric that we see in other aspects of Maison Margiela's collections, they demand the recovery and application of a knowledge of historical styles and techniques. The house refuses the force of now-time to make tabula rasa of fashion history on which conventional innovation is premised (Debo, 2008: 3).

TIME AND FASHION HISTORY

Barbara Vinken characterizes Margiela's resistance to the temporality of the fashion system as an intention to establish a counter-rhythm to the 'fashion of the seasons', an 'economic form in the grip of dizzying consumption-frenzy, manifesting itself in a particularly merciless form in the bi- or tri-annual collections of fashion' (Vinken, 2005: 143). Derrida's conception of time that emphasises paradox and double-movement that defers experience, provides the tools to make sense of an unconventional, non-linear temporality and an experience of being carried 'backwards towards the future' by Margiela's garments and collections (Evans, 2003: 14). Vinken (2005: 142–43) writes 'that time clings to Margiela's work' as it has created a paradoxical project of 'initiating a fashion based on duration, rather than change'. The conventional temporal pattern of change, in a dizzingly fast-paced fashion forward direction is an alchemy unfolding linearly by which the 'fashion of tomorrow turns today's fashion into yesterday's fashion' (143), premised on an insistent forgetting of today and yesterday. Instead, Margiela expresses duration, their 'clothes carry the traces which time leaves behind in the fabric' and the 'traces of the production process' (Vinken, 2005: 142), which mark changes in these clothes that are not driven by a fashion imperative to generate new looks, rather they are accretions in fabric and shape through age and use. Signs of wear and tear are conventionally effaced by an aesthetic idealism for seamlessness and refresh which rarely allows an opportunity to perceive 'use' in fashion design.

Evans (1998: 75) and Debo (2008: 8–9) concur that a distinctive use of second-hand materials that incorporate fabrics of different ages and provenance position the temporal rhythm of his garments at variance to a system which insistently celebrates the generation of the unworn. Because they literally introduce intervals of time, aged fabric, to trouble a forward movement of time, these references to clothing history exceed the citation of recontextualised motifs typical of historical quotation. As an expression of counter-rhythms, it is possible that any one garment is the convergence of multiple rhythms, uncertain duration, vestiges of production and provenance, as say the heels of woollen army socks are recycled as small puff sleeves and breast mounds on a pullover made of patchwork socks (Autumn–Winter 1991/2). The traces of past lives (perhaps not singular) are dispersed through the weave of a future for new pullover experiences.

An expression of duration and permanence can also be found in the design tendency to reproduce and recontextualize ideas from earlier collections, selecting garments and accessories as emblematic, permanent features across his collections. In sum, the Maison's recycling of linings, basting threads, fabrics, patterns, trench coats and whole iconic garments is a material expression of a temporal language introducing returns and deferring pauses to derail fashion's conventionally forward cycle of material and symbolic re-new.

CONCLUSION

In this chapter I have expanded on the features of an encounter of the contemporary fashion design of Maison Margiela with Derridean deconstruction's activation of the text. In spite of the central position Maison Margiela maintained within Parisian if not global fashion, even while it demanded a freedom to rethink its parameters (Debo, 2008: 3), its designs invite further thinking about the inter-relationship between the production of fashion and the everyday use of clothing. While there are other designers that can be included in such a dialogue about the counter-rhythms and embodied praxis of fashion use, for example Issey Miyake who believed that clothes need a wearer to complete them (see also chapter 7), the purpose of this chapter has been to point to the insights offered by Maison Margiela's designs to experiment with deconstructionist concerns about dominant binary logic and the presuppositions that hold texts together.

For Jacques Derrida, the act of thinking and writing is an encounter with the undecidable elements and logical impasses that affect not only philosophy but extend to, underpin and limit other cultures and everyday practices. There are interesting convergences between deconstructive thinking and Margiela's conceptual and material experiment, evident in the designs and the organisation of Maison Margiela, shown here through a discussion of authorship, innovation and temporality in fashion. I have pointed to the potential for fashion students and scholars to interpret the radical positioning of dressmaking elements, traces and techniques such as the seam to be read along deconstructive and transformative lines. There is ample potential to further explore the efforts of designers to push beyond the runway into the continuing life of everyday fashion as the promise of a creatively invigorating future, as a testing ground to explore innovation and design differently. Ultimately, the possibilities of further innovation are not to be found, from Margiela's perspective, in the effacement of the experience encapsulated in fashion history.

REFERENCES

Barthes, R. (1967) 'Death of the Author', reprinted in (1978) *Image, Music, Text*, S. Heath (trans), Glasgow: Fontana Collins.

Benjamin, A. (1988) 'Deconstruction and Art/The Art of Deconstruction' in C. Norris and A. Benjamin (eds) *What is Deconstruction?*, London and New York: Academy Editions/St Martins Press.

Brunette, P. and Wills. D. (1989) *Screen/Play: Derrida and Film Theory*, Princeton, NJ: Princeton University Press.

Butler, J. (2004) 'Jacques Derrida' in *London Review of Books*, 26 (21): 32.

Byrne, C. and Witte. M. (1990) 'A Brave New World: Understanding Deconstruction', Print 44 (6): 80–87, 203.

Caputo, J. (1997) *Deconstruction in a Nutshell*, New York: Fordham University Press.

Culler, J. (1983) *On Deconstruction: Theory and Criticism after Structuralism*, Ithaca, NY: Cornell University Press.

———(2008) 'Why Deconstruction Still Matters: A Conversation with Jonathon Culler', interview with Paul Sawyer in *Cornell Chronicle*, retrieved through http://www.news.cornell.edu/stories/2008/01/why-deconstruction-still-matters-according-jonathan-culler on 11 June 2014.

Debo, K. (2008) 'Maison Martin Margiela "20", The Exhibition' in *Maison Martin Margiela* [exhibition catalogue], Antwerp: ModeMuseum.

Derrida, J. (1976) *Of Grammatology*, G.C. Spivak (trans), Baltimore, MD: John Hopkins University Press.

———(1982) *Positions*, A. Bass (trans), Chicago: University of Chicago Press.

———(1988) 'Letter to a Japanese Friend' (dated 1983) in D. Wood and R. Bernasconi (eds), *Derrida and Différance*, Evanston, IL: North Western University Press.

Encyclopaedia Britannica (2014) 'Deconstruction', retrieved through http://www.britannica.com/EBchecked/topic/155306/deconstruction on 11 June 2014.

English, B. (2010) *Japanese Fashion Designers: The Work and Influence of Issey Miyake, Yohji Yamamoto, and Rei Kawakubo*, London: Berg.

Evans, C. (1998) 'The Golden Dustman: A Critical Evaluation of the Work of Martin Margiela' in *Fashion Theory*, 2 (1): 73–94.

——(2003) *Fashion at the Edge*, New Haven, CT and London: Yale University Press.

Foucault, M. (1969) 'What is an Author?', reprinted in J.D. Faubion (ed) (1994) *Aesthetics, Method and Epistemology*, London: Allen Lane.

Gill, A. (1998) 'Deconstruction Fashion: The Making of Unfinished, Decomposing and Re-assembled Clothes' in *Fashion Theory*, 2 (1): 25–50.

Lucy, N. (2004) *A Derrida Dictionary*, Oxford: Blackwell.

Lupton, E. and Abbott-Miller, J. (1996) 'Deconstruction and Graphic Design' in *Design, Writing, Research: Writing on Graphic Design*, New York: Princeton Architectural Press.

Lynge-Jorlén, A. (2010) 'When Silence Speaks Volumes: On Martin Margiela's Cult of Invisibility and the Deconstruction of the Fashion System' in *Vestoj*, 2 (winter): 134–55.

Martin, R. and Koda, H. (1993) *Infra-Apparel*, New York: Metropolitan Museum of Art/ Harry Abrams.

McCoy, K. and Frej, D. (1988) 'Typography as Discourse' in H. Armstrong (ed) (2009) *Graphic Design Theory: Readings from the Field*, New York: Princeton Architectural Press.

McCumber, J. (2011) *Time and Philosophy*, Durham, UK: Acumen.

Reynolds, J. (s.a.) 'Jacques Derrida 1930–2004' in *Internet Encyclopaedia of Philosophy*, retrieved through http://www.iep.utm.edu/derrida/#H3 on 8 May 2014.

Sawchuk, K. (2007 [1988]) 'A Tale of Inscription: Fashion Statements', reprinted in M. Barnard (ed), *Fashion Theory: A Reader*, Oxon: Routledge.

Silverman, H.J. (1994) *Textualities: Between Hermeneutics and Deconstruction*, New York and London: Routledge.

Spindler, A.M. (1993) 'Coming Apart' in *The New York Times*, 25 July, Styles Section: 1, 9.

Vinken, B. (2005) *Fashion Zeitgeist: Trends and Cycles in the Fashion System*, M. Hewson (trans), Oxford and New York: Berg.

——(2008) 'The New Nude' in *Maison Martin Margiela* [exhibition catalogue], Antwerp: ModeMuseum.

Warwick, A. and Cavallaro, D. (1998) *Fashioning the Frame: Boundaries, Dress and the Body*, Oxford and New York: Berg.

Wigley, M. (1993) *The Architecture of Deconstruction*, Cambridge, MA: MIT Press.

——and Johnson, P. (1988) *Deconstructivist Architecture*, New York/Boston, MA: Museum of Modern Art/Little Brown & Co.

Wortham, S.M. (2010) *Continuum Philosophy Dictionaries: Derrida Dictionary*, London: Continuum.

Zahm, O. (1995) 'Before and After Fashion' in *Artforum*, 33 (7): 74–77, 119.

16

BRUNO LATOUR
Actor-Network-Theory and Fashion

Joanne Entwistle

INTRODUCTION

Amongst the most significant sociological developments of the last 30 years or so has been the rise of science and technology studies (STS) and its associated method, actor-network-theory (ANT). One of the major proponents of STS has been the French intellectual Bruno Latour, whose early work has been highly influential far beyond thematic concern with science and technology. However, at first glance, these terms, with their focus on scientific practice and technologies, seem about as intellectually far away from fashion as is possible. Indeed, Latour and his immediate colleagues have not themselves focused any attention on fashion, but in this chapter I want to demonstrate the applicability of STS and ANT to the fashion system(s) and discuss some work that does draw on these ideas to understand fashion. To do so, it is necessary to understand Latour's project, so in the first part of this chapter, I introduce Latour's work on science and how it challenges conventional thinking within sociology. In the remainder of the chapter I want to demonstrate how his work might have implications for ways of thinking about and researching fashion.

LATOUR: SCIENCE AND TECHNOLOGY STUDIES AND BEYOND

Latour's early work sets out to observe and record science as it is practised by scientists in their various laboratories. As he argues, 'The only way to understand the reality of science studies is to follow what science studies do best, that is, paying close attention to the details of scientific practice' (1999: 24). His influential book (with Steve Woolgar) *Laboratory Life: The Social Construction of Scientific Facts* of 1979 (see also Latour, 1987 and 1999) aims to understand the organization and operations of scientific work and has its roots in ethnomethodology, which proposes that actors are accomplished experts that we can learn from, and which focuses attention on the minute, routine and ordinary aspects of daily life. The important point to note about an 'actor' in ANT is that it does not only designate a human subject with consciousness but can describe anything with the ability to act or produce action. For example, a microscope or computer programme like a spreadsheet can be an actor because they *do* things and enable us to do things we might otherwise not have been able to do. Both objects enable us to 'see' and calculate: microscopes enable us to see microscopic elements not visible to the naked eye while a spreadsheet enables us to 'see' at a glance profit and loss if used in a business setting. Both act on us, promoting all sorts of actions and interventions, so that we might think of these things as prosthetics or extensions of human bodies and minds. All of us are 'hooked' or 'networked' into many such devices, hence the conjunction, actor-network.

This early work challenged the conventional view of science that tends to see humans as actors with agency who deploy devices and instruments of observation for the purposes of recording particular objects (cells in a petri dish, for example; the HIV virus or bacteria), all of which are seen as inert matter. From these observations, as this conventional thinking goes, comes objective scientific knowledge which claims to know the natural world – a world entirely different to, and separate from, 'culture'. This view of the world is derived out of Enlightenment and Modernist thinking that draws a sharp distinction between human and non-human actors and between the social and natural world. In this view, nature is ontologically different from culture and we humans, armed with science, can exercise unique control and dominance over our environment. However, in *Laboratory Life* Latour and Woolgar provide an ethnographic study of a neuro-endocrinology scientific laboratory at the Salk Institute in California, famous for developing vaccines, to argue against this traditional view of culture and science as a superior and neutral form of knowledge. They begin by asking apparently basic questions about the practice of science: what are the aims of this practice, what objects and instruments are assembled, how do they make visible certain objects/elements that would otherwise be unseen? They argue that scientists derive their descriptions as a result of particular ways of working and training, as well as through the deployment of particular kinds of instrument and devices that actively shape their findings. What we discover is that science does not observe a world of independent objects from a neutral and objective distance, rather it assembles particular sorts of objects – Bunsen burners, microscopes, molecules and so on – and these *assemblages* (a key STS word) actively construct and perform the world they apparently describe. This might seem like a radical departure from our understandings of objects and agency and indeed it is: in STS and in actor-network-theory (ANT) that emerged out of it, scientific and technological instruments of measurement and calibration are seen to exert some sort of agency – they are non-human actors, in other words – in that they are 'enrolled' (another key STS/ANT word) into the construction of these observations they enable.

Latour's critique also goes far beyond science and technology and to the heart of our understandings of modern society, since our claims to be 'modern' have largely, if not wholly, depended upon the idea of the march of objective knowledge from science and the progress of technology to redefine and liberate 'culture' from 'nature'. In his later work in *We Have Never Been Modern* (1991), Latour argues that this notion of 'modern', which does not exist in pre-modern peoples,[1] is an artificial one; it is a fiction that we tell ourselves and which sustains the claims of science as a superior form of knowledge and human Culture as superior to passive Nature. However, if we examine objects that appear to be Nature, we find they are the result of our ways of seeing – our instruments as discussed above. Taken to its logical conclusion it means that modern objects of concern like global warming or HIV cannot be seen as merely natural events, but hybrids that are simultaneously natural and social: 'the very notion of culture is an artefact created by bracketing Nature off. Cultures – different or universal – do not exist, any more than Nature does. There are only *natures-cultures*' (Latour, 1991: 104; my emphasis). From this perspective Nature is not a separate sphere from Culture: Nature is no longer seen as merely 'out there' and different to us: we are enmeshed in Nature, a part of it ourselves, our apparently 'social' or 'cultural' world is in fact a hybrid of nature-culture. This way of thinking might be particularly useful and indeed politically very relevant now that we waking up to the environmental costs of our actions and the necessity of thinking about our co-dependency on 'nature', as will be discussed in more detail below.

APPLYING STS/ANT

We seem to be a long way from fashion, but the distance is not so great when we remember that fashion is very much a culture-nature hybrid itself. It is constructed out of natural materials like cotton and silk (as well as synthetics, of course) which are fashioned into garments through a long, complex design and distribution process. While fashion appears to us – in shops, in our wardrobes and so on – ready-made and finished, it is the end produce of complex interventions into the natural world, and entangled into networks of actors around the globe, human and non-human (from water and chemicals to grow cotton at one end of the process, through to hangers and other devices to display clothing on the shop-floor). Indeed, questions of design, energy usage and consumption practices have come to the fore of late as scientists and designers try to think through our relationships to the material world around us. This attention to materiality and practice has some roots in STS/ANT, and has been extended in the work of Shove and others (Shove et al., 2007) to focus attention on design and consumption practices. Shove (2003) has highlighted the way objects, like humble domestic appliances, for example, are utilized in everyday practice, often creatively so and in ways that can feed back into the design of objects. While this 'practice theory' work (see Shove, 2005) has not been widely extended to fashion – with the focus of Shove's attention on such things as domestic technologies and innovations as 'Nordic walking' (Shove, 2005, see also Pantzar and Shove, 2005) – there is certainly scope for thinking about fashion consumption in terms of practices that encompass the whole life history of clothes and our relationships to them as material objects. Academic work has still to be done to trace these connections, but adopting a broad STS/ANT approach means paying close attention to fashion design, production and consumption in terms of hybrid practices of culture-nature. They also attest to the importance of materiality and practice – central concepts in STS/ANT.

STS has thus spread its tentacles outside laboratories and this way of analysing the world has been influential within social sciences more widely. The STS/ANT method of working, involving close ethnographic observation of actors, has become a widely used method for understanding many aspects of social life, not just science. As a method, ANT is not particularly fancy or remarkable. It simply involves 'following the actors': observing what they do, where they go and what objects they 'enrol' into particular 'assemblages'. As with STS, an 'actor' can be any object enrolled in an assemblage, so tools, instruments, devices and technologies of calibration, observation and measurement can all be said to be actors in that they are actively involved in the making up or assembly of the world and shape how that world comes together.

One particularly strong strand of ANT has focused attention on markets of various kinds, championed by the French sociologist Michel Callon. For Callon (1998), the market is not simply the abstract theoretical concept of neo-liberal economics with abstract principals or 'laws', although this notion of 'the market' is 'real' in so far as it exists on Wall Street and the Square Mile, is frequently described in the newspapers and on TV and comes to be believed in and acted on. Indeed, this notion of 'the market', beloved of neo-liberal economics, is performative (another key STS/ANT word): it takes on a reality as a powerful construction that shapes how people behave or through the policies of the governments or inter-governmental agencies such as the World Bank or the International Monetary Fund (IMF). However, the point for Callon is that besides this much vaunted concept, we have a whole range of different, live markets that shape how particular objects are manufactured, retailed and sold to us. These are the markets we encounter daily – let's face it, most of us don't work in the City or on Wall Street – as in the supermarket, street market or car boot sale, to name but a few. As we all know, each of these markets is a very different sort of place, with different 'devices' for showing us the goods on sale – a supermarket shelf, a basket filled with carrots, the boot of someone's car. Behind the different devices for retailing in these different markets are a range of mechanisms for bringing the goods to market – supply chains that must be managed by various instruments and many different ways of accounting for stock and sales – from inventories to merchandising spreadsheets to notes on the back of an envelope (if you're selling a few old toys out of the back of your car boot and want to keep track of your total).

Callon draws on the work of Marie-France Garcia from 1986 (now Garcia-Parpet and published for the first time in English in 2007) in her analysis of the establishment of a new kind of strawberry market in Fontaines-en-Solonge in France. Where once strawberry sellers had been randomly distributed, this new market – which was the vision of a neo-liberal entrepreneur – brought a large number of strawberry sellers together in one place; a contained area for selling strawberries that also relied on a number of strategies for retailing the strawberries, such as standardised arrangements for display and price that allowed customers to examine the strawberries and make comparisons. This market then enabled new forms of interaction between strawberry sellers and their suppliers, and between sellers and customers. Markets, as this example illustrates and various ANT-inspired accounts have demonstrated (MacKenzie et al., 2007; Knorr Certina and Bruegger, 2004), are social arrangements, shaped by particular techniques and devices. By bringing particular sorts of actor together, markets encourage particular forms of 'testing', different strawberry stalls allow for presentation of the commodity that enables it to be tested – seen, felt, tasted.

The point for Callon is that all goods brought to market are put through various forms of tests, not stopping when they reach the consumer. Callon et al. (2005) refer to this process as 'qualification', which describes how the qualities of goods are evaluated, measured, exchanged through various tests, measurements, comparisons. Thus, the qualities of goods are not as secure as we might think they are, but always up for discussion and examination and must be constantly tested along the supply chain to the customer. Take, for example, the food scare in 2013 in the UK: in routine tests in laboratories conducted on ready meals it was discovered that beef products were contaminated with horse meat. In this case, the qualities of beef did not simply transfer from abattoir supplier to supermarket; testing provided evidence of different – and unwanted – qualities. The resulting scandal has apparently changed how supermarkets interact with their supply chain, with a new concern for the provenance of meat, and as a result some abattoirs closed down and, for a (perhaps limited) time, eating patterns in the UK changed as well, with the sale of ready meals dropping significantly in subsequent months. What this illustrates is that goods brought to market are not stable, secure entities we can take for granted, but unstable assemblages that are constantly made and remade, while the qualities of the goods transacted are always subject to a qualification process. This has implications for the ways in which we think about commodities and their production, distribution and consumption. We might think about how the quality of 'fashionability' is not stable, but subject to constant qualification by a whole multitude of different actors and, ultimately, by consumers, since only clothes and their sales fed back to retailers can be said to contribute to fashion – those items left on the rails in the sale have evidently 'failed' this important test. More on this testing and qualification of fashion below.

THINKING THROUGH FASHION: EXTENDING LATOUR

Returning to my brief summary of STS and ANT we might ask what, in practical terms, does this argument about scientific knowledge, modernity and markets have to do with fashion? We might note two things. The first is onto-logical, concerning the nature of things or objects and how we might think about objects in fashion. The second is epistemological, concerning the kind of knowledge we should aim to produce about fashion. However, in practice these two are not distinct – arguments about the nature of objects and actors lead naturally into considerations that are epistemological, involving our methodologies for studying fashion. Some of these ideas have already been developed in the literature, largely in relation to Callon's work on markets, while the full potential of Latour's work into cultural aspects (as opposed to science/laboratories) has not really been developed as yet, as Entwistle and Slater (2013) argue. Here I want to review the small amount of academic work on fashion that has already drawn upon STS/ANT, as well as suggest some new areas for future research.

First, the radical ontological claim as to the nature of objects and how agency may be non-human as well as human provides a different way of thinking about fashion. In terms of existing literature (Entwistle, 2009; Entwistle and Slater, 2012 and 2014; Sommerlund, 2008), there has been a growing interest in the way in which fashion is a kind of assemblage – as a market it arises out of the combination of human and non-human objects. In this way of thinking, fashion is not one 'thing' but a complex assemblage of a heterogeneous range of actors. Indeed, following Callon, we might think of fashion as a set of overlapping markets that bring many different actors – human and non-human – into play in order to sell particular sorts of goods, labelled 'fashion' or 'fashionable'. We can take a few examples to examine this further.

Fashion clothing is a very diverse and highly differentiated product that, in effect, is made up of different markets that produce, distribute and retail fashionable clothing, from 'fast fashion' on the high street, to second hand clothing markets, to 'high' or 'designer' fashion. These are simultaneously quite distinct markets that circulate clothing in relatively unconnected sup-ply chains, and also interconnected in various ways: high end designer fash-ion shown in Paris and London and retailing at high prices in exclusive stores is often copied and circulated in fast fashion retail outlets, while high end designers may produce cheaper, fast fashion collections for big high street stores like H&M. The second hand clothing market also follows fash-ion trends, with exclusive second hand shops retailing 'vintage' designer items. And all of these markets try to capture what they see as the prevail-ing 'trend' or mood of the season. Fashion magazines and journalism of various sorts – in Sunday supplements, blogs and online retail sites like net-a-porter.com – are important sources of information as to trends and are significant actors within these fashion networks. These markets are heterogeneous actor-networks made up of human and non-human elements that are assembled and reassembled continuously to define 'fashion'.

What does thinking about actor-networks as ontological entities mean in terms of our epistemological strategies? The second point which derives directly out of Latour's and Callon's work involves the importance of 'following the actors' through empirical observation. How else are we to see heterogeneous assemblage except through close observation? How else can we trace the connections between actors in the case of fashion markets? We need to observe how products make their journey, are selected, displayed, sold, and the qualities they take on through this process. My own research drew on this method to examine designer fashion at Selfridges, the high-end department store on London's Oxford Street (Entwistle, 2009). Through close observation I followed fashion buyers and merchandisers through a fashion cycle or season: on buying trips to designer studios and warehouses, observing how the buyers/merchandisers managed the stock once it arrived on the shop-floor and how they tracked sales through the season. This particular fashion market involves particular issues unique to designer-led fashion: buying in high fashion is risky as lead times are longer than in high street and fast fashion markets, which meet trends in season. Indeed, high fashion, which is shown on international 'catwalks', is previewed and ordered months before it arrives on the shop-floor and largely made to order, so there is a high degree of unpredictability and risk to be calculated by buyers as they try to predict future trends and can't adjust their orders once the season starts. These market conditions demand particular practices on the part of buyers and merchandisers to render the market calculable.

Bearing in mind Latour's and Callon's concepts of actor-network and assemblage, we can observe interactions and interfaces between human and non-human actors that are important to understanding how this market comes together, a point that is made by Sommerlund (2008) in her analysis of fashion mediations. As she notes, mediation occurs in particular ways, through particular spaces and devices – she examines three in particular: fashion fairs, showrooms and look-books. In her work, as with my own, there is a concern to examine the way particular actors meet one another and what happens in the interaction to shape the qualities of the product. Just like Garcia's point about strawberry markets we need to ask, how are garments displayed? What meanings and qualities do garments take on through these interactions? How is the fashionable commodity qualified – its qualities tested and re-tested through these interactions and ultimately by reaching the consumer? Perhaps these questions seem rather mundane, and yet, in the fashion literature, these simple questions have not been routinely asked until recently. The new economic sociology, much of it influenced by Callon and his close associates and inspired by STS, is now opening up these questions and providing new ways to think about the study of fashion.

We can apply ANT concepts to look at numerous interfaces between buyers and other actors. Firstly between buyers and sales reps on a fashion buy. Borrowing from the language of STS/ANT, our attention is drawn to a range of techniques and devices for selling that shape the interaction – from the 'fit' model in the studio who tries on the clothes for the buyer, to a rail of clothes or a presentation by the rep – and these different sales devices produce different results in terms of buying strategies. Further, Callon's concern with the specificity of markets as actual spaces can be useful: high fashion is promoted at various international 'fashion weeks' which are important trade events in real time that temporally organise the fashion cycle into distinct 'seasons' and bring together particular actors face-to-face. Although the shows themselves are not cost-effective they are nonetheless important devices for promoting the identities of those invested in the fashion system. Entwistle and Rocamora (2006) use Bourdieu (see chapter 14) to analyse fashion shows, but one could equally apply Callon to understand this spatial configuration of the market.

We can follow yet more interfaces and see what other sorts of actors get enrolled in these buying interactions to make sense of fashion. Once garments arrive in the store, their sale has to be constantly monitored by the buyers and, more significantly, by the merchandisers. Again, the STS/ANT's attention to the enrolment of various 'actors' in this market is very helpful for understanding the way this market is actively put together. Indeed, various devices, tools and instruments are employed to keep track of sales and ensure goods aren't left on the shop-floor at the end of the season. So the financial 'plan' of the store is devised by management ahead of season and drives the buyers towards particular strategies. Other tools, such as trend forecasts – the seasonal 'Directive' produced by the store – might aid them in their decisions as to what to look for on a buy, a strategy for store re-development or rebranding similarly directs their buying decisions. Of all the devices, the weekly merchandising spreadsheet is a critical device for 'seeing' their market, providing a snapshot of what is selling and what is not that buyers have to act on, as Law (2002) has previously shown in his analysis. It directs buyers and merchandisers to think about strategies for dealing with stock that isn't selling (a promotion or sale? move to another location on the shop-floor?) and whether to buy more stock that's selling fast, if that's possible (it usually isn't at this level in the market). Hence, the spreadsheet is an actor: once in place, human actors have to respond to spreadsheets as virtual read-outs of what is happening 'out there' on the shop-floor/in the market.

We can trace the flow of objects right through off the shop-floor and on to consumers as well. The recent rise within consumption studies towards 'practice theory' (Bourdieu, 1977, 1990; Shove, 2005; Shove et al., 2007; Ortner, 2006) has shown the way in which consumers and consumption are actively involved in the constitution of the objects they consume, so much so that producers now recognise the importance of consumers and there are multiple 'feedback loops' that enable producers to learn from consumers' practice. This idea has been championed in analyses of advertising (Moor, 2007), branding (Lury, 2004, 2009), design (Shove et al., 2007), although it has yet to be fully developed in fashion consumption.

In other work on fashion modelling (Entwistle, 2002, 2009), similar concerns with the trajectory of the fashion object are apparent, here the model's 'look'. How models are selected, qualified and re-qualified through their careers depends on the way they move through the fashion network and the various tests they are put through. This journey often begins with the device of the 'Polaroid' which is utilized to 'test' whether someone has model potential: since almost nobody looks good in Polaroids, if (s)he can shoot a great photo with this, they are probably quite 'photogenic'. After this initial 'test', the model will go on unpaid test shoots with photographers and, if the qualities seen by the agency are seen by photographers, the model is re-qualified as having 'potential' and may also be sent on 'go-sees' – meetings with potential casting agents and magazines. The other main device for managing and displaying the qualities of the model – the model portfolio or 'book' – is an object that assembles the model's best jobs and becomes a way of seeing the model's work as a whole and directs particular ways of managing the model's career – what clients to send him or her to, for example. Here the distinction between 'edgy/editorial' fashion models (the ones that shoot exclusive high fashion magazines), and 'commercial' models who do catalogue and other mainstream products, is partly formed through the assemblage of work in the model's book and becomes a way of seeing these qualities for further re-qualification.

In this way, models can be thought of in the same way as new thinking on the 'brand', as Entwistle and Slater (2014) have argued. Brands are not static semiotic signs or symbols with stable meanings, as some conventional brand literature has argued. Instead, the brand is an 'event' – a thing in time that is constantly evolving and has multiple and changing qualities. Moreover, as an event it is widely distributed – not existing in any one place at one time but dispersed over many spaces and places. This way of thinking about branding, associated particularly with Lury's work on brands, draws upon STS/ANT to demonstrate the mutable and mobile qualities of the brand which she also terms a 'new media object' (see Lury 2004). As Entwistle and Slater (2012, 2014) suggest, models, like brands, are mobile 'events' whose qualities are effervescent and fluid and whose career/image/status/qualities are in constant flux. It explains how, despite the flux in fortune, Kate Moss was able to re-qualify her status as a top model, following her drugs scandal: as a brand she successfully managed to adapt and capitalize on the scandal.

IMPLICATIONS FOR FUTURE FASHION RESEARCH

At this point it might be worth reflecting on where we have come to in terms of understanding what an STS/ANT way of thinking about fashion enables. What is different about an STS/ANT study of fashion? As before, let's recap some epistemological and ontological points about this way of analysing fashion.

First, from an epistemological perspective, it is evident that to do a study of fashion has real methodological implications: if you were to do this kind of study of the fashion industry you cannot sit back in your armchair and merely analyse fashion as it might be constructed in say, a magazine (Brooks, 1992; Jobling, 1999). If you were interested in fashion magazines and wanted to do an ANT analysis, you would have to 'get your hands dirty' by doing ethnographic empirical work that would involve observing the many processes that make up a fashion magazine – from editorial meetings to fashion shoots. Or to understand models and modelling, you could not merely look at photographic representations, but you would need to see how models are selected, cast, photographed and so on.

Some of this empirical work has, of course, already been undertaken, although not within an STS/ANT framework. For example, Ane Lynge-Jorlén's (2012a and b) work on the niche fashion magazine *Dansk* has involved interviews and some ethnographic study of how issues of the magazine are put together, and likewise, Aspers' (2001) study of fashion photography in Sweden has already shown the networked nature of this work. That said, what is the difference between doing this kind of ethnography as opposed to something more conventional? Perhaps not a lot – all good ethnography requires us to attend to the minutiae of our participants' world. However, there are ontological points of difference we might note. For one thing, the necessity of thinking about actor-networks as made up of human and non-human actors does perhaps shift some of our observations to things that perhaps ordinarily are not observed or are taken for granted. My own work on modelling and fashion buying, discussed above, highlights some of the advantages of looking at the non-human actors in a network for the significant way they shape actions and the role that devices play in shaping the qualification of goods like fashionable objects. I would suggest, therefore, that there is more to be gained from considering *all* the objects assembled in a fashion actor-network than would be in conventional research focused only on the distinctly 'social' or 'cultural' human actors. We might more usefully think about fashion in terms of a range of objects and activities and extend our notions of actor and agency beyond distinctly agentic qualities to humans.

What else might we gain from approaching fashion in an STS/ANT way? Attending to the specificities of markets as performative is useful, borrowing from Callon's work. Here we can see how markets are specific sorts of actor-network that are spatially located and actively constitute the qualities of the goods they sell. Indeed, we can think about fashion in terms of networks of actors, extending some important work within human geography which has tended to champion the idea of 'chains of production'. Metaphors like 'chains', 'circuits' or 'networks' (Crewe, 2004; Hughes and Reimer, 2004; Leslie and Reimer, 1999) have become popular in discussions about fashion provision in that they focus attention on the spatially dispersed but interconnected linkages between many different actors across production, distribution and consumption. Each term has advantages by emphasizing particular qualities of these linkages. In other words, the actual spatial configuration each metaphor invokes differs and therefore provides different ways of analysing 'vertical' relationships between parts within. The idea of a 'commodity chain', often referred to as 'global commodity chain' (or GCC), championed by Wallerstein (1979), usually acknowledges the power of particular actors within that chain and in fashion; this will tend to translate into accounts that focus on the power of particular large, Western/Northern fashion businesses to dictate the terms along the chain to producers in the East/South. A 'systems of provision' approach, which is best seen in the work of Leopold (1992, see also Fine and Leopold, 1993), is more sensitive to the historical contingencies and particularities of systems. However, according to Leslie and Reimer (1999, 2003), though preferable, this Marxist inspired approach tends to favour analysis of the production side of the system and focuses less attention on the other actors across the system, with the aim of 'unveiling' the power relations of production.

The metaphor of 'network', used in an STS/ANT sense, has a number of advantages over these two approaches. For one thing, it tends to 'flatten' out the network to examine actors across the entire network, not just those located at the production end. This analysis also allows us to examine the different sorts of non-human actors that are interconnected, and thus to connect up nature-culture. This is particularly pertinent today in an era of heightened awareness of sustainability, especially in recent years as concerns about the environmental cost of 'fast fashion' are growing. Future ANT research in this area can allow us to trace the nature-culture hybrid nature of fashion. Take, for example, something like water. Rather than thought of as an external, inert object, water is, in fact, an actor within the fashion industry. In recent years there has been environmental criticism levelled at the fashion industry's unsustainable use of water to grow cotton in countries with water shortage. Do we grow less cotton or develop genetically modified cotton that demands less water? These questions, apparently about something 'natural' and therefore outside 'fashion' are, in fact, going to shape the fashion systems of the future. Water, as this example shows, is entangled within our fashion systems and is not a separate 'natural' object. Following the example of the work of Shove (2003) and Shove et al. (2007), whose work examines everyday consumption and the daily practices of life that draw together 'stuff', we can begin to examine the 'stuff' of fashion in all its fullness within our everyday life.

CONCLUSION

Latour's work makes some radical departures from much vaunted concepts within sociology. His work entails an ontological and epistemological challenge to the very basis of modern forms of knowledge and its faith in the narrative of science as an objective, value-free form of knowledge, superior to that of pre-modern societies. Latour's methodological roots lie in ethnomethodology and he is committed to ethnographic observation as necessary to understand the social world. Ethnomethodology has placed emphasis on how people 'do' the social world – on the routine practices and activities that make up the everyday organization of life. To study how people 'do' the social world – the rules, routines, practices, habits of daily life, entails observation. We must observe these practical accomplishments in *situ*. In *situ* observing has methodological implications for the sorts of study we might do of fashion, namely ethnographic, observational studies that examine how fashion is made up or put together.

By examining the practicalities of approaching fashion in this way we can 'think through fashion' quite differently – as a network of actors, some of them non-human – and trace the connections across these spatially. Callon's work demonstrates one direction that this analysis moves in – towards understanding fashion markets as particular sorts of network, assembling in time and place particular actors whose job it is to qualify and re-qualify the sorts of goods made available in that market.

Some of this work is already underway, as discussed above, but the full potential of STS/ANT has yet to be fully explored in relation to fashion, as I hope I have also suggested in this chapter. In particular, thinking about fashion as a nature-culture hybrid provides us with really productive ways to consider the environmental issues that fashion raises.

NOTES

1   Latour refers to both 'pre-modern' and 'modern' as systems of thought or classification that organize things, often into binaries that draw distinctions between things of 'nature' and 'culture'. These different ways of thinking are separated, in Western thought, by a temporal 'Great Divide', with 'moderns' replacing 'pre-moderns' to produce an apparently superior knowledge of the world. However, the world that 'modern' denotes never properly existed since the distinctions are themselves artificial. It is in this way that, to quote the title of Latour's book, 'we have never been modern'. Latour proposes 'non-modern' as a way around this problematic distinction.

REFERENCES

Aspers, P. (2001) *Markets in Fashion: A Phenomenological Approach*, Stockholm: City University Press.

Bourdieu, P. (1977) *Outline of a Theory of Practice*, Cambridge: Cambridge University Press.

———(1990) *The Logic of Practice*, Cambridge: Polity Press.

Brooks, R. (1992) 'Fashion Photography, The Double-Page Spread: Helmut Newton, Guy Bourdin and Deborah Turberville' in J. Ash and E. Wilson (eds), *Chic Thrills: A Fashion Reader*, London: Pandora Press.

Callon, M. (1998) 'Introduction' in *The Laws of the Markets*, Oxford: Blackwell.

————Meadel, C. and Rabeharisoa, V. (2005) 'The Economy of Qualities' in A. Barry and D. Slater (eds), *The Technological Economy*, London: Routledge.

Crewe, L. (2004) 'Unravelling Fashion's Commodity Chains' in A. Hughes and S. Reimer (eds), *Geographies of Commodity Chains*, London: Routledge.

Entwistle, J. (2002) 'The Aesthetic Economy: The Production of Value in the Field of Fashion Modelling' in *Journal of Consumer Culture*, 2 (3): 317–40.

————(2009) *The Aesthetic Economy of Fashion: Markets and Value in Clothing and Modelling*, Oxford: Berg.

————(2012) 'Models as Brands: Critical Thinking about Bodies and Images' in J. Entwistle and E. Wissinger (eds), *Fashioning Models: Image, Text and Industry*. Oxford: Berg.

————(2014) 'Reassembling the Cultural: Fashion Models, Brands and the Meaning of "Culture" after ANT' in *Journal of Cultural Economy*, 7 (2): 161–77.

———— and Rocamora, A. (2006) 'The Field of Fashion Materialized: A Study of London Fashion Week' in *Sociology*, 40 (4): 735–51.

———— and Slater, D. (2014) '(2014) 'Reassembling the Cultural: Fashion Models, Brands and the Meaning of "Culture" after ANT.' *Journal of Cultural Economy* 7 (2). 161–177 (2012)

Fine, B. and Leopold, E. (1993) *The World of Consumption*, London: Routledge.

Garcia-Parpet, M.F. (2007) 'The Social Construction of a Perfect Market: The Strawberry Auction at Fontaines-en-Sologne' in D. MacKenzie, F. Muniesa and L. Sui (eds), *Do Economists Make Markets?: On the Performativity of Economics*, Princeton, NJ: Princeton University Press.

Hughes, A. and Reimer, S. (eds) (2004) *Geographies of Commodity Chains*, London: Routledge.

Jobling, P. (1999) *Fashion Spreads: Word and Image in Fashion Photography since 1980*, Oxford: Berg.

Knorr Certina, K. and Bruegger, U. (2004) 'Traders' Engagement with Markets: A Postsocial Relationship' in A. Amin and N. Thrift (eds), *The Blackwell Cultural Economy Reader*, Oxford: Blackwell.

Latour, B. (1987) *Science in Action: How to Follow Scientists and Engineers Through Society*, Milton Keynes: Open University Press.

————(1991) *We Have Never Been Modern*, Hertfordshire: Harvester Wheatsheaf.

————(1999) *Pandora's Hope*, Cambridge, MA: Harvard University Press.

————(2005) *Reassembling the Social: An Introduction to Actor-Network-Theory*, Oxford: Oxford University Press.

———— and Woolgar, S. (1979) *Laboratory Life: The Social Construction of Scientific Facts*, Princeton, NJ: Princeton University Press.

Law, J. (2002) 'Economics as Interference' in P. du Gay and M. Pryke (eds), *Cultural Economy*, London: Sage.

Leopold, E. (1992) 'The Manufacture of the Fashion System' in J. Ash and E. Wilson (eds), *Chic Thrills: A Fashion Reader*, London: Pandora.

Leslie, D. and Reimer, S. (1999) 'Spatializing Commodity Chains' in *Progress in Human Geography*, 23 (3): 401–20.

————(2003) 'Fashioning Furniture: Restructuring the Furniture Commodity Chain' in *Area*, 35 (4): 427–37.

Lury, C. (2004) *Brands: The Logos of the Global Economy*, London: Routledge.

————(2009) 'BRAND AS ASSEMBLAGE: Assembling Culture' in *Journal of Cultural Economy*, 2 (1): 67–82.

Lynge-Jorlén, A. (2012a) 'Between Frivolity and Art: Contemporary Niche Fashion Magazines' in *Fashion Theory: The Journal of Dress, Body and Culture*, 16 (1): 7–28.

————(2012b) 'Preaching to the Already Converted' in P. McNeill and L. Wallenberg (eds), Nordic Fashion Studies, Stockholm: Axl Books.

MacKenzie, D., Muniesa, F. and Sui, L. (eds) (2007) Do Economists Make Markets?: On the Performativity of Economics, Princeton, NJ: Princeton University Press.

Moor, L. (2007) The Rise of Brands, Oxford: Berg.

Ortner, S.B. (2006) Anthropology and Social Theory: Culture, Power, and the Acting Subject, Durham, NC: Duke University Press.

Pantzar, M. and Shove, E. (2005) 'Understanding Innovation in Practice: A Discussion of the Production and Reproduction of Nordic Walking' in Technology Analysis and Strategic Management, 22 (4): 447–62.

Shove, E. (2003) Comfort, Cleanliness and Convenience: The Social Organization of Normality, Oxford: Berg.

————(2005) 'Consumers, Producers and Practices: Understanding the Invention and Reinvention of Nordic Walking' in Journal of Consumer Culture, 5 (1): 43–64.

————, Watson, M. et al. (2007) The Design of Everyday Life, Oxford: Berg.

Sommerlund, J. (2008) 'Mediations in Fashion' in Journal of Cultural Economy, 1 (2): 165–80.

Wallerstein, I. (1979) The Capitalist World-Economy, Cambridge: Cambridge University Press.

17

JUDITH BUTLER
Fashion and Performativity

Elizabeth Wissinger

INTRODUCTION

Something radical happened to fashion studies in the 1990s: as post-modern and post-structural disruptions ripped through many academic fields, fashion studies experienced a new kind of energy. Feminism, formerly rejecting fashion as a patriarchal conceit, started looking at it with fresh eyes, amidst the rumblings of third wave feminist ideas that gave birth to riot grrrrl culture and a re-appropriation of the joys of lipstick and lingerie, re-cast as feminine practices to be wielded at the wearer's will. As HIV/AIDS forced a formerly closeted culture to fight for life, and in so doing, raised mainstream awareness of gay culture, transgender became more visible, as well. This new awareness trickled through celebrity turns from David Bowie, Grace Jones and Michael Jackson's sleek evocations of playful androgyny, to Boy George's eyeliner and Madonna's gender-bending. As the rise of biotechnology burst through formerly sacrosanct divisions between the living and inert, elevating the cyborg as a new cultural ideal, Judith Butler's work emerged amidst disintegrating binaries of all sorts.

Fashion's continuous interrogation of existing boundaries in search of the new, combined with its history of androgyny and gender play, lent itself well to the nascent movement of queer studies, for which Butler's work eventually became central. By arguing for more than just the categories 'male' and 'female' to describe the human experience, queer studies ventured into a new kind of academic analysis of sexuality aimed at challenging the heteronormative order by critiquing forms of power that marginalized anything but heterosexual practices. Judith Butler's feminist analysis of gender dovetailed well with these concerns, and conferred a new status on the study of style, asking, as it did, deeply philosophical questions about the body and how it is stylized into existence within predominant structures of culture and power, not the least of which is fashion.

By moving the focus from the role of clothes in creating or monitoring identities, to the role of clothes in fashioning the body itself, her work radically interrogated the idea of subjectivity, questioning every aspect of how identities are formed, stabilized and naturalized by social practices. Questioning the given-ness of just two sexes, male/female, Butler pushed her analysis toward questioning the divide between the material and the psychic, theorizing how the body itself is not something that just naturally occurs, but is in fact made through interactions constrained by existing power structures. As such, Butler brought fashion into the conversation about bodies, as a form of discourse in which the clothed body is an utterance reflecting existing relations of power.

By laying this kind of conceptual groundwork Butler opened up new realms of possibility in fashion studies. While previous analysis had focused on clothing and its social implications, such as Valerie Steele's seminal work on the fetish, handbag and corset (1997, 2003; Steele and Borelli, 2000), or Christopher Breward's (1995) *The Culture of Fashion*, a 600-year survey of fashion's cultural and social meanings, Butler provided fashion studies a new direction, questioning the very categories of gender and psychological meaning fashion supposedly represented. Rather than focus on men's or women's fashion as given types, Butler's work revealed how tenuous these distinctions can be, and made it possible to look instead to clothes as deployments in the game of shifting social forces, gendered, queer or otherwise.

Scholars of queer culture were quick to embrace this fluidity. The use of the word 'queer' linked directly with 'fashion' or 'style' in fashion studies book titles, however, has been less common, as authors have preferred to associate their work with gender, sex, particular gay and lesbian subcultures or historic moments in gay and lesbian life (with titles such as Shaun Cole's *Don We Now our Gay Apparel* (2000), or Joanie Erickson and Jeanine Cogan's *Lesbians, Levis, and Lipstick: The Meaning of Beauty in Our Lives* (1999)). The recent publication of two volumes, *Queer Style* (2013) by Adam Geczy and Vicki Karaminas, and *A Queer History of Fashion* (2013), edited by Valerie Steele, evidence a new foregrounding of Butler's ideas in the field of fashion studies. While always in the background of cultural studies approaches to fashion, these new works in the field will no doubt cement her place in the fashion studies canon. At times criticized for her inscrutable writing style, Butler's major contribution was, in fact, her theoretical heavy lifting. By writing deeply through difficult philosophical concepts, she brought together strands of thought from Freud, Althusser, Lacan, De Beauvoir and Foucault in novel ways, shedding new light on the implications of analyses for understanding gender, the body and power.

PERFORMAVITY: GENDER PERFORMANCE OR PRESCRIPTION?

Judith Butler is perhaps best known for her notion of performativity, yet it is a term that is often misconstrued. Confusing the concept of performance with performativity, casual readers assume that Butler's notion of gender as a 'stylized repetition of acts' (1990: 140) refers to conscious choices we make about gesture, clothing and style. While affording a key set of ideas for thinking about the role of fashion in producing and stylizing gendered bodies, Butler's notion of 'gender performativity' describes far more than just the act of putting on a dress or tying a necktie.

Butler used the concept of 'performativity' to analyse the ontological origins of gender itself, not just what gender means, but what gender is.[1] For Butler, 'gender is always a doing' (1990: 25); by this she means that no *de facto* gender or gendered bodies exist outside practices that bring them into being. To paraphrase one of Butler's more famous sources of inspiration, Simone De Beauvoir, we are not born female or male, but rather *become* a woman or man, for example when we are sexed by the doctor's proclamation, 'It's a boy', or, 'It's a girl!' Even though some bodies are not clearly either one, we rarely, if ever, hear the doctor say, 'I'm not sure what it is, but we'll manage anyway!' Yet Butler (1990) argues that in the very sexing of bodies themselves, language and discourse come into play, pulling the 'naturalness' of sexed attributes into question. Relying on Foucault's notion of discourse (see chapter 11), that is, culturally constructed representations of reality governed by rules that give meaning, Butler argues, 'gender is not a noun' (1990: 24). It does not exist in and of itself, but only in the expressions of gender aimed at giving it coherence. Gender becomes something only in the practices of gendering that iterate and reiterate the body, that repeatedly make, do or utter it, into existence.

For Butler, then, the body is not a pre-given anatomy about which we have ideas, but rather the result of a tension between the psychic and the material in which an imaginary schema, a framework that helps organize and interpret information from the world around us, is laid over the material to make it available to our psyches. In other words, bodies are unintelligible without the imaginary schema that makes them available to us. This imaginary schema is imbued with cultural ideas and images, learned through interaction and socialized into us via punishment and discipline.

Since it is only available through this schema, the body is hopelessly caught up in language, signification and the cultural realm. Even scientific descriptions of the body take place through a circulation and validation of imaginary schemas, which underlie knowledge systems and their acceptable evidence. Beneath any such schema, Butler argues, lie the gender instituting prohibitions that allow language to have meaning at all (1990: 35 ff). From this perspective, the body is a mode of appearance whose boundaries are conferred upon it by psychic projections in a series of repeating iterations. Since the body exists only in this repetition, however, it is not fixed in form or meaning, and there are temporal gaps in between, in which the moments of the structure that give it its meaning are instantiated.

Butler argues that these temporal gaps leave the body open to re-signification, a repetition with a difference, since the body's anatomy always exceeds the terms with which it is given. The body is always moving beyond, through or around the schemas of discourse, meaning or production into which it is put, or within which it interacts. The body's reach into the virtual realm that surrounds it may be thought in terms of excess. It is in this moment of escape where the variability may be found. As she explains: 'The injunction to be a given gender produces necessary failures, a variety of incoherent configurations that in their multiplicity exceed and defy the injunction by which they are generated' (1990: 145). For Butler, this excess is the source of compulsive repetition of acts on and in the body, a compulsion to bring what we experience as a body as close as possible to idealized projections of it. Thus, each time the body is delimited, it gets sedimented with a history of norms (among which norms of the sexed morphology are the most important).

These norms also include fashion's dictates, and speak in some ways to the difficulty of determining or maintaining a body that is 'fashionable', especially with respect to the dynamism of that term. Butler's ideas speak to this dynamism, as she argues that the sedimentation of the history of norms is not inflexible; there is always the possibility that the world and the bodies in it will change in an instant, when an impossible action could slip in during one of the temporal gaps between instantiations of the structure.

Contingent upon dynamic forces, the body is neither psychic nor material, but a mixture of both, existing *as* the tension between the psychic and material.

In this sense, her work laid out the idea that gender is performative, established through repeating iterations or instantiations, and this repetition leaves open some room for variation in the compulsory categories of male or female. Part of this openness stems from the fact that there isn't really a 'there' there. On the one hand, 'gender is the repeated stylization of the body', but this stylization takes place as a 'set of acts' within a 'highly rigid regulatory frame that congeal over time to produce the appearance of substance, of a natural sort of being' (1990: 33) which is anything but natural, as it is just the repetition of the iteration that makes it seems to be so. For Butler, the crux of the difference between performance and performativity lies in the fact that 'performance presumes a subject, but performativity contests the very notion of the subject' (Butler et al., 1994: 33) and thereby, any re-articulation that occurs is not a conscious choice. In this way, we may understand fashion's iterations as constructing the body within regimes of value that grid its intelligibility, mattering bodies through various cultural codes, policing gender boundaries in the process. Bodily instantiations repeat, with a difference, with every fashion cycle, offering possibilities for slippage outside accepted norms, a view that speaks to the notion of a body contingent upon social forces for its existence.

PERFORMATIVITY AND DRAG

Separating performativity from performance is crucial to understanding Butler's argument that we cannot just put on any gender performance we please, as if donning or doffing a new dress or bespoke suit. While some seem to have missed this point in her writing, Butler has been careful to note the compulsory nature of this process, explaining that entry into the repetitive practices that make up the 'terrain of signification is not a choice' (1990: 148), but rather the 'forcible citation of a norm' (1993: 232). The possibility of variation exists in the fact that the 'girling' of a 'girl', for instance, demands a 'formation of a corporeally enacted femininity that never fully approximates the norm' (1993: 232). No matter how many frills and ruffles you put on her, a girl is still an iteration, a shadowing of social forces that seek to define and tie down the essence of girlness, but which never succeed, as the coherence of what makes a girl a girl is imaginary.

As such, the set of ontological presuppositions at work in the 'embodied life of individuals' can be 'open to rearticulation' (2004: 214). This openness has led to some confusion about Butler's ideas. Misinterpretations of her discussion of performances of gender with regard to drag, or cross dressing (two terms she uses interchangeably), advanced in her 1990 work Gender Trouble, occasioned Butler's subsequent attempts to nuance them throughout the following decade. After her 1990 statement, 'in imitating gender, drag implicitly reveals the imitative structure of gender itself – as well as its contingency' (1990: 187), casual readers of Butler found it hard to resist the temptation to take the performative nature of drag at face value, elevating it to an action capable of subverting the existing gendered order, stylizing the body in presumably political ways. In 1993, however, Butler was careful to point out that:

> Although many readers understood Gender Trouble to be arguing for the proliferation of drag performances as a way of subverting dominant gender norms, I want to underscore that there is no necessary relation between drag and subversion, and that drag may well be used in the service of both the denaturalization and reidealization of hyberbolic heterosexual gender norms.
>
> (1993: 125)

Butler has since pointed out that she did not intend to construct drag as a 'model for resistance or for political intervention' (2004: 214–15). Rather, due to the 'unchosen' nature of 'social categories', drag is not 'subversive of gender norms', as much as it points out 'implicit accounts of ontology, which determine what kinds of bodies and sexualities will be considered real and true, and which kind will not' (2004: 214–15). In other words, drag, by copying signs and symbols of the dominant norms, may, depending on its stylization, reinforce the idea that there is a 'right' and 'real' way of being either masculine or feminine. Important to note, however, is how it uncovers implicit assumptions in the order of being, assumptions that, once revealed, might be interrogated.

Reducing the concept of gender performativity to cross-dressing misses a crucial aspect of Butler's unique contribution to fashion studies. Cross-dressing, reconceived as a discursive act, whether or not the intent is explicitly political, highlights the fabrication of gender identity, by revealing the parody behind the essentialist categories of 'male' and 'female'. As gender scholar Rosemary Hennessy has observed:

> Drag for Butler is not merely a matter of clothing or cross-dressing. It is a
> discursive practice that discloses the fabrication of identity through par-
> odic repetitions of the heterosexual gender system. As parody, drag belies
> the myth *of a stable self, preexisting* cultural codes or signifying systems.
>
> (Hennessy, 1994–95: 28)

Thus, rather than celebrating drag or cross-dressing as a way to climb out of
the heterosexual matrix, seeking a deeper understanding of performativity
demands exploring the role that fashion plays in bringing forth the sexed
body. This occurs through a process of disavowals that create 'bodies that
matter' (Butler, 1993).

Fashion is among the regimes that give bodies intelligibility, that is, make
it possible for them to be known. Thus, bodies become part of reality in
part through fashion, forming identities and subjectivities along the way.
Fashionable binaries of what's hot or not, in or out, organize bodies along
axes that facilitate or deny certain types of bodies, and in so doing, define
what a body is in contemporary culture. While the simplest interpretations
of performativity point merely to the idea that the body is used to perform
gender as we make choices about what to wear, Butler's ideas in fact question
the idea of the sexed body as something that exists outside the practices of
wearing clothing itself.

BUTLER'S IMPLICATIONS FOR FASHION STUDIES

While psychology is one of the most common regimes of intelligibility used
to delimit the body, for Butler, it is a paradigm that is limited at best. In the
1930s, J.C. Flügel produced what has now become a canonical text in fashion studies, *The Psychology of Clothes*, a psychoanalytic analysis of why we wear
clothing and what it means. Decoding the meaning of the garment itself
has been a common theme in fashion studies ever since, from deconstructing the social significance of hemlines to taking apart the duelling impulses
toward adornment or asceticism. For Butler, the connection between clothing and psychoanalysis was problematic, however, especially when it comes
to sexual perversion as reflected in forms of dress, such as the fetish. In an
interview with anthropologist Gayle Rubin, she explained:

> For me, the explanatory potency of psychoanalysis seemed [...] limited
> with regard to sexual variation [...]. For example, to look at something

like fetishism and say it has to do with castration and the lack [...] when I think about fetishism I want to know about many other things. I do not see how one can talk about fetishism, or sadomasochism, without thinking about the production of rubber, the techniques and gear used for controlling and riding horses, the high polished gleam of military footwear, the history of silk stockings, the cold authoritative qualities of medical equipment, or the allure of motorcycles and the elusive liberties of leaving the city for the open road. For that matter, how can we think of fetishism without the impact of cities, or certain streets and parks, of red-light districts and 'cheap amusements', or the seductions of department counters, piled high with desirable and glamorous goods? To me, fetishism raises all sorts of issues concerning shifts in the manufacture of objects, the historical and social specificities of control and skin and social etiquette, or ambiguously experienced body invasions and minutely graduated hierarchies. If all of this complex social information is reduced to castration or the Oedipus complex or knowing or not knowing what one is not supposed to know, I think something important has been lost.

(Rubin, 1994: 79)

That 'something important' threads through Butler's attempts to situate bodily practices in the specific social and historical environments in which they emerge. From this angle, categories such as 'gay dress', 'lesbian chic' or the meaning of clothes themselves demand nuance, to achieve a more detailed analysis of the complex social formations in which they are wrought. The history of clothing production, qualities of materials, the networks governing their availability, all must become part of the analysis. In addition, Butler consistently questions the basic understandings of sexuality, whether expressed through clothes or otherwise, underlined by Freud's theories (see chapter 3). Desire and attraction, so often threaded through analysis of fashion, demand radical interrogation. Butler particularly questions Freud's relatively clear cut notions of the Oedipus complex, and the aims and objects related to fetishism, for instance, which have become Freud's, so to speak, 'greatest hits', arguing instead for a proliferation of categories for understanding the complexities of sexuality.[2]

In the same vein, Butler's work has implications for another major player in the fashion canon, Roland Barthes (see chapter 8), whose work posited that clothing is a language with a grammar he carefully laid out in the mother of all fashion studies, *The Fashion System*. Using a semiotic analysis, the study of how meaning is produced and put into circulation, he argued that fashion is a linguistic structure, and clothing is its expression. According to this structuralist logic, anything can be fashionable; its fashionable nature is determined not by what it is, but rather its place in the fashion system. Once a series of signs is established, they confer meaning consistently, even though the objects serving as vehicles for the sign may change. Thus, while various objects rotate in and out of the 'it' position (Fendi baguette bags, Jil Sander's leather lunch bag purses, nail art) the 'it' position remains constant within the system's logic.

While she does not critique Barthes directly in her main body of work, for Butler, language is a two edged sword, and far more fluid and difficult to map out than Barthes' early work implied. Butler calls for insisting on 'the disjunction between utterance and meaning', which she calls 'the condition of possibility' for 'the performative' (Shulman, 2011: 230). From her perspective, linguistic vulnerability has two meanings. While we become active agents in our lives (subjects) through the constitutive power of language, at the same time, we are not fully contained by this power. Since signification is imperfect, there is always a chance for re-signifying, especially when language is injurious. Taking control of words such as 'bitch', 'nigger' and 'queer', for example, defuses their pejorative power, giving back some sense of self-definition to groups formerly defiled by these terms. While fashion's power to dictate styles may seem absolute, it is in fact in the very nature of the slippages between high and low style, street and couture, that we find the space for fashion's dynamism. With regard to gender, as cultural critic Alison Bancroft has observed:

> fashion ignores the very idea of men and women from the outset, and it puts men in the place of women, women in the place of men, and trans becomes the default, the norm, rather than an oddity or an abasement. This disregard for the usual categories of man and woman is evidence firstly that gender binaries are irrelevant in fashion, and more generally that gender identity is not located in the anatomical body anyway. For anyone familiar with the development of Queer Theory in the last twenty years, this second point is no surprise.
>
> (Bancroft, 2013: n.p.)

Fashion may be a language to which we are vulnerable, but from Butler's perspective, we may also be empowered by it, a view that is spelled out in this next example.

REVEALING THE NATURAL BODY AS ALREADY CLOTHED: DE BEAUVOIR, BUTLER AND BIG BOTTOMS

In a playful riff on a photo of De Beauvoir in the nude, taken by a lover, presumably without her knowledge, De Beauvoir's naked bottom provides philosopher Kyoo Lee a vehicle for analysing Butler's take on De Beauvoir's thinking about gendering the body, as elaborated in *The Second Sex* (Lee, 2013). Lee suggests that Butler has found, in the 'psychopolitical tragicomedy of [...] glamorized victimization', evidence that this 'oppression, despite the appearance and weight of inevitability, is essentially contingent' (Butler, 1986: 41 as cited in Lee, 2013: 189). Within the rhythms of fashion, we can see how a 'necessary contingency coupled with ritualized vicissitude gets coded into a weighty imperative' (2013: 189). That is to say, one can never *be* in fashion, as it is always becoming something else, just as one can never arrive at being a woman, as one is always becoming one in the process of doing gender. As Lee trenchantly observed, if a woman's biology is purportedly her destiny, 'she is already a woman before or after she "chooses" to become one, and yet she can only be properly woman by choosing to become one' (2013: 189). In Butler's terms:

> to 'choose' a gender in this context is not to move in upon gender from a disembodied locale, but to reinterpret the cultural history which the body already wears. The body becomes a choice, a mode of enacting and reacting received gender norms which surface as so many styles of the flesh.
>
> (Butler 1986: 48)

The body always already wears a cultural history, because the cultural world is incorporated 'incessantly and actively', in a process so continuous and easy, 'it seems a natural fact' (Butler, 1986: 49). Lee sees in the nude body of De Beauvoir an intensification of the complexity of its gendered sociality, a 'quasi-sartorial complexity of gender identity', in which 'naked bottoms "reveal the natural body as already clothed", almost instantly and irreversibly coded' (Lee, 2013: 190). Thus, even in nudity, fashion plays a role as one of the 'compulsory frames set by the various forces that police the social appearance of gender' (Butler, 1990: 33), since its codes are part of the many in play that stylize bodies.

Thinking through fashion via Butler blurs the line between clothing and the body, an idea that has become critical within fashion studies today.

Despite this impact on the study of fashion, specific aspects of clothing itself have seemed less of a concern in Butler's most influential works. Her analysis of the documentary film *Paris Is Burning*, which treats drag ball culture and makes up a significant segment of her book *Bodies That Matter*, engaged fashion somewhat obliquely, without discussing particular styles of dress as such. Similarly, while discussing the performative ramifications of pronouncing a couple 'man and wife', she paid scant attention to the attire of those involved (1993: 229 ff). In the same vein, while the rustle of satin and the click of pearls is almost audible in De Beauvoir's text, Butler's discussion of De Beauvoir's idea of 'becoming' a woman in *Gender Trouble* leaves the details of the transformation to the reader's imagination (1990). Despite leaving dress itself in the background, by showing us how the naked body is already clothed, Butler's work carved a path for clothing to became part of the study of identity construction and embodiment. Yet, it goes far beyond identity politics. Although her work tends to stay focused on processes informing the gendering of human bodies, it raises questions about the processes of becoming for bodies in general, both human and non-human.

BUTLER'S THEORY IN ACTION

Because studying the performativity of the body includes studying the place where inside meets outside, in the fold where the body/skin becomes bodily experience, and the lived body incorporates the mind, Butler's work is extremely useful for questioning what a body is and does. The symbolic and the material are not merely intertwined, they are one and the same, emerging only as one or the other according to social and historical forces. Butler would most likely deny, for instance, that there is any separate symbolic structure of fashion that explains all fashion everywhere; rather, she would argue that whatever we call fashion is defined in dynamic power relations shaped by material and social contingencies.

Tying Butler so closely to ideas of material constraints might seem strange to some. According to many readings of her work, she was among the main architects of the 'linguistic turn', a notion born of post-modernism that claims reality exists only in discourse, echoing French philosopher Jacques Derrida's famous declaration that 'there is nothing outside of the text' (Derrida, 1997 [1976]: 158; see also chapter 15 in this book). From some passages in Butler's writing, it seems that discourse is all there is, matter only becomes real in the form of utterance, and culture is all that matters (pun intended). From this point of view, fashion is a discourse that confers reality on bodies.

Recent re-readings of her work by new materialist feminists, however, have nuanced this position. As gender scholar Iris van der Tuin has pointed out, this is an ongoing debate, in which some feminists 'simply deny' Butler's materialism, while others claim that 'the paradox that [...] forms the ultimate characterization of Butler's work – we are not outside of language, and yet not determined by it either – is the best starting point for a new materialism' (Van der Tuin, 2011: 273). In Butler's work, in concert with other feminist thinkers, such as Karen Barad (2003), Rosi Braidotti (2002, 2011), Elizabeth Grosz (1994), Donna Haraway (1991), bodily materiality is clearly at stake.[3] As Elizabeth Grosz observed of this group of thinkers, they were neither social constructionists nor egalitarians. For them, the body was not a tabula rasa written upon by culture but rather, a lived body that was always sexed/gendered. As such, this group 'shares a notion of the fundamental irreducible differences between the sexes' (Grosz, 1994: 17–18)[4] in which the body is both subject and object, a source of agency within processes of cultural marking or inscription.

This perspective allows for analysing the body within fashion studies in new ways. As feminist theorist Ilya Parkins has argued, looking at agency within a totalizing system such as fashion demands thinking of fashion 'both at the level of individual negotiations of fashion [...] and the fashion industry as a site of mass consumption, making possible a nuanced discussion of agency' (Parkins, 2008: 510). As Parkins has pointed out, this reading of fashion as both intimate encounter and mass manipulation has been made possible in part by Butler's theory of performativity, which had a 'massive impact' on feminist concepts of agency, allowing, as it did, for understanding agency as separate from conscious intention (510). In this sense, fashion is what Butler would call a 'matrix of intelligibility' (1990), in which the body is both that which is intelligible, and that which escapes intelligibility, within what Braidotti might describe as tensions between the dynamic structure of the body and 'processes of becoming' (Braidotti, 2011: 17). The body's dynamic materiality exceeds the compulsive repetitions through which the body is sedimented. This excess leads to heavy policing of the body, in efforts to bring it into alignment with the threshold of intelligibility given by culture.

This insight has been crucial to my own research on fashion modelling. In modelling's everyday practices, I found instances of this 'heavy policing' in terms of the control and modulation of models' bodies, personalities and their overall 'look' (Wissinger, 2009). Models' agents, for example, made their girls into models by dictating their clothing and hairstyles, living circumstances, travel arrangements, schedules and social activities.[5] They told their models to lie about their age to fit with the feminine ideals of pliability and youth. Similarly, many models were encouraged to wear high heels to castings, to embody the feminine look, and submit to coercive measuring and strict personal management to monitor diet, weight and body size (Wissinger, 2013, and forthcoming). The intense vigilance implies a constant threat to the body's integrity. The fashionable body is made, and remade, in repetitious acts that never quite secure it, partly because of fashion's inconstancy, and partly because of the body's tendency to exceed the limits of the norms through which it is lived, never quite coming under absolute control.

CONCLUSION

In sum, I want to argue that Judith Butler's insights provide a critically informed point of view from which to assess central and ongoing issues surrounding the body, clothing and power. By queering notions about sexuality through radically destabilizing the naturalized categories of male and female, she paved the way for critically assessing fashion's allure, identifying subversive forces not formally acknowledged, yet integral to fashion's processes. Questioning the naturalness of the body also revealed the body to be always already clothed, even in nudity. This blurring of lines helped bring the body back into the analysis of clothing. As such, Butler's theoretical stance facilitated examining both fashion as system and as intimate encounter on a lived body. Showing us how the body is instantiated every time it is iterated in the discourse that is fashion, Butler's work has become foundational for any account of fashion that seeks to go further than merely skin deep.

NOTES

1   'Ontological', or having to do with ontology, the branch of metaphysics that studies being or existence.
2   It is fascinating to note that despite her thorough going critiques of Freud's analyses, Butler was also a huge admirer of his work, as evidenced in this later remark in the same interview:

At some point, I went back and read some of the early sexology and realized that Freud's comments on the sexual aberrations were a brilliant, but limited, intervention into a preexisting literature that was very dense, rich, and interesting. His brilliance and fame, and the role of psychoanalytic explanation with psychiatry, have given his comments on sexual variation a kind of canonical status.

(1994: 80)

3   See also the interviews with Karen Barad and Rosi Braidotti in *New Materialism: Interviews and Cartographies*, by Rick Dolphijn and Iris van der Tuin (eds) (2012).

4   Here, Grosz is referring to the work of Luce Irigaray, Hélène Cixous, Gayatri Spivak, Jane Gallop, Moira Gatens, Vicki Kirby, Naomi Schor and Monique Wittig, among others.

5   In the modelling industry, to call a model a 'woman' is an insult, implying she is too old for the job.

REFERENCES

Bancroft, A. (2013) 'How Fashion Is Queer' in *The Quouch*, 14 March, retrieved through http://theqouch.com/category/gender-studies/ on 8 January 2014.

Barad, K. (2003) 'Posthumanist Performativity: How Matter Comes to Matter' in *Signs: Journal of Women in Culture and Society*, 28 (3): 801–31.

Barthes, R. (1990 [1963]) *The Fashion System*, Berkeley: University of California Press.

Braidotti, R. (2002) *Metamorphoses: Towards a Materialist Theory of Becoming*, Oxford: Polity Press.

———(2011, 2nd ed) *Nomadic Subjects: Embodiment and Sexual Difference in Contemporary Feminist Theory*, New York: Columbia University Press.

Breward, C. (1995) *The Culture of Fashion*, Manchester: Manchester University Press.

Butler, J. (1986) 'Sex and Gender in Simone de De Beauvoir's Second Sex' in *Yale French Studies*, (72): 35–49.

———(1990) *Gender Trouble: Feminism and the Subversion of Identity*, New York, London: Routledge.

———(1993) *Bodies that Matter: On the Discursive Limits of Sex*, New York, London: Routledge.

———(2004) *Undoing Gender*, New York, London: Routledge.

——— Osborne, P. and Segal, L. (1994) 'Gender as Performance: An Interview with Judith Butler' in *Radical Philosophy*, 67: 32–39.

Cole, S. (2000) *Don We Now Our Gay Apparel*, London: Bloomsbury.

De Beauvoir, S. (1953) *The Second Sex*, H.M. Parshley (trans and ed), New York: Alfred A. Knopf.

Derrida, J. (1997 [1976]) *Of Grammatology*, Baltimore, MD: Johns Hopkins University Press.

Dolphijn, R. and Van der Tuin, I. (2012) *New Materialism: Interviews and Cartographies*, Open Humanities Press.

Erickson, J. and Cogan, J. (1999) *Lesbians, Levis, and Lipstick: The Meaning of Beauty in Our Lives*, New York: Routledge Press.

Flügel, J.C. (1976 [1930]) *The Psychology of Clothes*, Brooklyn, NY: AMS Press.

Geczy, A. and Karaminas, V. (2013) *Queer Style*, London: Bloomsbury.

Grosz, E. (1994) *Volatile Bodies: Toward a Corporeal Feminism*, Indianapolis: Indiana University Press.

Haraway, D. (1991) *Simians, Cyborgs and Women: The Reinvention of Nature*, London: Free Association Books.

Hennessy, R. (1994–95) 'Queer Visibility in Commodity Culture' in *Cultural Critique*, winter, 29: 31–76.

Lee, K. (2013) 'Should my Bum Look Bigger in This? Re-dressing the De Beauvoirean Femme' in E. Paulicelli and E. Wissinger (eds), *WSQ:Fashion*, 41 (1–2): 184–93.

Parkins, I. (2008) 'Building a Feminist Theory of Fashion' in *Australian Feminist Studies*, 23 (58): 501–15.

Rubin, G. (1994) 'Sexual Traffic: Interview with Judith Butler' in *Differences: A Journal of Feminist Cultural Studies*, 6 (2–3): 62–99.

Shulman, G. (2011) 'On Vulnerability as Judith Butler's Language of Politics: From Excitable Speech to Precarious Life' in *WSQ*, 39 (1–2): 227–35.

Steele, V. (1997) *Fetish: Fashion, Sex, and Power*, New York: Oxford University Press.

——(2003) *The Corset, A Cultural History*, New Haven, CT: Yale University Press.

——(2013) *A Queer History of Fashion: From the Closet to the Catwalk*, New Haven, CT: Yale University Press.

—— and Borelli, L. (2000) *Handbags: A Lexicon of Style*, New York: Rizzoli.

Van der Tuin, I. (2011) 'New Feminist Materialisms: Review Essay' in *Women's Studies International Forum*, 34 (4): 271–77.

Wissinger, E. (2009) 'Modeling Consumption: Fashion Modeling Work in Contemporary Society' in *Journal of Consumer Culture*, 9 (2): 273–96.

——(2013) 'Fashion Modeling, Blink Technologies and New Imaging Regimes' in D. Bartlett, S. Cole and A. Rocamora (eds), *Fashion Media: Past and Present*, London: Bloomsbury.

——(forthcoming) *Fashion Modeling in the Age of the Blink*, New York: New York University Press.

CONTRIBUTORS

Joanne Entwistle is Senior Lecturer in culture, media and creative industries at King's College, London. She has published widely on fashion, dress and the body, and is author of *The Fashioned Body: Fashion, Dress and Modern Social Theory* and The *Aesthetic Economy: Markets and Value in Clothing and Modelling*. Her latest research, 'Configuring Light', is focused on light as material culture.

Adam Geczy is an artist and writer who is Senior Lecturer and Chair of the Faculty Board of Sydney College of the Arts, at the University of Sydney, Australia. With 20 years of artistic practice, his videos, sculptural installations and performance-based works have been exhibited throughout Australasia, Asia and Europe to considerable critical acclaim. He is co-author with Dr Michael Carter of *Reframing Art*. His *Art: Histories, Theories and Exceptions* won the Choice Award for best academic title in art in 2009. With Vicki Karaminas he has co-edited *Fashion and Art*, and co-written *Queer Style*. His *Fashion and Orientalism* (Bloomsbury) was also released in 2013. Upcoming titles include (with Jacqueline Millner) *Fashionable Art* and (with Vicki Karaminas) *Fashion's Double: Representations of Fashion in Painting, Photography and Film*. His next project is on models, mannequins and marionettes.

Alison Gill is Design Educator in the School of Humanities and Communication Arts at the University of Western Sydney, Australia. Her research interests in design philosophy, critical theory, material culture and the social lives of design are evident in key publications about sports product advertising, deconstruction fashion, audiences/user practices and sustainable material cultures including clothing. A co-authored publication with Mellick Lopes titled 'Recoding Abandoned Products' (2012) analyses the pedagogical setting of a sustainable design project for visual designers. This project emerged from ongoing collaborative research that draws on social practice theory to investigate 'wearing and the worn' as related to multimodal design concepts (titled 'On Wearing', Gill and Mellick Lopes, 2011). A co-edited journal issue on design and social practice theory was published in 2014.

Francesca Granata is Director of the MA Fashion Studies and Assistant Professor in the School of Art and Design History and Theory at Parsons School of Design in New York. She is founder and editor of the non-profit journal *Fashion Projects* (fashion-projects.org). A New York Foundation for the Arts sponsored project, it has received grants from the Lower Manhattan Cultural Council and the New York City Department of Cultural Affairs. She holds a PhD from Central Saint Martins University of the Arts London and is the recipient of fellowships from the University of the Arts London and the Metropolitan Museum of Art. Her work has been published in *Fashion Theory*, *Fashion Practice* and *The Journal of Design History* as well as in a number of books and exhibition catalogues. Her monograph, *Experimental Fashion: Carnival, Performance Art, and the Grotesque Body*, is forthcoming from I.B. Tauris in 2015.

Paul Jobling lectures and researches in the School of Humanities at the University of Brighton. Among his publications are *Fashion Spreads: Word and Image in Fashion Photography since 1980*; *Man Appeal: Advertising, Menswear and Modernism*; and *Advertising Menswear: Masculinities and Menswear in the British Mass Media Since 1945*.

Vicki Karaminas is Professor and Deputy Director of Doctoral Research at the College of Creative Arts, Massey University, Wellington, New Zealand. With Adam Geczy she has co-edited *Fashion and Art*, co-written *Queer Style* and the soon-to-appear *Fashion's Double: Representations of Fashion in Painting, Photography and Film*. She is the author of *Shanghai Street Style* (with Toni Johnson Woods), *Sydney Street Style* (with Toni Johnson Woods and Justine Taylor) and *Fashion in Popular Culture* (with Joseph Hancock and Toni Johnson Woods). Other book projects include *The Men's Fashion Reader* and *Fashion in Fiction. Text and Clothing in Literature, Film and Television*. She is the Editor (with Adam Geczy) of the *Australasian Journal of Popular Culture*.

Peter McNeil is Professor of Design History and Associate Dean, Research, at the University of Technology Sydney and Professor of Fashion Studies at Stockholm University. His research interests are primarily the cultural history of fashion and its interaction with other aspects of art, design and material culture. He has published numerous works on fashion, including the best-selling *Shoes: A History from Sandals to Sneakers* (with Giorgio Riello, 2006, 2011; Italian translation, 2009). Recent book-length projects include the 'long' history of luxury, supported by the Leverhulme Trust (with Riello for Oxford University Press); and 'Fashion Writing and Criticism' (with Sanda Miller). He is also currently working with the Los Angeles County Museum of Art on 'Reigning Men', the largest exhibition of men's fashion ever assembled. In June 2014 he was appointed a Distinguished Professor by the Academy of Finland for Aalto University, in the area of costume.

Janice Miller is Senior Lecturer in Cultural and Historical Studies at London College of Fashion, University of the Arts, London. Her publications include chapters, reviews and journal articles on the significance of fashion to performances of various kinds and a monograph, *Fashion and Music*. Recent work has focused on the relationship between makeup, embodiment and identity, including the article 'Making Up is Masculine' which explores the increasing cultural connections between masculinity and makeup for the journal *Critical Studies in Men's Fashion* in 2014. She is currently developing research projects that explore further the cultural significance of makeup and ones that also examine the relationship between fashion and social class.

Llewellyn Negrin is Head of and Senior Lecturer in Art and Design Theory at the Tasmanian College of the Arts, University of Tasmania, Australia. She has published widely in the area of fashion theory including her book *Appearance and Identity: Fashioning the Body in Postmodernity* and in various anthologies on fashion. She has also published articles in journals such as *Theory, Culture & Society*, *Body & Society*, *Philosophy & Social Criticism*, *European Journal of Cultural Studies* and *Feminist Theory* on topics related to the role of art and art institutions in post-modern culture and the function of aesthetics in everyday life, as well as on theories of fashion and the body.

Aurélie Van de Peer received her doctoral degree in Philosophy at Ghent University and in Sociology at the University of Leuven, Belgium. Her research explores the politics invested in written fashion journalism in the twentieth and early twenty-first centuries. Her articles have appeared or are forthcoming in such journals as *Fashion Theory*, *Cultural Sociology*, *The International Journal of Cultural Studies* and *Poetics*.

Agnès Rocamora is Reader in Social and Cultural Studies at the London College of Fashion, University of the Arts, London. She is the author of *Fashioning the City: Paris, Fashion and the Media* (I.B. Tauris, 2009). Her writing on the field of fashion and on the fashion media has appeared in various journals, including *Fashion Theory*, *Journalism Practice*, *Sociology* and the *Journal of Consumer Culture*. She is a co-editor of *The Handbook of Fashion Studies* and of *Fashion Media: Past and Present* and a contributor to *Fashion's World Cities* and *Fashion as Photograph*. She is also a co-editor of the *International Journal of Fashion Studies* and is currently developing her work on fashion and digital media.

Anneke Smelik is Professor of Visual Culture on the Katrien van Munster chair at the Radboud University Nijmegen, Netherlands. She is coordinator of the MA programme 'Creative Industries'. She (co-)edited *From Delft Blue to Denim Blue, Contemporary Dutch Fashion* (I.B. Tauris, 2016); *Performing Memory in Art and Popular Culture*; *The Scientific Imaginary in Visual Culture*; *Technologies of Memory in the Arts*; and *Bits of Life: Feminism at the Intersections of Media, Bioscience, and Technology*. She is author of *And the Mirror Cracked: Feminist Cinema and Film Theory* and several books in Dutch on issues of visual culture, including a book on cyborgs in popular culture. Anneke Smelik is project leader of the research programme 'Crafting Wearables; Fashionable Technology' (2013–2018), funded by the Netherlands Organization for Scientific Research.

Anthony Sullivan is Senior Lecturer in Cultural and Historical Studies at the London College of Fashion. He has written and presented a number of papers on issues such as the role of brands in the UK summer riots of 2011 and the influence of class on late teenagers' branded consumption. He is also a contributor to *The Wiley Blackwell Encyclopaedia of Consumption and Consumer Studies* (edited by Tim Cook and Michael Ryan). His book *Branding Fashion: Bridging the Self and the Social Consumer* will be published by I.B. Tauris in 2016.

Efrat Tseëlon is Chair of Fashion Theory at the School of Design, University of Leeds. Since receiving her PhD from Oxford on *Communicating via Clothing* she has developed the perspective of Critical Fashion. She has contributed to fashion scholarship in extending the research agenda from designer fashion to ordinary clothes, shifting the focus from the stereotype approach of ceremonial costumes to the wardrobe approach of everyday clothes, and challenging the notion of the *language of clothes* of objects with fixed meanings, showing it as a process where meanings are negotiated and not fixed. Tseëlon instigated the *Intellect Books* series of fashion studies, and is the Editor in Chief of *Critical Studies in Fashion & Beauty*. In her books *The Masque of Femininity* (1995) and *Masquerade & Identities* (2001) she developed the theory of fashion as an ideology of gender construction, and of masquerade as a technology of identity critique. In *Fashion Ethics* (2013) she analyzed ethical fashion as ideological discourse.

Jane Tynan is a lecturer at Central Saint Martins, University of the Arts, London. She has published on aspects of art, design, fashion and the body. In her recent book *British Army Uniform and the First World War: Men in Khaki* she explores the social meaning of uniforms worn by British combatants on the Western Front; how khaki embodied gender, social class and ethnicity, impacted the tailoring trade and became a touchstone for pacifist resistance. Her current research concerns aesthetic practices created by and for civil disobedience and insurgency, which is the subject of her forthcoming book, *Images of Insurgency*.

Elizabeth Wissinger is an associate professor of Sociology at BMCC/City University of New York, and teaches Fashion Studies at the Graduate School of CUNY. She studies fashion, technology and embodiment, and her work has earned several grants and awards, including two Mellon Fellowships, in the Centre for the Humanities, and in the Centre for Interdisciplinary Science Studies, at the Graduate School of CUNY. Among her various publications, she discusses fashion and imaging regimes in *Fashion Media: Past and Present*; and fashion and branding in 'Modeling Consumption: Fashion Modeling Work in Contemporary Society', in the *Journal of Consumer Culture*. She has co-edited an anthology, with Joanne Entwistle, entitled *Fashioning Models: Image, Text, and Industry*. Recent projects include *WSQ's* issue on *Fashion*, co-edited with Eugenia Paulicelli, and her book on the glamour labour of fashion models. Wissinger's next focus is wearable technology and the issues it raises about bodily optimization and enhancement.

INDEX

References to images are in *italics*; references to notes are indicated by n.

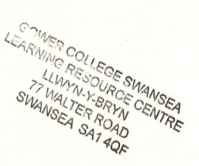